Translating
Buddhist Medicine
in Medieval China

ENCOUNTERS WITH ASIA

Victor H. Mair, Series Editor

Encounters with Asia is an interdisciplinary series dedicated
to the exploration of all the major regions and cultures of this
vast continent. Its time frame extends from the prehistoric to
the contemporary; its geographic scope ranges from the Urals
and the Caucasus to the Pacific. A particular focus of the series
is the Silk Road in all of its ramifications: religion, art, music,
medicine, science, trade, and so forth. Among the disciplines
represented in this series are history, archaeology, anthropology,
ethnography, and linguistics. The series aims particularly to
clarify the complex interrelationships among various peoples
within Asia, and also with societies beyond Asia.

A complete list of books in the series
is available from the publisher.

TRANSLATING
BUDDHIST MEDICINE
IN MEDIEVAL CHINA

C. Pierce Salguero

PENN

UNIVERSITY OF PENNSYLVANIA PRESS

PHILADELPHIA

Published by
University of Pennsylvania Press
Philadelphia, Pennsylvania 19104-4112
www.upenn.edu/pennpress

Printed in the United States of America on acid-free paper
2 4 6 8 10 9 7 5 3 1

A Cataloging-in-Publication record is available from the
Library of Congress
ISBN 978-0-8122-4611-7

For Maxine and Simone

CONTENTS

Introduction

With translation there is transmission; without translation there is but obscurity.

—Sengyou (445–518)[1]

The transmission of Buddhism from India to China in the first millennium of the Common Era ranks among the most significant and most well documented examples of cross-cultural exchange in the premodern world. Although the study of the global spread of Buddhism is most commonly undertaken by scholars of religion, this cross-cultural encounter involved much more than simply the transmission of religious or philosophical knowledge. Buddhism influenced many other aspects of Chinese life, including contributing to the economy, inspiring changes in the sociopolitical order, and spurring the adoption of foreign material culture. This book is a study of one, often-overlooked facet of this Indo-Sinitic exchange: the introduction of Indian medicine to China.[2]

Knowledge about health and illness held a central place within Buddhist thought from the earliest times.[3] Anatomical and physiological terminology was frequently invoked in early Indian Buddhist texts, particularly in descriptions of meditation practices and other ascetic discourses. Medical similes and metaphors were utilized in order to make accessible many aspects of the Dharma, including the most abstruse philosophical positions. Narratives of the healing exploits of deities, monks, and other heroes were a feature of the Buddhist hagiographic literature of all periods. Rites to dispel disease were central to the ritual repertoires of Buddhist clerics across Asia. Many Buddhist scriptures even go so far as to suggest that fully understanding the body is the very essence of the Buddha's teachings. Taken collectively, such Buddhist perspectives on health, illness, healers, patients, therapies, and bodies are today often spoken of by East Asian scholars and devotees as "Buddhist medicine" (Ch. *foyi* or *fojiao yixue*; Jp. *bukkyō igaku*).

Buddhist medicine, if I may employ that term here for purposes of convenience, is a moving target. It represents a loose collection of ideas and practices that originated in the Indo-European context in the latter centuries B.C.E., but that was modified and expanded as a result of cross-cultural interactions during the vigorous geographical expansion of Buddhism. Transmitted along the networks of land and sea trade routes, the core doctrines and perspectives of Buddhist medicine came to exert a powerful influence on medical thought and practice across a large swath of Eurasia. To this day, they continue to form the basis of traditional medicine in Sri Lanka, Thailand, and Tibet, among other places. However, the history of how the tradition was locally received, understood, and transformed differed greatly from place to place.

The Chinese reception of Buddhist medicine was complex and multi-faceted. Medieval China was culturally diverse and politically fractured, and therefore it—like virtually all other facets of Buddhism—was subject to multiple interpretations in different contexts.[4] Importantly, China had long-standing and prestigious traditions of learned medicine that were objects of official patronage and that looked to a corpus of ancient classics for authority.[5] China also had long-established repertoires of ritual healing, bodily self-cultivation, and alchemical experimentation that claimed to be able to heal, to prevent illness, and even to confer immortality. Over the long term, the impact of some aspects of Buddhist medicine on the Chinese medical world was profound: Indian-inspired healing deities, rituals, occult practices, and hagiography, for example, all proved to be enormously popular and permanent contributions to Chinese culture. At the same time, some doctrines that lay at the very center of Buddhist medical thought and practice were perceived as conflicting with indigenous precedents. In the long run, these failed to catch on and were ultimately either ignored or actively replaced by homegrown models within Buddhist discourses.

I am planning future publications that will provide in-depth analysis of the medical content of Chinese Buddhist texts, the relationship between this medical system and others throughout Eurasia, and the historical development of Buddhist medicine in a global context. The present book focuses on understanding the local reception of Buddhist medical ideas in China. While it starts with an overview of the transmission of Buddhist medical knowledge to China, the majority of its pages are dedicated to exploring the processes of translation involved in this historic episode of cross-cultural exchange. The many Chinese Buddhist writings under consideration in this book demonstrate that foreign medical ideas introduced along with Buddhism were voluminously translated, enthusiastically commented upon, and widely disseminated in China. At the same time, however, they show that translators went to great lengths to adapt Indian ideas and practices to domestic cultural and social contexts. Far from passively being influenced by transmitted knowledge from abroad, they actively retooled these imports to fit with Chinese intellectual concerns, to mesh with preexisting literary and cultural conventions, and to forward their own political and economic interests.

The examination of these dynamics of cross-cultural transmission and reception will bring into sharper focus several important facets of religious and medical history that are worth highlighting from the outset. In the first place, Chinese Buddhist texts dealing with medicine throw into question some of the basic assumptions about the history of Indian medicine, not least of which is the tendency to label all ancient Indian medical knowledge as "Āyurveda." Clearly, there were significant currents of medical thought outside of the Āyurvedic context. Second, and from a more global standpoint, these texts showcase the centrality of healing as one of the most important mechanisms by which Buddhism gained prominence outside of India. They demonstrate how the body and its processes of health and illness could be used as effective tools for translating Buddhist doctrines across geographic, ethnic, and linguistic divides, and how engaging with medical knowledge helped Buddhists position themselves as cross-cultural mediators.

At the same time, the study of these texts also greatly enhances our understanding of the local religious and medical context in medieval China. That is the main focus of the current book. Focusing on the Chinese reception of Buddhist medicine underscores how the history of Chinese medicine is inseparable from that of Chinese religion, and vice versa. It helps us to understand the medieval Chinese religious and medical landscape, and the roles of Buddhist ideas, practices, and practitioners in that world. It sheds light on the multivalence of healing knowledge in medieval society and its significance as a site of political and social contestation. It highlights the importance of clerics as health-care practitioners, the tensions between them and other groups of healing specialists, and the role of religion in their processes of differentiation. And, at a more fundamental level, this study strongly urges us to think of historical processes of cross-cultural exchange as creative moments that hinged on the translational activities of individual historical actors.

Cultural Exchange and Translation Theory

While it is familiar territory for scholars of religion, medieval China has received far less attention from historians of medicine. Those who have studied the period have shown that healing was a major facet of contemporary religion, and their findings have suggested that the Indian contributions to Chinese medicine should be analyzed in much more detail than thus far has been the case. To date, however, only a handful of scholarly books have been published in Western languages that concentrate on the interaction between religion and medicine in the period.[6] Moreover, much of this scholarship has focused on a single cache of documents from the remote Silk Road oasis town of Dunhuang (in present-day Gansu Province), on the far periphery of Chinese civilization.

The scholarly assessment of Buddhism's contributions to medieval Chinese medicine has not been unanimous. The majority has focused on those medical ideas from the Indian context that were influential in China and has enumerated many concrete references to foreign doctrines in the writings of medieval Chinese physicians.[7] A vocal minority has instead emphasized that the core doctrines of Indian medicine were misunderstood, misconstrued, and mistranslated in China.[8] Whatever side they have taken in this debate, however, scholars have tended to focus on the similarities (or lack thereof) between the writings of Chinese physicians and the extant Indian texts from the Āyurvedic tradition, rather than systematically examining the corpus of Chinese Buddhist literature on its own terms.

In my view, this interest in charting the correlations between Indian and Chinese medical traditions parallels the overriding concern in twentieth-century religious studies scholarship with measuring the "influence" versus the "sinicization" of Buddhism in China more generally. The prevailing approach to Chinese Buddhism until the past quarter century or so, this model emphasized identifying which Indian ideas and practices were transmitted to China, how these exerted an impact on native thought and social structures, and how they were absorbed, transformed, and eventually assimilated into the Chinese culture.[9] In this type of scholarship, comparing Indian and Chinese writings to find similarities is understandably a common theme.

As criticisms of this "influence versus sinicization" approach began to take root in the 1990s and 2000s, however, scholars increasingly tended not to treat Indian and Chinese cultures as reified entities that came into contact with one another, but rather began to understand cross-cultural exchange at a more granular level. Explicitly or implicitly drawing on the theory of cultural systems as developed in the field of cultural anthropology, a significant body of scholarship has emerged in the past twenty years that emphasizes the complexity of the processes whereby foreign and indigenous practices, beliefs, and symbols interacted and intermixed.[10] This approach has led to an increasingly nuanced appreciation of Chinese Buddhism as a syncretic composite of both Indian and Chinese cultural elements, as well as to a reevaluation of the many subtle Buddhist influences on medieval Daoism. Such a way of approaching the topic has led to seismic shifts in the study of Chinese religion. Rather than Indian influence and Chinese sinicization, many scholars now prefer to think in terms of "Buddho-Daoism," and almost all emphasize the syncretism of Chinese religions.[11]

Though syncretism remains a valuable tool for thinking about cross-cultural exchange, a radically different approach to the problem has also gained currency since the turn of the twenty-first century. Inspired by the cross-disciplinary "linguistic turn" prioritizing discourse analysis, many prominent North American scholars have abandoned thinking of culture as a "thing" or collection of "things" with the ability to influence or intermix. Drawing on models of culture as performance developed in the social sciences, many scholars have now begun to speak about Buddhism (or, often, "Buddhisms") as a multiplicity of rhetorical categories that were continually and situationally negotiated by individual historical actors. They have spoken of Buddhism as a collection of "repertoires" or "strategies," and have promoted the investigation of religious discourse as a site for the social and literary performance of identity.[12] Robert Sharf perhaps articulated this position as clearly as anyone when he wrote the following lines:

> The problem is that the category of syncretism presupposes the existence of distinct religious entities that predate the syncretic amalgam, precisely what is absent, or at least unrecoverable, in the case of Buddhism. . . . In the final analysis, pure or unadulterated Buddhism is little more than an analytic abstraction posited by Buddhist polemicists, apologists, reformers, and now scholars. . . . The authority

of the word "Buddhism" lies not in its normative signification(s) so much as in its rhetorical deployments.[13]

Although some scholars, including Sharf, have vocally rejected the idea of syncretism, it is important to emphasize that both modes of current scholarship outlined above—what I call the "cultural-systems approach" on the one hand, and the "discourse-centered approach" on the other—have now developed in dialogue and in mutual interaction over the past decade or more.[14] What is more, while approaches emphasizing influence, sinicization, hybridity, and syncretism may now be considered unfashionable in certain circles, acclaimed works unapologetically touting the "impact" of Indian culture on China continue to appear, and older studies in this mold continue to be counted among the most engaging and worthwhile contributions to the field.[15] In short, multiple approaches now coexist side by side as distinct methodological orientations available to scholars interested in the Indo-Sinitic cross-cultural encounter.

In a sign that old dichotomies are moving toward a new synthesis, in the past few years a number of innovative scholars have begun to explore ways of bridging the gap between the cultural-systems and discourse-centered approaches. For example, several recent studies have provided methodologically rich analyses of how cross-culturally exchanged Buddhist iconographic elements were self-consciously and strategically deployed in order to negotiate site-specific political circumstances.[16] Rather than collapse their analyses into any single framework, these scholars have explored the dialectic between transregional traditions and local reception, and have explicitly focused on the unstable and symbiotic nature of this relationship.

Like those other studies, my approach to Buddhist medicine is also interested in forging a "Middle Path" between the local and the translocal. Rather than focus on iconography, however, this book focuses squarely on the cross-cultural transmission and reception of ideas. The underlying theoretical model I employ is to approach this process primarily through the lens of translation.[17] I am attracted to translation theory as a conceptual tool for bridging the gap between the cultural-systems and discourse-centered approaches because even the most basic analysis of translation necessitates integrating both.

Translation, of course, lies at the very heart of the Indo-Sinitic cross-cultural encounter given that it was primarily through translated texts (both written and oral) that Buddhist knowledge was imported into China. While a good portion of this book is about "translation proper" (i.e., the reencoding of foreign language texts in Chinese), however, I am following the common practice in translation studies of using "translation" as a heuristic device or organizing metaphor to talk about a wide spectrum of processes of intercultural communication. Here, I use the term to refer to any and all practices of mediating, negotiating, or explaining cultural differences through literature.[18] I explicitly intend to include both interlingual translations (i.e., texts transferred between languages) as well as the wide range of intralingual translations of Indian knowledge (i.e., writings that further explained and interpreted interlingual translations for Chinese audiences).[19]

One of the most basic premises of translation studies is that acts of translation are much more complex than simply the transfer of a text encoded in one language (the "source text") to an equivalent text in a second language (the "target text"). Figure 1 presents a simplified version of a widely known model of translation introduced in the 1960s by one of the godfathers of translation studies, Eugene Nida. Nida's model is by no means the final word on translation, and it has been expanded, refined, and rejected by many scholars since. Be that as it may, precisely because of its simplicity, this diagram serves as a useful starting point to discuss some of the central concerns of this book.

In the first place, the diagram draws attention to the intermittent steps in translation in between the source and target texts, in which the translator analyzes the meaning of the text in its original cultural and linguistic milieu,

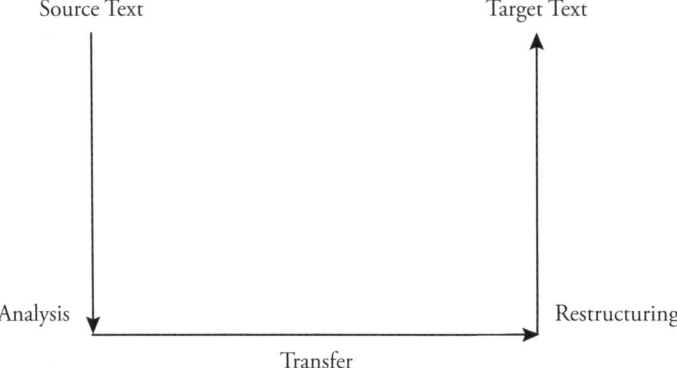

Figure 1. A simple model of a translational act. Adapted from Nida and Taber 2003 [1969]: 33.

mentally transfers this meaning from the source language to the target language, and restructures his[20] understanding of the text in this new context. Following the diagram's flow from left to right, one way to think of Indo-Sinitic cross-cultural exchange is as the movement of a constellation of words, concepts, metaphors, symbols, ideas, tropes, and other structures horizontally across the diagram from the Indian cultural-linguistic system to the Chinese. From this perspective, Buddhist translators can be thought of as occupying an intercultural space: through each act of transfer, they imagined and built conceptual bridges between two distinct semantic worlds. They adapted foreign ideas to fit into new linguistic structures and cultural categories, and expanded domestic systems to accommodate fresh inputs. That is to say, one way to look at the practice of translation is to see the translator as an active mediator between cultural-linguistic systems.[21]

An important issue that arises in this way of thinking about translation is the problem of equivalence. Can a text or passage or word mean the same in its source and target contexts? How do meanings shift in the process of transfer? Are there certain ideas that simply cannot be translated? There is a long tradition of asking these sorts of questions in European translation theory, and of making distinctions such as "word-for-word" versus "sense-for-sense" equivalence, going back as far as Cicero (106–43 B.C.E.) and St. Jerome (ca. 347–420 C.E.).[22] Nida himself differentiated between what he called "formal" and "dynamic" equivalence—the former referring to the literal translation of terminology that prioritizes the semantics of the source text, and the latter referring to looser translations that recreate the source text's social or cultural function in the new setting.[23] As we will see in Chapter 2, similar distinctions were made by medieval Chinese translators.

While not necessarily couching their work in translation studies terminology, it is precisely on questions of equivalence that most of the existing scholarship on Buddhist translation and cultural exchange has concentrated. The "influence versus sinicization" approach mentioned above, for example, is in large part a debate over to what extent Buddhist ideas were expressed in formal versus dynamic terms in Chinese texts.[24] I will discuss the translation of Buddhist medicine from this perspective in more detail below. However, scholars of translation have long argued that a fuller understanding of translation necessitates shifting focus from the movement of cultural-linguistic elements horizontally across Nida's diagram to also examining in as much detail as possible the processes taking place at the bottom of the chart.

One of the thorniest problems in the study of translation is that while the structural aspects of the translation process—the textual inputs and outputs, as well as the larger systems texts are embedded within—can in most cases be studied extensively, the interpretive acts performed during the transfer take place within the black box of an individual human mind. While scholars of translation have interrogated living translators, tracked their eyeballs while they worked, and subjected them to neurological study in order to gain a sense of their understandings and procedures, this is obviously impossible with historical translators.[25] Specifically in the case of medieval China, we are even further constrained by a paucity of records written by translators reflecting on their craft. The limitations of the sources prevent us from gaining anything near a complete picture of medieval translation practice. Despite the obvious challenges, however, the field of translation studies provides a wide range of tools to think about the myriad factors that inform the decisions of translators, and I argue that we can use some of these approaches to think more deeply about the medieval materials.[26]

For example, rather than concentrating only on the equivalence or lack thereof between source and target cultural-linguistic structures, we might gain an even better appreciation for translation as an active and creative process if we borrow from translation theorists the ideas of "foreignizing" versus "domesticating" translation strategies.[27] Though perhaps seemingly similar to the formal-dynamic distinction, this approach does not hold up the source text as the authoritative point of reference by which the target text is measured. Rather than focus on how much of the original is transferred and how well, the latter approach is concerned with the translators' strategic crafting of their target texts. The questions that now draw our attention include: How do translators actively mold translations in order to fit with certain expectations, achieve certain rhetorical goals, or elicit certain responses in their intended audience? When and why does a translator invoke the source context through the use of unfamiliar "foreignizing" words, grammatical structures, or imagery? When and why does he deploy "domesticating" terms with indigenous resonances that might signal to his readers that a foreign text is compatible with the target cultural-linguistic system? Of course, "foreignizing" and "domesticating" are themselves not fixed entities, but ever-evolving registers of expression. They are the products of the norms (including the assumptions, imaginations, and rhetorical practices) of the recipient culture, which also must be explored.[28]

The study of historical instances of translation thus requires understanding not only the source and target texts and cultural-linguistic systems, but also as much of the local social situation as possible, including the translator's intended audience and interpretive communities, the prevailing conventions and expectations of these groups, the sociopolitical and ideological environment, the intellectual and economic stakes, and so on. I need not belabor this excursus into translation studies any further than I already have. The long and short of it is that, taking Nida's simple schematic of an act of translation as our point of departure, we rapidly arrive at the conclusion that an adequate account of the reception of Buddhist medicine in China involves a number of factors beyond simply an evaluation of how accurate Chinese translators were in capturing Indian ideas.

This study integrates the various aspects of translation introduced above, concentrating on the following:

1. The texts: an exploration of the range of literature by which Buddhist medicine was explained and introduced to Chinese audiences, and how Buddhist medicine was presented in different genres.
2. Influence and syncretism: an account of the foreign ideas transmitted, as well as to the short- and long-term changes in the target cultural and linguistic repertoires brought about by their introduction.
3. Equivalence: a discussion of the relevant cultural and linguistic systems prevailing prior to the introduction of Buddhism, and how translators used these to construct equivalents.
4. Norms: an analysis of why certain types of equivalence were employed in certain Ideological or social settings, and the force of translation norms in guiding translation decisions.
5. Performative value: an accounting for the status of "the foreign" and "the domestic" as rhetorical categories, as well as how and why knowledge was marked as one or the other.
6. Translation strategies: an analysis of the broader goals and historical contexts of the individuals and groups involved in this project of cross-cultural medical exchange, including biographical data, contemporary translation institutions, and prevailing patterns of patronage.

7. Translation tactics: an examination of how translators pursued their broader strategic aims through particular choices of words and phrases.

With this list, we find ourselves in the midst of a massive undertaking that extends well beyond the confines of translation proper. Nevertheless, stitching together these manifold facets seems to be critical for our understanding of medieval Chinese Buddhist medicine. Of course, it would be folly to think that one could say everything there is to say about all of the above points in one book, or even in one scholar's career. My goal here is to survey this territory, to outline some of its major contours, and to stake out some ground for future research. I have already mentioned that future publications will more closely concentrate on the texts themselves, their contents, and their global contexts, all of which will receive short shrift here. In this book, I am most interested in examining what translational choices were made in the introduction of Buddhist medicine to China, and what these decisions tell us about the cultural and social worlds in which these translators lived and worked.

Let me acknowledge clearly here that we cannot ever gain complete access to the black box and definitively determine what our medieval translators and authors were thinking when they took up their ink and brushes. However, I will argue in the chapters to come that we can indeed peek inside and come to some reasonably solid conclusions about translators' intentions, concerns, and thought processes. As I will show, an analysis of the above factors, read against the social and cultural contexts in which translation took place, can tell us much about the multivalent meanings of religion and medicine for medieval Chinese people.

Contents of This Book

The body of this book is divided into seven thematic units. The introduction you are currently reading sets up the basic frameworks for my analysis and contains a few preliminary notes about the sources, terminology, and translation conventions I employ. This is followed by Chapter 1, which opens by describing the religious and medical vocabularies that prevailed in China prior to the introduction of Buddhism. These cultural-linguistic elements represent the raw materials available to translators from which they could construct equivalence, as well as important interpretive lenses through which translated Buddhist medical knowledge could be understood and explained. However, the bulk of the chapter is concerned with broadly introducing the range of Indian medical ideas, practices, and institutions imported from abroad and the texts that introduced these to China. I also summarize the widespread influence of Indian medical ideas on medieval Chinese medical texts, ranging from the writings of medical officials to Silk Road manuscripts.

Chapter 2 shifts from a focus on the transmission to one on translation practice. It opens with a discussion of the translators and the environment in which they worked. I then provide an overview of how translators used foreignizing and domesticating terminology in order to both draw their readers into a foreign world and fit their target texts into the Chinese context. I also introduce in this chapter what I call the "religiomedical marketplace," or the competitive social environment in which healing specialists contended for patronage and cultural capital. I show that choices about how to translate Buddhist medical ideas helped to position Buddhist clerics vis-à-vis their competition, and that seemingly small translation decisions could carry an inordinate amount of weight in how well they could negotiate the medieval Chinese social and political landscape.

Next, Chapter 3 outlines in broad strokes the norms that emerged in the Chinese translation of the medical content contained in Buddhist scriptures. I discuss a large corpus of extant scriptures, focusing on how they translate five core medical metaphors that are found in Buddhist literature across multiple languages worldwide. In China, I argue, these metaphors were translated in different ways in order to appeal to different domestic audiences. Translators writing texts for the internal consumption of the monastic community, the sangha (Skt. *saṃgha*; Ch. *seng* or *sengjia*), utilized more formally equivalent or foreignizing language, while those writing for wider audiences relied heavily on dynamic equivalents that tapped into domestic vocabularies. I suggest that such differences are not accidental but relate to the strategic purposes of the translators, which I examine in some detail.

Following this discussion of the broader corpus of translated scriptures, Chapter 4 moves to consider how individual authors reinterpreted translated Buddhist knowledge in indigenous Chinese compositions. Though examples of intralingual translation rather than translation proper, these authors played just as important a role in the Chinese reception of Buddhist medicine. Throughout this chapter, I focus on the relationship between an author's social and intellectual context and his translation decisions, demonstrating that even the same individual might modulate his strategies when writing for different audiences. I also identify a series of historical shifts in strategy that took place between the sixth and ninth centuries. As contact with India deepened and China became more familiar with Buddhist ideas, interpreters of Buddhist medicine began to utilize more foreignizing vocabularies that marked Buddhist medical knowledge as authentic, unique, and even incompatible with Chinese knowledge.

Chapter 5 switches gears and tells a diametrically opposed story about another genre of Buddhist literature. This chapter explores how Buddhist medical ideas and ideals were incorporated into popular narratives. In these tales, rather than emphasize the source context, authors worked to resituate Buddhist healers within the domestic Chinese literary world. In the hands of these intralingual translators, foreign healers were recreated as familiar characters from indigenous genres. Monks offering healing services to the laity were represented as important actors in contemporary society, and their therapies were molded to appear highly compatible with indigenous Chinese cultural expectations. Such narratives circulated widely and ultimately played a larger role than any other form of literature in introducing the Chinese populace to Buddhist healing. These stories contributed to making certain aspects of Buddhist medicine universally known and enduring parts of the Chinese religiomedical landscape.

Finally, a short conclusion briefly discusses the decline of Buddhist medicine as a vital doctrinal system in China. I identify shifts in the reception environment as a principal reason why Buddhist medical knowledge became less important for elite physicians outside of Buddhist circles in the ninth to twelfth centuries and beyond. This section also wraps up with a summary of the basic arguments forwarded here. At the back of the book, I have provided a list of Chinese and Japanese characters, bibliographies of historical sources and references, and an index.

From the above synopsis, it should be apparent that this book is not a social history of healing in medieval China, an exegesis of Buddhist medical thought, or a word-by-word analysis of translation technique—although it does a little of each. Rather, it represents an initial foray into a broad range of Chinese Buddhist texts on medicine, the language and rhetorical strategies employed in their translation and authorship, the goals of the people who produced them, and the contexts in which such writing was undertaken. I will probably spend less time discussing the translation of specific passages or specific words than the reader might expect, preferring to pay attention to a wider spectrum of translation practices. Because my analysis and conclusions are framed broadly, many individual stones have been left unturned, and I intend to return to a number of these in future publications. For now, my chief goal is to reconstruct something of the vibrant medical world of medieval China and of the place of translated Buddhist knowledge within that milieu.

Sources for This Book

Historical sources consulted in the preparation of this book include both canonical and extracanonical Buddhist literature, as well as a number of Indian and Chinese medical texts that lie outside the Buddhist sphere altogether. My focus, however, is the *Taishō-Era Newly Revised Tripitaka* (Jp. *Taishō shinshū daizōkyō*), a one-hundred-volume compilation well known to all scholars of East Asian Buddhism.[29] My analysis includes primarily those texts that were composed or translated in China between the second and the midninth centuries C.E.—which constitutes the main period of translation activity that introduced Buddhist medicine to East Asia.

My choice to focus on the *Taishō Tripitaka* perhaps requires some explanation. Assembled by scholars in Japan in the 1920s and 1930s, this compilation of texts includes a selection of historical sources that were gathered from all over East Asia. Though it has the word "Tripitaka" in its title, which is most commonly translated into English as "canon," it does not constitute a proper historical canon as it was never recognized as an authoritative compilation by any premodern group of Buddhists. In recent years, many scholars have turned away from this heterogeneous collection as they have become increasingly excited about recovered manuscripts, local temple gazetteers, stone inscriptions, and other newly excavated or rediscovered sources. Scholarly excursions into this virgin territory have had a reinvigorating effect on the field of Buddhist studies, and in many cases have overturned long-held assumptions. At the same time that these new directions are being explored, however, the *Taishō Tripitaka* still remains an invaluable source for certain types of research. For a study of the history of Chinese translation strategies across a wide expanse of geography and time, for example, this collection is the natural starting point. Not only does it contain a broad sample of premodern Chinese Buddhist literature, but it is fully digitized, allowing for accessible corpus-level analysis. Ranging from major sutras and commentaries to relatively obscure texts, the *Taishō Tripitaka* includes virtually all of the most historically influential writings of the Chinese Buddhist tradition that are extant today as well as a cross-section of other less influential pieces. While there is much work to be done on the history of Buddhist healing in any number of local contexts across China, a study of the medical knowledge in this particular collection is a necessary undertaking in order to provide both a baseline and point of departure for any such scholarship.

Received Buddhist texts do raise some potential sticking points that are worth contemplating, however. For one, this study must proceed under different assumptions about how texts work than studies of contemporary translation might. We must recognize that Chinese Buddhist texts belong to a world in which notions of authorship operated differently than they do in the modern West. Persistent borrowing and adaptation of material among writers (whether from the same or from rival groups) without attribution was the norm. In addition, our received texts come down to us via generations of copyists and editors who thought nothing of adjusting texts to suit the prevailing ideologies of their times. While some scholars have decried such activities as "plagiarism" and "censorship," it is simply how authorship worked in premodern China.[30] Consequently, in this book, I use the term "author" *cum grano salis*, intending to refer to the name attached to a particular version of a text. I do not mean to infer that this individual was the sole person who contributed to its composition, or that the text we have today is necessarily a fully faithful copy of his original.

The idea of "the translator" of these sources is just as problematic. An unknown but significant percentage of Chinese Buddhist translations were anonymously done, although these texts were often backdated and given false attributions retroactively for polemical purposes.[31] Even when we are confident about the name and date, we must bear in mind that most texts were not translated by a single individual. Rather, as I will discuss in more detail in Chapter 2, Buddhist texts were most frequently the output of a committee: symbolically headed by that individual, but in actuality composed of numerous individuals with varying linguistic and literary expertise. When I talk about the "translator" of a text in this book, I do not mean to exclude all of the other individuals involved in the translation, reinterpreting, and rewriting of a text. While I ascribe certain motives to Chinese Buddhist translators, I am fully aware that we cannot reconstruct the deliberations of translation assemblies or separate out the intentions of the individuals who constituted them.

Another issue that confronts us is the one-sidedness of the corpus available to us in the present day. The vast majority of Chinese Buddhist scriptures are today available only as target texts, the source texts having been lost long ago. Even when there are recensions of these texts still extant in Indian languages, these represent different, usually much later, editions rather than source texts in the strict sense. In only extremely rare cases were the Indic texts from which Chinese translators worked preserved to the present day.[32] While this lacuna might on its face seem to present an insurmountable obstacle for a project such as this one, in actuality, a focus on a monolingual corpus is not that unusual in translation studies. While it would be nice to have our translators' sources, enough comparable Buddhist and medical literature exists from the Indian sphere that we often can make informed estimates of what missing source texts may have said when appropriate. In my research, I have most frequently used for these sorts of comparisons the Pāli Buddhist Canon[33] and the three most influential classics from the Āyurvedic tradition.[34] In fact, however, this book does not spend any time comparing source and target texts. I am most interested in examining Chinese translations as examples of Chinese literature written in the Chinese target context. That is to say, the lack of Indic source texts sharpens our focus on the reception end of the translation process and underscores our commitment to treating translations as "facts of target cultures."[35]

One final consideration worth mentioning is that, due to the lack of source texts, what does and does not constitute "translation" is not always clear from our historical remove. Many of the writings associated with Chinese Buddhism are known or suspected to be pseudotranslations (often called "apocrypha"), texts that were newly composed in China but were passed off as translations from Indian languages.[36] As I will discuss in detail below, it is impossible to make clear categorical distinctions between texts or parts thereof that adhere closely to the source texts, those that represent creative reinterpretation, and those that are all-out fabrications. Most Chinese Buddhist texts combine the whole gamut of approaches, and, because we have no source texts to compare them against, we are often unsure what portions of a text are examples of what kind of approaches.

In fact, however, the issue of what does and does not constitute translation is easily settled when we think of translation in broader terms. Once we include both inter- and intralingual translation in our definition, then all medieval Chinese Buddhist texts count as translations. Even if they are not translations proper, all are the product of authors' attempts to explain, elucidate, and engage with foreign knowledge. All Chinese Buddhist exegetes and thinkers grappled with how to understand, explain, and mobilize foreign ideas in ways that were meaningful to their readers. Anthologizers, catalogers, collectors, and other "rewriters" of preexisting material were no less involved in translational activity.[37] Far from mindlessly compiling they selected from existing sources, extracting texts from one context and recasting them to fit another. Even cases of outright appropriation—for example, when a Daoist author lifts passages or entire texts from Buddhist scriptures—can similarly be understood as a type of translation. By adapting existing material or redeploying it in new compositions, all of these authors infused borrowed materials with new meaning and resituated them in new frameworks, in effect translating them into new social, ideological, and intellectual contexts.

All of these translational acts—whether translation proper, pseudotranslation, rewriting, adaptation, or a mix of all—involved similar processes of extracting an idea from a source context and restructuring it in a new target context. But how translators derived meaning from the sources available to them and how they chose to express those ideas in new linguistic, cultural, and ideological frameworks varied greatly. While Chinese Buddhist target texts invariably are intricate mosaics of Indian and Chinese cultural-linguistic elements, as we will see below, there are important patterns that emerge upon closer inspection. It is precisely on reading these patterns to see what they reveal that we will focus in the pages to come.

Some Notes on Terminology and Translations

The anthropologist Joseph Alter has written that the broad categories commonly used by scholars to compare different cultures, such as "religion," "economics," "philosophy," and "science," reflect reality only partially. Their usage, he argues, "produces frameworks of analysis . . . that are completely at odds with histories of contact and sustained cultural communication."[38] This mismatch between scholarly categories and historical realities is especially problematic in a study of the history of Buddhist medicine.

In the first place, we must ask ourselves, just what do we mean by the term "medicine" in the context of medieval China? Historians of Chinese medicine have given the lion's share of their attention to the learned strands of healing historically associated with the members of a particular social group called in Chinese *yi* (conventionally translated into English as "physicians").

This focus is perhaps understandable given that the healing system advocated by physicians—itself also called *yi* (in this context conventionally translated as "medicine") or *yifang* ("medical techniques")—enjoyed increasing official favor and eventually became the dominant learned medical discourse from the eleventh century onward. The doctrines and practices associated with the word *yi* also constitute the basis of Traditional Chinese Medicine (TCM), a modern hybrid therapeutic system that is increasingly popular across the globe today.[39] Nevertheless, it is a mistake to assume that the *yi* were the only practitioners in the long history of China that were taken seriously by patients or that produced sophisticated treatises on health, illness, and the body. If we aim to gain a more comprehensive picture of the Chinese medical world, it is imperative to investigate the history of other groups of healers—despite the fact that they may not fit neatly into the modern understanding of the word "medicine."[40]

In the medieval period, one obvious area needing further research is the activities of religious healers. In China prior to the eleventh century, "religion" was not a thoroughly separate category from "medicine." (I use the word "religiomedical" when I want to explicitly flag this overlap for the reader.) The origin of the medical system of the *yi*, it might be noted, was commonly attributed to the deified culture hero known as the Yellow Emperor (*Huangdi*), who was a figure of widespread philosophical and religious importance in early China. It centered on understanding the intricacies of the ethereal cosmic vapor called "qi" and the resonances of yin and yang, which were the same concerns that undergirded multiple Chinese religious, divinatory, and cosmological traditions.

If "religion" thus lay at the heart of "medicine," then, conversely, every school of thought we might want to identify as "religious" in early China forwarded its own systematic model of how the body worked, what one needed to do to keep it functioning optimally, and how to respond when it broke down. Healing fell well within the realm of expertise that the clerics, priests, religious leaders, and ritual specialists of all persuasions arrogated to themselves. Moreover, judging by the huge volume of popular medieval literature about healing and healers, it was also one of the chief social functions that was expected of them by the laity.

If it is not the case that there was a systematic and secular "medicine" opposed to doctrinally unsophisticated traditions of "religious" healing in the medieval period, it is also not a question of "elite" versus "folk" therapies. As I will discuss below in detail, Buddhist monks actively competed against physicians, Daoists, spirit healers, and other religiomedical practitioners for patients of all social classes. Their competitions played out on a field that was largely unified by shared expectations, conventions, and assumptions. There are many indications in the historical record that healers of all of these types were taken seriously across all levels of society, and that their therapies were recognized as legitimate and prestigious even by emperors.

Given these facts, I am of the opinion that historians of the medieval period lose more than they gain if they reserve the category of "medicine" for the *yi,* and relegate other groups to the residual category of "healing." This bifurcation seems anachronistic in that it grants physicians more authority than they probably enjoyed in the medieval era and sets them off too distinctly from their contemporaries. In this book, I would rather use the English word "medicine" in an intentionally broad and fuzzy way in order to encompass the whole range of practitioners and to draw attention to the fluidity and interactions between them. When I want to refer to the *yi* in particular, I will use the term "physicians," and I will refer to their ideas and practices as "classical Chinese medicine."[41]

Since this volume is primarily a study of translation practices, there are many aspects of medicine I will not have the opportunity to discuss here, no matter how expansively I use that term. I will not have much to say about medical institutions, material culture, or artistic representations, for example, which I will leave to future publications. Out of necessity, I am also limiting the scope of this book to medicine associated with the physical body. Though there is an argument to be made that mental health should be included as well, if I were to attempt to do so, I would have to consider virtually every Buddhist text, as the vast majority of them claim to be intervening precisely in that arena. Other realms of Buddhist knowledge that connect closely or overlap with medicine but have also been omitted from this discussion include pharmacology, astrology, divination, calendrical sciences, alchemy, martial arts, hygiene, and longevity practices. Each of these constitutes a distinct field of study with its own large body of literature, and in my opinion they are best taken up in separate projects.

Building on this discussion of the scope of the term "medicine," my use of the term "Buddhist medicine" requires additional clarification. I am aware of only one example where medieval Chinese writers use a term that might be translated as "Buddhist medicine" (*foyi*)—and it is unlikely that that is what is meant in this particular case.[42] There is no equivalent term in Indian Buddhist texts, suggesting that this was not thought of as a distinct field of knowledge in the original cultural context. Not all Indian medical knowledge transmitted to China was associated with Buddhism, either. As I will discuss in the next chapter, texts about "Brahmanical" medicine (presumably meaning Āyurveda, but this is not certain) were also introduced into the Middle Kingdom. When I use the term "Buddhist medicine" here, I do not mean to clump all transmitted Indian medicine together nor to suggest that the ideas under discussion here were exclusively Buddhist. Rather, I use the term as a convenient label for discourses about medicine that were introduced to China via Buddhist translations and that were elaborated upon in Chinese Buddhist compositions. As will become clear below, I am not interested in retrospectively reifying the category of Buddhist medicine, but rather in exploring its construction and continual renegotiation in medieval China.

That being said, though the use of the term *foyi* did not come into common currency until the middle of the twentieth century, it is clear that Chinese authors in the medieval period did think of the medical knowledge contained in Buddhist scriptures and commentaries and practiced among the sangha as patently Buddhist. Most often, Buddhist writers discussed medical knowledge under generic headings such as "treating illness" (*zhibing*), "the suffering of illness" (*bingku*), and "nursing the sick" (*zhanbing*), but they make abundantly clear that the knowledge contained within is meant to be understood as Buddhist through both the context and the paratext of their compositions. In fact, as I will examine rather closely in the remainder of this book, over the course of the medieval period, authors were increasingly concerned with marking out what constituted Buddhist medical knowledge, with presenting it as superior to contemporary alternatives, and with policing these boundaries against unorthodox intrusions.

The examination of such writings reveals the changing contemporary understandings of what medical ideas counted as "Buddhist." Frequently, medieval Chinese Buddhist writings on medicine are characterized by their engagement with doctrines and practices that originated in the Indo-European cultural sphere and that were introduced into China as part of the transregional transmission of Buddhism. This was not a unified or homogeneous body of knowledge, however, since Buddhist texts entered China from any number of South, Central, and Southeast Asian territories over the span of centuries. At the same time, Buddhist authors also frequently worked indigenous Chinese vocabularies, ideas, and practices into their compositions. This book will not dedicate any significant amount of space to explicating the doctrines and practices that make up medieval Buddhist medicine, as this will be done in future publications. Rather, it is those processes of negotiation, inclusion, and exclusion that are our central concern here.

Moving now to a discussion of the translation conventions employed in this book, I am acutely aware of the ironies of writing about cross-cultural translation while simultaneously engaging in it. I will be the first to admit that I am, by the very nature of this project, translating the medieval Chinese historical experience in order to bring it under the gaze of the Euro-American academy.[43] In order to write as contextualized an account as possible, throughout the book I have made an effort to try to describe the medieval Chinese cultural and social world in my own words rather than by performing a series of acts of translation proper. On the occasions that I do engage in translation proper, I have often defaulted to the translation terms listed in the *Digital Dictionary of Buddhism* (below, *DDB*), a collaborative scholarly work that is now beginning to set translation norms in the field of Buddhist studies. However, though I have striven for a certain level of consistency with my colleagues, like most translators, in the end I present the reader with an idiosyncratic mishmash of equivalents of various types.

For the most part, I have tried to use English whenever possible so that this book will be accessible to nonspecialists. The first time I bring up a technical term, I give the most commonly occurring Chinese and Sanskrit equivalents, leading with the language that is most pertinent to the context I am speaking about. In discussions of the Chinese context, I only provide the Sanskrit if a Chinese term is clearly to be understood as a translation of a specific Indian word. Where such connections are not immediately apparent, I do not provide speculative back-translations that privilege the source over the target context.

Some sinologists object to the use of Sanskrit in discussions of Chinese Buddhism altogether, and I think there is much to commend that position. For example, I agree in principle with the argument that the word "Tripitaka" (Skt. *tripiṭaka*; Ch. *sanzang*; lit."three storehouses" or "three treasuries") is not literally applicable to the Chinese canon, as the Sanskrit implies a collection that is divisible into three parts but such divisions never were strictly adhered to in China.[44] Likewise, I agree that the word "sutra" (Skt. *sūtra*) is not interchangeable with the common Chinese translation $jing_1$, as the first refers to a specific subcategory of Indian Buddhist literature and the latter is a catchall word for a variety of genres of scripture and secular classics. Nevertheless, for the purposes of clarity and dialogue with scholars of Buddhism across Asia, I have used the Sanskrit in these and similar cases.

Throughout this book, I have normally translated medical terminology, whether Indian or Chinese, into English. When doing so, I have capitalized technical terms to distinguish them from their everyday English usage (e.g., Great Elements, Wind, Liver). However, I have left important keywords such as *tridoṣa* untranslated because of the lack of concrete translation equivalents in English. In all cases, I have briefly defined these terms when they are first mentioned. When using Sanskrit and Chinese words that have entered common English usage (e.g., qi, yin-yang, sutra), I leave them unitalicized and without diacriticals.

Like most scholars today, I use Hanyu pinyin to romanize Chinese characters. This transcription system reflects the modern Mandarin Chinese pronunciation, which has strayed far from the prevailing modes of speech in the medieval period. The historical drift in the pronunciation of characters becomes an issue in this study when speaking of the Chinese transliteration of Sanskrit. For example, when I give the Chinese transliteration of the name of the legendary Buddhist physician Jīvaka as "Qiyu" or "Qipo," the reader must keep in mind that the Early Middle Chinese pronunciation would have been much closer to the Sanskrit than the pinyin suggests.[45]

Finally, I have been flexible on whether individual people should be identified by Chinese or Sanskrit names, deciding on a case-by-case basis and defaulting to their most commonly known appellations. I have applied this same logic to names of deities, using English, Chinese, or Sanskrit terms as the case may be.

I hope by making the above choices I have made this book more readable and more accessible for a general audience. Of course I recognize that, like in all instances of translation discussed throughout this book (and, indeed, in all translations anywhere), there are both gains and losses that result from my decisions.

CHAPTER I

The Buddhist Medical Transmission

With the preliminaries behind us, we can begin our analysis by exploring the transmission and influence of Buddhist medicine. The arrival of Buddhist medicine in China represents the moment in world history that two relatively distinct Indo-European and Chinese medical models were brought into direct, sustained contact for the first time. This chapter begins by outlining the religiomedical vocabularies and ideas (i.e., the indigenous cultural-linguistic system) that prevailed in China prior to the arrival of Buddhism. These had an essential role to play in the reception of Buddhist medicine in China, as they provided both the linguistic backdrop against which translation activities took place and the font of cultural resonances translators could tap into when interpreting and explaining Indian medical ideas. The bulk of the chapter then focuses on a discussion of the medical ideas, practices, and institutions that were transmitted to China via Buddhism. These made notable contributions to medieval Chinese medical thought and culture as they were absorbed into the writings of elite physicians, into the political culture, and into the everyday lives of ordinary people.

The Indigenous Chinese Religiomedical System

In pre-Buddhist Chinese discourses about healing, two main modes of talking about health, illness, and the body predominated: a vocabulary that focused on the effects of spirits on the human world and one that revolved around the patterns of cosmic energies.[1] The first of these idioms, the more ancient of the two, posited a world teeming with gods, ghosts, ancestors, and other spiritual entities (known as *shen*, *gui*, and so on) that could affect the health and well-being of human beings.[2] This model appears in the Chinese historical record as early as the emergence of writing itself. Oracle bones from the Shang dynasty (ca. 1600–1046 B.C.E.) demonstrate that corporeal afflictions as varied as toothaches, headaches, bloated abdomen, and leg pains were blamed on the interference of ancestors or pernicious spirits.[3] Once the source of illness had been identified through ritual pyromancy using the plastrons of tortoises or the scapula of oxen, the Shang kings would make sacrifices to the offended spirits to atone for their transgressions in hopes of being granted a cure. Texts from the Eastern Zhou (770–256 B.C.E.) through the Han (206 B.C.E.–220 C.E.) show that rituals for managing pestilential demons remained a top priority in the maintenance of health and treatment of illness in the classical period. They also show that fears of divine retribution (*bao*) and desire for spiritual favor (*fu*) continued to be a focal point of religious practice of all kinds.[4]

Daoist movements emerging in the late Han and early medieval period employed this vocabulary of spirit retribution and ritual intervention to describe their techniques for warding off or curing illnesses.[5] For example, when illness struck followers of Celestial Masters Daoist (*tianshi dao*) sect, victims eschewed conventional medical therapies and instead entered into an oratory (*jingshi*), within which they contemplated their transgressions and repented in hopes of being granted a cure. While in many cases illness was characterized as a personal or familial moral failing, they could enlist the help of the spirit world by drinking consecrated water to exorcize evil demons, and by writing letters seeking clemency addressed to the spirits of Heaven, Earth, and Water. For followers of Shangqing Daoism, on the other hand, maintaining health involved caring for a pantheon of gods that lived within the human body. When disaster befell, patients could visit a priest who held official rank in the celestial bureaucracy and could negotiate on their behalf by sending official missives to the spirit world. The practice of sealing (what the scholar Michel Strickmann dubbed "ensigillation") also mimicked the routines of government officials: ritual officiants applied inked seals (*fuyin*) to pieces of paper that were consumed or worn by the patient as talismans, or placed directly on specific locations on the body in order to drive out disease-causing demons and other baleful influences.

Throughout the ancient and early medieval period, exorcisms, talismans, incantations (*zhou*), and other techniques to communicate with spirits were also proffered by ritualists who operated outside institutional religious organizations, and who were known to contemporaries as *wu*. Modern scholars writing in English have usually referred to these practitioners as "shamans" or "spirit mediums," although the applicability of these terms has been debated.[6] While entering the historical record only infrequently in the medieval period, scattered references to such healers are found in collections of narratives, dynastic histories, Buddhist and Daoist texts, and other sources. The medieval authors of such texts often go to great lengths to differentiate themselves from any association with the *wu*. However, although we are limited to reading between the lines of unflattering polemics, there is every indication that spirit healers of all sorts provided an important source of health care for much of the population in the medieval period, as continued to be the case throughout later Chinese history.

The practices of spirit medicine were by no means limited to the fringes of society or to the lower classes. The available sources suggest that spirit healing was used to treat a wide range of physical and mental disorders, and that commoners, members of the elite, and even emperors were interested in such therapies. Exorcistic spells and incantations have been found, for example, in the manuscripts unearthed at elite Han burial sites such as Shuihudi (217 B.C.E.) and Mawangdui (186–168 B.C.E.).[7] The "spellbinding" (*jie*) texts from Shuihudi, for example, are instructional manuals providing practical advice on how to perform exorcisms with everyday objects such as shoes, eggs, and pig excrement, and their presence in tombs suggests that knowledge of such things was highly valued.

The public exorcism of pestilential demons was also an important part of the official repertoire of responses to epidemics and was integral to the state ritual calendar.[8] The Great Exorcism (*danuo*) was an annual purification rite for the expulsion of a variety of evils. Among the demons expelled were numerous agents of disease, and, as a consequence, the ritual was sometimes referred to as "the expulsion of pestilences" (*zhuyi*). Performed within the imperial residences each New Year as early as the Zhou, the Great Exorcism remained an important means of keeping the spirit world at bay throughout the first millennium of the Common Era. It was closely associated with the state cult in the Han, enjoyed imperial sponsorship in the Sui (581–618) and Tang (618–907), and was still being performed at Dunhuang in the ninth and tenth centuries.

Spirit healing also continued to be influential among the medical officials attached to rulers' courts throughout the medieval period. Medical administration was a relatively unorganized affair in the Period of Division that stretched between the collapse of the Han dynasty and the reunification in the Sui. However, the Imperial Medical Office (*taiyi shu*) of the reunified Sui dynasty included four Erudites of Apotropaics (*zhoujin boshi*) who specialized in spells, talismans, exorcisms, and other ritual healing techniques.[9] The title given to these masters of ritual medicine, "Erudite," tells us that their knowledge was considered as respectable and as worthy of being taught in the imperial palace as any other aspect of medicine. Such ritualists continued to fill official posts in the state medical bureaucracies of the Tang and Song (960–1279) dynasties as well. A massive encyclopedia of medicine compiled at imperial behest at the height of the Song dynasty contains three fascicles (*juan*) cataloging talismans, rituals, and other interdictions, an indication of the continuing high value placed on spirit-based medicine in the loftier echelons of society.[10]

Disease-causing demons and the techniques to control them would remain pervasive topics of discussion throughout the remainder of Chinese history. However, beginning as early as the Warring States period (475–221 B.C.E.), certain authors began to argue that the cosmos was governed by cosmic patterns instead of capricious unseen beings.[11] By the early third century C.E., some members of the elite, such as the poet Cao Zhi (192–232), could consider their contemporaries' practices of hanging talismans and performing exorcisms to protect against epidemics to be "ridiculous."[12] While not all (or even most) were as quick to jettison their beliefs in spirits, the Han was a formative period for a new understanding of health, politics, and cosmology based on cosmic cycles that were predictable and impersonal.

According to this model, which is commonly called "correlative cosmology" or "sympathetic resonance," the cosmos was a homology of Heaven (*tian*), Earth (*di*), and Mankind (*ren*), united by qi. This universal substance, which permeated—and in fact made up—all things, was molded and influenced by the great polarity of yin and yang and by the Five Phases of transformation (*wuxing*, i.e., Wood, Fire, Earth, Metal, and Water).[13] The interconnected and holistic universe was governed by a principle that was as simple as it was profoundly explanatory: objects of the same category or nature were thought to spontaneously resonate with each other at a distance, just as when a note is struck on a lute, a nearby lute will reverberate at the same pitch.[14] This resonance was spoken of in terms of "stimulus and response" (*ganying*): events in one realm "stimulated" the qi of the entire cosmos, and the cosmos "responded" with parallel transformations in other realms.

The idea of a resonant connection between the qi of the body and that of the cosmos undergirded several currents of literature that began to proliferate in elite circles in the Han. Self-cultivation treatises taught how to "nourish life" (*yangsheng*) and manipulate qi with breathing exercises, therapeutic movements (*daoyin*, lit. "guiding and pulling"), and sexual practices (*fangzhong shu*, lit. "bedroom arts"). Other techniques included specialized dietary regimens, alchemical experimentation, and the consumption of drugs—all of which could lead to perfect health and extreme longevity.[15]

One of the most influential expressions of this idiom of cosmic energies and patterns is the seminal *Inner Canon of the Yellow Emperor* (*Huangdi neijing*).[16] While this first-century B.C.E. compilation is a composite text representing a range of divergent opinions, its unknown authors agree that the human body exists in a homologous relationship with the cosmos. A well-known and often-cited passage makes these connections explicit by correlating each anatomical or physiological feature of the human body with the spatiotemporal features of Heaven and Earth. In this passage, the shape of the head and feet corresponds with the round Heaven and square Earth, the eyes with the sun and moon, the emotions with the weather, the number of bones in the body with the number of days in the year, and so forth.[17]

In the *Inner Canon*, the human body is also compared to the ideal state, a homology that ensured medicine's key role in the legitimization and naturalization of the workings of the imperial government.[18] A network of circulation vessels (*mai* or *mo*) connected the extremities of the body with the five yin and six yang Viscera (*wuzang* and *liufu*). One's allotted quantity of qi flowed through these vessels and was shared among the Viscera, just as foodstuffs and other goods were effectively transported from granaries to depots along the waterways of the unified empire. The various systems operated in harmony within the body, just as the officials did within the ideal state. The Heart was the monarch, the Lungs were the ministers, the Liver was the general, and so forth, each one embodying the imperial values of efficiency, interdependence, and accountability.[19] Just as the government needed organization for its continuity, the body's offices needed to operate in concert in order to preserve health—with no one system failing in its duties or exceeding its bounds.

According to this harmonious ideal, cosmic patterns governed physiological processes in an orderly and efficient way that could be understood by the well-educated physician. The entire corporeal system was continually in flux and flow as it resonated with the changes of the seasons, the astral cycles, and the cosmic patterns of yin-yang and the Five Phases, but these changes were methodical and predictable. Medicine, like governance, was about discovering the natural order of the universe and adjusting one's behavior to accord with it. Illness meant not that the gods or spirits had been offended by one's moral failing, but that the natural cycles had been interrupted, impeded, or disturbed by an external agent or by one's own improper regimen. Healing involved the restoration of systemic balance through the manipulation of the body's qi with acupuncture, moxibustion, specialized regimen, bathing, exercise, and other therapies.[20] Even more important than cure, however, was prevention. Like the officials who advised the state on avoiding calamity by means of preemptive action, the physician doled out advice on preventing Internal Calamity (*neizai*) by adjusting to the seasonal shifts in qi before illness had a chance to arise.[21]

Although presented as discrete above, these two basic modes of talking about the body and its place in the cosmos—the idiom of spirits and that of cosmic energies—were never static and were in the medieval period usually closely intertwined. Different groups or individuals posited and defended unique blends in their writings that occasionally seem to favor one set of concepts at the expense of the other, but in actuality both were inseparable in the clinical and ritual practice of virtually every religiomedical group. Physicians steeped in classical Chinese medical models readily discussed therapies against demon infestation (*guizhu*, among other terms), while ritualists commonly understood disease-causing spirits as being composed of malefic qi.[22] In the popular consciousness, the human and the unseen worlds were unified by manifold spiritual and natural connections, and metamorphosis or transformation (*hua*, *bianhua*) between states was expected.

The spirit healers, Daoists, and physicians mentioned in this section are the practitioners that appear most often in the historical record, but they were far from the only healers around. If the popular genres of literature from the classical and medieval periods are any indication, immortals (*xian*), sages (*sheng*₁), ritual technicians (*fangshi*, lit. "gentlemen with techniques"), and other adepts possessing all sorts of transformative and healing knowledge were regularly sought for ailments of all sorts.[23] Lesser-attained practitioners were virtually ubiquitous—including pharmacists, herb gatherers, sellers of potions and nostrums, astrologers, diviners, and a panoply of others. The scholar of Chinese religion Erik Zürcher once described medieval Chinese Buddhism and Daoism as the professionalized tops of two pyramids rising from a shared base representing "an indistinct mass of popular beliefs and practices."[24] One might think of the Chinese health-care world as consisting of a similar spectrum. The tops of the pyramids are the syntheses developed by physicians, clerics, and other learned practitioners, which were promulgated in their texts and authorized by government institutions. Descending the pyramids, distinct syntheses fade into the communal reservoir from which all of these groups and individuals drew inspiration for their doctrines, practices, and explanatory narratives. The nebulous and constantly changing currents of popular medicine at the bottom of the pyramids had no all-encompassing name and, due to their oral nature, are difficult for historians to study in depth. Nevertheless, it is clear that this vernacular medical knowledge in all of its diversity also revolved around the dual themes of spirits and cosmic patterns. Thus the core vocabulary of the two idioms introduced in this section (*fu*, *bao*, *shen*, *ganying*, *bianhua*, qi, yin-yang, *wuxing*, and so on) represented the indigenous religiomedical cultural-linguistic system, the normative lexicon that bound together Chinese religion and medicine at all levels of society. When Buddhist specialists began to promulgate Indian models of disease and healing in China, this is the conversation into which they were inserting themselves.

The Introduction of Buddhist Medicine to China

Though rudimentary trade routes cutting across Central and Southeast Asia had allowed for some amount of Indo-Sinitic exchange in the ancient period, the Indo-European and East Asian medical worlds were largely separate before the second century B.C.E.[25] The vast desert sands, dense malarial jungles, and formidable altitudes of the Tibetan plateau represented significant barriers to extensive intercourse. Direct trade and diplomatic links between the two lands began to be established only in the year 138 B.C.E., when an emissary of the Han dynasty court named Zhang Qian (d. 114 B.C.E.) led a Chinese expedition west into Central Asia.[26] Zhang's mission, to secure an alliance with the Yuezhi people against their mutual foe, the Xiongnu, was unsuccessful. He was captured by the enemy and held for about a decade. However, his reports to the emperor upon his eventual return to China stoked the Han dynasty's enthusiasm for penetrating further into the "Western Regions" (*xiyu*).

As Emperor Wudi (r. 141–87 B.C.E.) extended the Great Wall and the network of military garrisons westward into what today is the province of Xinjiang, China began to project power deeper into the Central Asian steppe. Mirror images of this Chinese expansion also took place on the southern and western ends of Central Asia, as both the Parthian (247 B.C.E.–224 C.E.) and later the Kushan (first to third centuries C.E.) empires also expanded into the region. The eventual occupation of the steppe by these three major land empires stabilized and enhanced the network of ancient trade routes crossing the region. Dubbed the "Silk Roads" in the nineteenth century, these overland routes were further developed by Parthian and Sogdian traders over the ensuing centuries, allowing for China's increased trade and communication with India, Persia, Rome, Egypt, and beyond.[27] In the second to third centuries C.E., advances in maritime technology meant that this overland traffic could be supplemented with a burgeoning "Southern Seas" (nanhai) trade via the kingdoms of Southeast Asia. Over the ensuing centuries, while the volume of trade over land and sea fluctuated in response to political and economic vicissitudes at various nodes throughout the network, the integration of Eurasia was inexorable and China came to be increasingly connected with other parts of the world.

Along with the increase in transregional economic interactions, the establishment of these cross-cultural connections also facilitated exchanges of a much more nefarious kind. Carried across the newly opened trade networks, foreign pathogens such as smallpox and measles were unleashed upon the immunologically unprepared Chinese.[28] In the opinion of some historians, the virulent epidemics unleashed by cross-cultural contact in fact played a role in destabilizing both the Han dynasty and Rome, on the opposite ends of the trade system.[29] Certainly, the onslaught of strange new illnesses contributed to the sense of uncertainty and social upheaval that marked the late Han and medieval period. Contemporary accounts testify to the personal and social toll of these epidemics and indicate that medical thinkers were desperate to develop new approaches in response. For example, the influential medical classic *Treatise on Cold Damage* (*Shanghan lun*), written by the physician Zhang Ji in response to an epidemic fever in 196 C.E. that killed two-thirds of his family, formed the basis for a new branch of medicine that specialized in febrile diseases and represented a significant departure from the models found in previous medical writings.[30]

In addition to epidemics, the late Han was also plagued by a resurgent nomadic alliance on its western frontier as the dynasty began to lose control over its outlying territories. The state finally collapsed from a complex combination of internal and external strains in 220. While a series of successor states vied for dominance, invaders from the steppe made increasingly deep incursions into China proper, eventually seizing the territory north of the

Yangzi River in 311. The new overlords were members of the Tuoba branch of the Xianbei, who like all peoples from beyond the frontier were routinely characterized by Han Chinese as barbarian and demonic.[31] Their invasion and occupation sparked a mass exodus of the Chinese elite to the southern side of the Yangzi. Large numbers of Han people settled deep in areas they had long noted only for noxious malarial swamps and disease-causing miasmas.[32]

The combined blows of epidemics, war, and mass displacement resulted in heavy death tolls and a sense of total economic and cultural devastation.[33] Because the state and cosmos were homologous in classical Chinese thinking, such monumental disruption of the sociopolitical realm could only signal that the harmony of Heaven, Earth, and Mankind had been rent asunder. For some of the elite, the only attractive alternative was to withdraw from politics in favor of a reclusive life of contemplation.[34] Others remained active in government and intellectual pursuits, struggling to reconcile an idealized past with the realpolitik of the present. Philosophers and administrators alike questioned whether the wisdom of the ancients still held viable solutions in such turbulent times and they actively sought a range of new approaches.[35] The questioning of classical models—including medical models—presented an unprecedented opening for new domestic religiomedical syntheses to arise and for the acceptance of novel ideas from abroad.

In the grim and uncertain environment of the Period of Division, it is not difficult to understand the psychological appeal of "Heavenly India" (*tian-zhu*).[36] As the Chinese subcontinent was engulfed in chaos and violence, the Indian one was flourishing. The Gupta dynasty (ca. 320–550 C.E.) is often called the "Golden Age" of Indian history. Across the transregional web of oasis towns and seaports, Indian merchants played a key role in a thriving trade of luxury goods such as glass, perfumes, indigo, textiles, tortoise shells, horses, silks, and the precious substances known as the "seven treasures" (Skt. *sapta-ratna*; Ch. *qibao*).[37] Indian agricultural, technological, architectural, artistic, and scientific knowledge were considered state-of-the-art and were emulated throughout Asia. Much of the stimulus for India's major exports can be attributed to practices associated with Buddhism, which was now beginning to spread along the same trade routes.

Tradition holds that the first Buddhist missionaries to arrive in China were the Indian monks Kāśyapa Mātaṅga and Zhu Falan in 67 C.E.[38] While the story has been shown to be legendary, aspects of Buddhism had indeed arrived in several parts of China by the end of Han dynasty.[39] At first, the new religion was largely limited to enclaves of foreigners and merchants, and elite Chinese, when they noticed it, seem to have taken it as some form of Daoism. By the fourth century, though, continuing contact with India and the rest of the Buddhist world via the land and sea routes had strengthened the religion's presence in China. Eventually, as its teachings were translated into ever more intelligible—and eventually even elegant—Chinese, Buddhism began to penetrate all levels of Chinese society.

In the medieval period, China was on the receiving end of a diverse array of Buddhist missionaries from across the Asian continent.[40] The first wave to arrive in the period from the mid-second century to about 270 hailed from Parthia. For the next century or so, monks from Kucha and Khotan predominated. At the peak of the Gupta period (ca. 380 to the mid-fifth century), monks from northern India began to represent the majority. From the middle of the fifth century onward, Indian missionaries continued to arrive, now supplemented by those from Southeast Asia. As one scholar has aptly put it, the geographic diversity of these Buddhist missionaries made for a "bewildering mass" of contradictory teachings in China.[41] Multiple schools of Buddhism that had developed over centuries in India entered China simultaneously alongside variants of the religion that had evolved in other localities. The confusion was made worse by the fact that the translation of Buddhist texts was piecemeal and haphazard. The absence of a centralized authority organizing translation projects across the disunited realm meant that the choices of which texts to translate were made arbitrarily or in response to local needs.[42] Often, such decisions were dictated by the chance appearance of foreign monks who previously had memorized certain texts or who happened to have possession of certain manuscripts. With the reunification of China in the Sui-Tang era, the importation of Buddhist texts became a much more organized affair. Chinese monks in this period sought out specific texts that were missing or that they perceived had been poorly translated in the past. Foreign monks specializing in particular types of Buddhist knowledge residing as far away as India and Southeast Asia were often "head-hunted"—personally sought out and called to the Chinese court to head up translation projects.[43] Translation activities were supported and overseen by the central government, and target texts were often tailored to bolster the ideologies of the current regime.

While there were thousands of Indians and Central Asians living in Chinese cities, the total number of named foreign missionaries in the medieval period remains limited to no more than 117 individuals.[44] Despite their sparse numbers, these people were responsible for the introduction of a dispropor-tionately large wave of Buddhist literature. Estimates place the total quantity of Indian literature imported into China at approximately 46 million charac-ters for scriptures and 26 million for related texts.[45] Zhisheng (669–740), compiler of the *Kaiyuan-Era Catalog of Buddhist Teachings* (*Kaiyuan shijiao lu*, T. 2154), reckoned that 3,136 scrolls (*juan*) of Buddhist scripture had been translated by his lifetime.[46] While such numbers are staggering, they account neither for the many Buddhist writings that went unrecorded in the catalog, nor for the oral aspects of the tradition that were never written down at all.[47]

The Indo-Sinitic transmission was not concerned only with topics we moderns would characterize as "religious." It introduced China to Indian ways of knowing the entire cosmos and everything in it. China was on the receiving end of Indian science and technology, agricultural knowledge, as-tronomy, calendrical sciences, mathematics, sugar making, alchemy, and many other fields of inquiry, as well as medicine. While the introduction of Buddhist philosophies, devotional practices, and monastic culture to China have received much scholarly attention, the impact of this scientific and techni-cal transmission on Chinese thought has remained woefully understudied.[48]

Not all examples of Indo-Sinitic exchange occurred in the context of Buddhism; nevertheless, much of the extant evidence of this transmission is today to be found within Buddhist literature. For example, many different strands of medical knowledge are embedded within the Buddhist scriptures imported into China. Of the Buddhist translations from this period that are extant, the number of texts that are relevant to the topic is huge. Though counting characters is a crude measure, the graph *bing* (meaning "illness," "disease," or "ailment") appears over 40,000 times in the Chinese portion of the *Taishō Tripitaka*.[49] One may object that *bing*'s semantic range is too wide as it can also mean "imperfection" or, more rarely, as a verb, "to injure." But *yao* (the most common term for medicinal substances) appears more than 26,000 times. Likewise, *yi* (meaning "medicine" or "physician," as discussed in the in-troduction) appears almost 7,000 times. Notably, the sources in which these characters appear include every genre and were composed in every era repre-sented in the collection. By any measure, medicine was clearly a topic of great concern.

A good percentage of the references to medical topics appears in narra-tives. Occasionally Buddhist stories hint at practices that are not adequately recorded in other types of literature. For example, the medical historian is tantalized upon reading an episode from the *King Aśoka Sutra* (*Ayuwang jing*,

T. 2043) translated into Chinese in 512 by Saṃghabhara (460–524), a monk from Funan (present-day Cambodia).[50] In this narrative, King Aśoka falls ill and his physicians are unable to cure him. However, the queen finds a sick man with similar symptoms and has him cut open. She discovers a parasite (Ch. *chong*; Skt. *kṛmi*) inside him and, by applying different substances, determines that garlic is effective in killing it.[51] She convinces the king to take garlic and thereby saves his life. While of course the historicity of the events depicted in this story cannot be taken for granted, tales detailing such procedures raise important questions about experimental anatomy and diagnostic procedures in early India.

Narratives provide a vista onto contemporary medical practices and the broader cultural meanings of healing, and I will discuss these types of sources in more detail in Chapter 5. However, the Chinese Buddhist corpus also includes many prescriptive texts that purport to teach Buddhist medical doctrines and practices. Such writings exist in large numbers and span multiple genres. As early as the third century, both translations and pseudotranslations began to appear that explained Buddhist ideas about anatomy, physiology, and embryological development; that discussed rituals for invoking the medical assistance of particular deities; and that gave instructions for healing disease and maintaining one's health with meditation, regimen, and dietary therapy. Monastic disciplinary texts translated and composed in the fifth and sixth centuries detailed the regulations concerning the handling, storage, and allowable use of medicinal substances. Spell texts outlining how to cure a host of maladies caused by demons and other malicious influences were in wide circulation by the early sixth century. Commentaries and compilations composed from the sixth to eighth centuries collated and interpreted the knowledge found throughout the Tripiṭaka, while travelogues gave detailed accounts of Indian monastic medical and hygienic practices to inspire the Chinese sangha. Together with the abovementioned narratives, these texts collectively make up the corpus at the center of this book.

The contents of such texts introduced Chinese audiences to doctrines and perspectives that were characteristic of Indo-European medical thought. Some of the basic principles of Buddhist medicine—encountered frequently in texts written in Sanskrit, Pāli, Tibetan, and other languages, as well as in Chinese—were fundamentally at odds with native Chinese medical discourses. For example, whereas Chinese writings tended to hold that the natural state of humanity was one of health and harmony, Buddhist texts stressed that suffering, including illness, is inevitable for all unenlightened beings. The human body is made up of Great Elements (Skt. *mahābhūta*), sometimes numbering four, five, six, or more, but always including Earth, Water, Fire, and Wind. These Elements are inherently antagonistic, and the resulting instability means that disease and discomfort are the default settings of the human body. Other basic Buddhist perspectives include the idea that it is ultimately karma that determines one's experience of suffering in this life. Also, negative mental or emotional states, particularly greed, hatred, and delusion, are major (often the primary) factors that lead to specific disorders. In addition to these broader philosophical positions, Buddhist writings also engage in detail or in passing with Indian anatomical and physiological concepts, etiological doctrines, and therapeutics.

Buddhism also introduced a new pantheon of all-powerful deities, and texts describing their healing powers became extremely popular in China. The most celebrated healing buddhas and bodhisattvas, especially noted for their abilities to heal the sick, included:

1. Master of Medicines Buddha (Ch. Yaoshi Fo; Skt. Bhaiṣajyaguru);
2. King of Medicine Bodhisattva (Ch. Yaowang; Skt. Bhaiṣajyarāja);
3. his brother, Supreme Medicine Bodhisattva (Ch. Yaoshang; Skt. Bhaiṣajyasamudgata);
4. Guanyin Bodhisattva (also Guanshiyin, i.e., "Perceiver of the World's Sounds"; Skt. Avalokiteśvara);
5. the deity known alternately as the Buddha of Infinite Light (Ch. Amituo Fo; Skt. Amitābha) or the Buddha of Infinite Life (Ch. Wuliangshou Fo; Skt. Amitāyus); and
6. Samantabhadra Bodhisattva (i.e., "Universal Worthiness"; Ch. Puxian).[52]

These Buddhist deities became increasingly important in both devotional practice and literary representation over the course of the medieval period. Such figures served many functions—including bringing salvation to the faithful, protecting individuals and the state from harm, and intervening in other this-worldly concerns—and were not exclusively, or even primarily, concerned with healing. However, major scriptures circulating throughout Asia, such as the

Lotus Sutra (*Fahua jing*, T. 262–264) and the *Sutra on the Master of Medicines Buddha* (*Yaoshi fo jing*, T. 449–451, T. 1331.12), often specifically promised that they would protect against epidemics and compassionately intervene in cases of illness on behalf of devotees who called upon them.[53] In addition, minor deities with names suggesting powers of healing—such as the bodhisattvas Bestower of Medicine (Shiyao) and Healer of Troublesome Ailments (Liao Zhu Fannao Bing)—frequently are named in Buddhist scriptures as part of the Buddha's assembly, or as overseers of particular paradises or Pure Lands.[54] Unlike the major deities listed above, these figures had little ritual or literary importance in China, but they still contributed in a more general way to a close association between Buddhist practice and intercessory healing powers.

In addition to buddhas and bodhisattvas, various other categories of superhuman beings from the Indian tradition—such as devas (*tian*), *vidyārāja* (*mingwang*), rakṣa (*luocha*), yakṣa (*yecha*), and other spirits—were also introduced to China as agents of healing. One example of this class of beings, Ucchuṣma (Ch. Wushusemo or Wuchushamo), also known as the Vajra-Being of Impurities (Ch. Bujing Jin'gang), became an important deity in esoteric healing rites in the late medieval period.[55] In Indian texts, some of these demigods were said to have originally been malevolent spirits that had been pacified and converted to Buddhism.[56] Others were appropriated from Vedic religion or local Indian cults, or else were personifications of asterisms, spells, or other esoterica. Chinese Buddhist authors soon followed suit, composing texts that purported to tame indigenous ghosts and ghouls as well, co-opting them into the ranks of beneficial protectors of the Dharma.[57] By incorporating local spirits in this way, Buddhist authors claimed dominion over the indigenous Chinese spirit world and made Buddhism more relevant to daily life in China.

Finally, Buddhist texts also introduced a range of heroes that were revered as wise healers. Jīvaka Kumārabhṛta (Ch. Qipo or Qiyu), the lay doctor known as the King of Physicians (Ch. *yiwang*; Skt. *vaidyarāja*), is one such figure. As I will discuss in more detail in Chapter 5, his biography was amended during its translation in order to transform the protagonist into a model healer that could rival the celebrated physicians of Chinese tradition. Nāgārjuna (Ch. Longshu) underwent a process of transformation from a human philosopher, tantric master, and teacher of esoterica to a superhuman bodhisattva. He would also be widely propitiated in the Tang and Song as a healing deity.[58]

In addition to medical doctrines, deities, and heroes, Buddhism also introduced to China novel social practices associated with healing disease and maintaining health. Merit making—which involved caring for the sick and poor in order to improve one's own karma—came to be an important part of everyday devotional practice in China.[59] Buddhist monastic institutions promoted and organized such charitable activities. Through donations, investment, and economic activity, temples amassed repositories of wealth in Inexhaustible Treasuries (*wujinzang*) that were used to orchestrate the storage of food for famine relief, nursing and hospice care for the sick, leprosariums, and dispensaries of medicines in times of epidemics.[60]

Meanwhile, local mutual aid groups (*fahui, yiyi, yihui,* and so on) promoted popularized versions of Buddhist morality, self-discipline, and charity among the laity.[61] Such organizations were not new with the introduction of Buddhism, and were modeled on societies for local deities that were active in the Han. In the Period of Division, however, mutual aid groups such as the famous White Lotus Society (*bailian she*) established in 402 by Huiyuan (334–416) became a major part of the Buddhist proselytizing effort across China. These societies ranged in size from a few members to thousands. They were usually led by members of the sangha and financed by subscription payments from the laity. Members pooled their resources to contribute to a range of communal merit-making and charitable efforts, including epidemic and famine relief. Such projects also included the inscription of medicinal formulas in the walls of a cave at Longmen, as well as establishing communal baths and hot springs at temples for the benefit of the local monastic and lay communities.[62]

As the medieval period progressed, Buddhism made continual inroads into Chinese political life as well.[63] Although it developed differently in different areas, the religion eventually became an inextricable part of the exercise of power across China. In the South, Emperor Wu of the Liang dynasty (r. 502–49) conspicuously renounced Daoism, took bodhisattva vows, hosted vegetarian feasts catering to thousands of monks, and patronized Buddhist charities in an effort to style himself as a Wheel-Turning Buddhist Sage-King (Ch. *zhuanlun shengwan*; Skt. *cakravartin*).[64] Meanwhile, in the North, the Tuoba emperors fashioned themselves as incarnated buddhas in their own right. Charitable projects in this part of China, such as devotional steles, colossal sculptures, and the inscription of Buddhist sutras in stone, emphasized the linkage between merit making, the good fortune of the state, and the personal well-being of its rulers.[65]

In the absence of centralized state control, the monastic order became an increasingly elaborate and sophisticated institution in the early medieval period. There always was a strand of society that criticized Buddhism on various grounds, including that it was inappropriate for the Han people to adopt any foreign religion. Occasionally, efforts by local rulers to curb rising ecclesiastical power involved the closure of temples and defrocking of Buddhist clerics.[66] Nevertheless, even the two largest campaigns against the sangha in the Period of Division, carried out in 446–52 and 574–78, had little effect on Buddhism's ascendancy. When China was reunited in the late sixth century by the Sui dynasty, the founding emperor Wen distributed relics across the land, built stupas, and established Buddhist charities for the poor and sick in magnanimous gestures modeled after the legendary Indian king Aśoka.[67] Such public devotion ensured that Buddhism—and Buddhist medical charity—became ideologically integrated with the reunification project. Although several emperors of the subsequent Tang dynasty on the whole favored Daoism, they continued to patronize Buddhist institutions across the growing empire as a matter of policy. Enthusiasm for Buddhist institutions reached new heights in the reign of Empress Wu Zetian (de facto ruler of China from 660 to 705), who mobilized the considerable symbolic, rhetorical, and ritual repertoire of Buddhism in order to legitimize the usurpation of power by a woman for the first time in Chinese history.[68] In the last years of her reign, she conspicuously used the network of imperial temples to promote medical charity throughout the realm.

The sixth to eighth centuries represented the height of Indian influence in China, and it was also the high point of the impact of Buddhist medical ideas and practices. By the mid-eighth century, almost all of the main texts on Buddhist medicine that were going to reach China had already been translated, and the major commentaries collecting and organizing this knowledge had already been composed. Emperors and commoners alike knew to call upon Buddhist specialists to deal with their ailments, and Buddhist medical charities were operational throughout the land. Government officials and the elite were organizing the recopying of the texts associated with healing deities to earn karmic merit for themselves and for the realm. Conducted with imperial grandeur, the Master of Medicines Buddha rites were being staged on a scale that involved a thousand monks and spanning as many days in order to protect the country against epidemics and other calamities.[69] On a more pedestrian level, healing rites became integrated with the annual Lantern

Festival and came to be celebrated by individuals, families, and communities across virtually all segments of society. Narratives about Buddhist healing were in wide circulation, and Buddhism had found a place in the popular religiomedical imagination.

Influence and Syncretism

When scholars have examined the question of the influence of Indian ideas on Chinese medicine, they have identified three main areas where the impact is especially clear. In the first place, medieval dynastic records show that texts containing Indian healing knowledge were housed within imperial libraries, which indicates they were collected by the most highly placed physicians in Chinese society. The medical section of the catalog of the Sui dynasty, for example, includes the following unapologetically foreign titles right alongside the indigenous medical classics:

> *Classic on the Sangha's Restorative Acupuncture and Moxibustion*
> (*Shiseng kuang zhenjiu jing*), one fascicle (*juan*)
> *Medical Formulas of Nāgārjuna Bodhisattva* (*Longshu pusa yaofang*),
> four fascicles
> *Medical Formulas Taught by Various Rishis of the Western Regions*
> (*Xiyu zhuxian suoshuo yaofang*), twenty-three fascicles
> *Medical Formulas of the Rishis of Gandhamādana Mountain*
> (*Xiangshan xianren yaofang*), ten fascicles
> *Formulas of the Brahman Rishis of the Western Regions* (*Xiyu boluo
> xianren fang*), three fascicles
> *Essential Formulas Compiled by the Famous Physicians of the Western
> Regions* (*Xiyu mingyi suoji yaofang*), four fascicles
> *Medical Formulas of Various Brahman Rishis* (*Poluomen zhuxian
> yaofang*), twenty fascicles
> *Brahman Medical Formulas* (*Poluomen yaofang*), five fascicles
> *Divinatory Methods of the Rishis, Practiced by Jīvaka* (*Qipo suoshu
> xianren minglun fang*), two fascicles[70]

By virtue of their inclusion in this catalog, these diverse writings on Indian medicine, Buddhist and otherwise, clearly were accorded a high level of regard by contemporary medical officials.

Second, and in a related vein, Indian medical doctrines and procedures are frequently discussed in the writings of some of the leading Chinese medical authors of the medieval period. For example, a materia medica compilation by the polymath Tao Hongjing (456–536), an encyclopedic handbook of etiology and symptomology by the court physician Chao Yuanfang (550–630), a seminal formulary by the celebrated Sun Simiao (581–682), and a treatise by the official Wang Tao (670–755) all incorporate Indian ideas.[71] These four authors employ the doctrine of the Four Elements, describe "Brahmanical" massage practices, promote Buddhist ethics, and attribute pharmaceutical preparations to legendary Indian healers. They advocate rituals, incantations, and other therapies drawn from Buddhist texts, and borrow terminology from the sutras. They describe Indian ophthalmological procedures for the treatment of glaucoma, cataracts, and other eye disorders, and redeploy Indian ideas about fetal development in their discussions of embryology.

Third, pharmaceuticals from South Asia—which were major items both of tribute and of commerce—exerted a formative impact on medieval Chinese pharmacological literature.[72] The foundational text of this tradition was the *Materia Medica of the Divine Husbandman* (*Shennong bencao jing*), compiled in the first or second century C.E. and featuring only 365 medicinal substances.[73] The influx of new medicines via the Silk Roads and maritime routes sparked a dramatic increase in the number of drugs, prescriptions, and pharmacological texts circulating in the medieval period. The *Newly Revised Materia Medica* (*Xinxiu bencao*) edited in 659 and the *Supplement to the Materia Medica* (*Bencao shiyi*) written in 739, for example, both included large numbers of new foreign drugs. The ninth-century *Foreign Materia Medica* (*Hu bencao*) and the ninth- to tenth-century *Overseas Materia Medica* (*Haiyao bencao*) were entirely dedicated to cataloging imported drugs. By the Song, some materia medica compilations included up to 1,700 different substances, including a large proportion that were introduced from abroad.[74]

While these three aspects of India's influence on Chinese medicine are compelling, the cross-cultural encounter seems to have had an even more profound impact outside of official medical circles. Historians have gained a glimpse of the extent of this influence thanks to a large cache of manuscripts discovered in a sealed room in the Mogao Buddhist cave temple at Dunhuang. This trove, which has received much attention of late from historians of Chinese medicine, comprises tens of thousands of manuscripts and parts thereof dating from the fourth through the tenth centuries C.E.[75] These manuscripts include local copies of the best known medical treatises of the time—

including multiple copies of Zhang Ji's *Treatise on Cold Damage*, copies of the *Newly Revised Materia Medica*, and excerpts from the *Inner Canon*—as well as commentaries upon them. The collection also contains a number of texts advocating self-cultivation practices such as breathing exercises, grain avoidance, sexual alchemy, and a range of other indigenous Chinese traditions based on the regulation of qi. In addition, a number of the Dunhuang medical manuscripts also have an overtly Buddhist character. These include previously unknown distillations of or commentaries upon texts in the received Tripitaka, liturgical manuals that outline the performance of Buddhist healing rites, and unique treatises on Buddhist healing and wisdom not attested elsewhere.[76]

The Dunhuang collection is not only eclectic, however, it is also highly syncretic. Many of the manuscripts explicitly position themselves within particular sectarian discourses, but the actual contents of these texts often defy easy categorization. They often freely mix themes, practices, and vocabularies from a number of medical and religious contexts, both foreign and domestic. A text known as *Buddhist Formulas for Grain Avoidance* (*Fojia bigu fang*, P. 2637), for example, places dietary restrictions typically associated with indigenous traditions of transcendence in the context of devotion to the bodhisattva Guanyin.[77] Likewise, a number of spell texts and instructions for the making of talismans present typical Chinese healing techniques as the teachings of legendary Indian masters.[78] Many other manuscripts combine Buddhist ideas with elements of iatromancy, physiognomy, self-cultivation, dietary regimes, love magic, and the ritual management of pestilential demons that overlapped sectarian divides and were the common cultural heritage of all Chinese traditions.

The syncretism of this cache of manuscripts is evidence that there was no dominant system of medical thought at Dunhuang during the medieval period. The texts also show us that there was a rich repertoire of techniques and explanatory frameworks available from which any individual patient, practitioner, or medical author could draw. While the manuscripts reflect the local situation at Dunhuang and cannot be taken as being representative of China as a whole, their syncretism and eclecticism throw into doubt some of our basic assumptions about how medical knowledge circulated in medieval China. Different facets of medical knowledge seem to have traveled separately and in unique combinations and to have been employed in locally specific ways. Moreover, distinctions between "religion" and "medicine"—while perhaps operative in other social settings—seem to have been all but irrelevant for the authors and collectors of these manuscripts. The boundaries between foreign and indigenous healing traditions were likewise porous in the extreme. Just as scholars of Chinese religion have emphasized that Confucianism, Daoism, and Buddhism were not "hard-sided, clearly demarcated containers" in the medieval period, the inescapable conclusion is that healing traditions were just as fluid.[79]

As the historian of Chinese science Nathan Sivin once pointedly said: even though Daoists ate rice, we do not say that rice is Daoist.[80] Like rice, many medical doctrines and therapeutic practices circulated so widely in medieval Chinese society that they became disconnected from their original context—whatever that may have been—and became diffused throughout the popular culture. To use an anachronistic phrase, therapeutic ideas and practices often do not appear to have been the exclusive "intellectual property" of any one particular group. The intensive borrowing, sharing, and adaptation of texts, doctrines, terminology, rituals, material culture, and other aspects of healing knowledge among all types of religiomedical practitioners were the norm rather than the exception. Once introduced into China, as demonstrated by the Dunhuang manuscripts, Buddhist ideas and practices came to be liberally mixed together with indigenous healing knowledge of all kinds. The result of this syncretism was both that Chinese Buddhist texts came to espouse hybrid forms of therapy that were unknown in India and that many Indian medical ideas became part of Chinese religiomedical culture.

* * *

Speaking of the Buddhist contributions to the Chinese medical world, as we have been doing in this chapter, focuses us on the transmission of Indian cultural-linguistic structures and their integration into Chinese culture. This approach emphasizes the fluidity of the boundaries between different religiomedical traditions and allows us to appreciate how many foreign elements entered that mix. So far, however, we have only been discussing the upper portion of Nida's diagram. This focus on the interplay between domestic and foreign cultural-linguistic systems is only one part of the story of cross-cultural exchange. It tells us what ideas were introduced from abroad and what cultural resources healers could draw upon in formulating their unique syntheses of texts and practices. But it does not explain why certain choices were made by individuals or groups of practitioners in particular historical contexts. It does not reveal the human agency and interactions that brought the medieval medical world to life. In the chapters that come, I will show that integrating the lower half of Nida's diagram into our discussion allows for a richer analysis of the medieval medical world than focusing on the questions of influence and syncretism alone. I will show that an analysis of the translation of Buddhist texts can provide a starting point to begin to reconstruct the motivations, goals, and priorities of historical actors. And, I will show that understanding cross-cultural exchange as an active process undertaken by individual people allows us to see it as dynamic, full of human agency and creative potential.

CHAPTER 2

Translators and Translation Practice

Though it is often convenient to discuss cross-cultural exchange from the perspective of transmission and influence, cultures are not historical actors and they do not impact one another directly.[1] The crucial catalyst is always the translational activity of individual people. This chapter thus shifts from discussing the elements of Buddhist medical knowledge introduced into China to analyzing how, why, and by whom these were translated. We will identify the individuals involved with the translation project, examine their strategic goals, and illuminate the sociopolitical contexts for their translation decisions. In the process, we will also investigate how medical ideas could become touchstones for boundary building and competition, and explore how translation helped the sangha to negotiate contemporary tensions with other religiomedical practitioners. Rather than limiting our understanding of Indo-Sinitic medical exchange to the interaction between disembodied cultural-linguistic systems, this type of analysis allows us to place human decision making at the center of our story.

The Translators

Few of the Buddhist ideas, social practices, and institutions mentioned in the previous chapter would have been able to take root in medieval China were it not for the mobility made possible by the consolidation of the Silk Road and maritime routes. Merchants and adventurers from Sri Lanka to Japan and from Persia to Indonesia plied the trade routes in far greater numbers than ever before, picking up and leaving behind texts, ideas, and material items wherever they went. Likewise, Buddhist monks crisscrossed their interconnected world in order to propagate the Dharma, collect scriptures, gain education, and find patronage.[2] While the exploits of a handful of famous Chinese travelers are well known, uncounted numbers of voyagers from all parts of Eurasia embarked on lesser-known sojourns of crosscultural discovery and exchange. Just as important as the people, goods, and ideas moving along the trade routes, however, were the translators who facilitated all of the communication along these "roads of dialogue."[3] While the individuals who served as translators often remain invisible in historical narratives, intercultural dialogue on such a scale could not happen without massive amounts of work on their part.[4] By one scholar's count, crosscultural exchanges throughout the region were transacted in "Old Turkic, Chinese, Sanskrit, Sogdian, Middle Persian, New Persian, Parthian, Tibetan, Mongolian, Prakrit, Tumshuqese, Tocharian A and B, Bactrian, Khotanese, Hebrew, Syriac, Arabic, Tangut, Greek and Khitan," and were written in at least twenty different scripts from all over Eurasia.[5] Manuscripts have been found recording all manners of Daoist, Confucian, Zoroastrian, Nestorian Christian, and Manichaean wisdom, as well as secular knowledge including divination, literature, music, dance, history, and, of course, medicine. However, judging from our extant texts, much of the conversation taking place along the medieval trade routes revolved around Buddhism.

Translators played an indispensable role in spreading Buddhism around the trade networks, and translation projects got under way as soon as Buddhism made inroads in China. These endeavored both to make sense of Buddhist teachings and to repackage the Dharma in ways that were compatible with Chinese literary conventions.[6] Who were these translators? Although I refer to the "Chinese translators" of Buddhist texts, I mean this in the sense that they translated the texts into Chinese—not that they themselves were necessarily of Han ethnicity. The individuals involved in the Buddhist translation effort exemplified the multicultural, multiethnic, and multilingual character of medieval Buddhism itself.[7] The majority of the individuals known to us were foreigners living in China. Others were Chinese-born pilgrims who trekked to the ends of the known world and returned back home again to share their stories.[8]

Some of the best-known translators of Buddhism were also significant translators of Buddhist medicine.[9] Allow me to briefly introduce just a few of them here.

An Shigao

An Shigao (d. ca. 170) hailed from Parthia, in what is now northeastern Iran.[10] Although there is some controversy over the identity of this enigmatic figure, and his actual life story may have differed greatly from the traditional accounts thereof, the standard legend is that he renounced his claim to the Parthian throne to become a monk. He arrived in the Han capital at Luoyang in 148, and under the patronage of local donors set to work translating scriptures for a nascent community of foreign and Chinese devotees. Scholars have debunked many of the attributions to An Shigao that crept into Buddhist catalogs over the centuries.[11] Nevertheless, he is still the earliest reliably dated Buddhist translator in Chinese history, the founder of the first translation assembly, and also the earliest translator to grapple with rendering Indian medicine in Chinese. Confirmed translations by An Shigao with medical content include the *Sutra on the Stages of the Path of Cultivation* (*Daodi jing*, T. 607) and a short Āgama text (*Foshuo qichu sanguan jing*, T. 150A: 882a). A commentary he wrote on dependent origination (*Ahan koujie shi'er yinyuan jing*, T. 1508) also contains some relevant passages.[12]

Dharmarakṣa

Dharmarakṣa, or Zhu Fahu (ca. 233–311), was born of Indian and Yuezhi parents in Dunhuang.[13] He studied with an Indian master and traveled in Central Asia before arriving in China around 266. At the city of Chang'an, where he enjoyed the financial support of several thousand lay disciples from both common and elite backgrounds, Dharmarakṣa collaborated with a multiethnic assortment of individuals in translating Buddhist scriptures. Their output amounted to over 150 texts, among which the most celebrated is the earliest Chinese edition of the *Lotus Sutra* (*Zheng fahua jing*, T. 263). For our purposes, his translations of the *Sutra on the Embryo* (*Foshuo baotai jing*, T. 317) and the *Sutra on the Stages of the Path of Cultivation* (*Xiuxing daodi jing*, T. 606) are just as notable. He also should be credited with the translation of the *Sutra on Bathing the Sangha in the Bathhouse* (*Foshuo wenshi xiyu zhong-seng jing*, T. 701) and some portion of the *Jivaka Sutra* (*Foshuo Nainü Qiyu yinyuan jing*, T. 553; *Foshuo Nainü Qipo jing*, T. 554), both texts that are erroneously attributed to An Shigao.[14]

Kumārajīva

Kumārajīva (344–413), whose name is transliterated as "Jiumoluoshi" in Chinese, is said to have been born in Kucha to a Brahman from India and a Kuchean princess.[15] His mother became a nun and took her son to be educated in Kashmir at the age of nine, where among other things, he studied the Five Indian Sciences (Skt. *pañcavidyā*; Ch. *wuming*), which included medicine. At some point early in his life he converted to the Mahayana and became well known for his skill in debate. A noted scholar from a young age, he came to the attention of Kuchean and Chinese rulers, who began to vie for his services. Caught up in a regional power struggle, he was captured and imprisoned for some time. Eventually, he was brought to Chang'an in 401 by the ruler of the Later Qin (384–417), where his translation activity was supported by the ruling family. Kumārajīva is most notable in the history of Buddhism for his role in establishing durable translation norms that influenced his successors for centuries after his death. Many of the translation terms he introduced are still in use today as standard Chinese Buddhist vocabulary. Several texts I discuss in this book that are attributed to him have been shown to be pseudotranslations (i.e., domestic compositions by others that were passed off as translations by Kumārajīva). His authentic translations include the most well-known editions of the *Lotus Sutra* (*Miaofa lianhua jing*, T. 262) and *Vimalakīrti Sutra* (*Weimojie suoshuo jing*, T. 475), sections of which introduce major healing deities and provide important explanations of the Buddhist perspective on the illusory nature of illness.

Yijing

Yijing (635–713), of Han Chinese ethnicity, was both one of the most prolific translators and one of the most renowned pilgrims in Chinese history.[16] Perceiving deficiencies in the availability of Buddhist texts in China, this Shandong native departed in 671 and spent the next twenty-four years in Southeast

Asia and India. He lived nine years at Nālandā (fl. fourth to twelfth centuries), one of the great international monastic "universities" of the medieval world. In 695, he returned to Luoyang and began to work on translating the texts he had brought back under the patronage of Empress Wu. His translation output focused on monastic disciplinary texts, but also included scriptures with medical importance, such as the *Sutra on Entering the Womb* (*Foshuo ru taizang hui*, T. 310.14, T. 1451: 251a–262a), the *Sutra on the Treatment of Sores* (*Foshuo liao zhibing jing*, T. 1325),[17] and the *Sutra of Golden Light* (*Jin guangming zuisheng wang jing*, T. 665). Yijing's reflections on his time spent abroad, which he compiled in a travelogue called *Record of Buddhist Practices Sent Home from the Southern Seas* (*Nanhai jigui neifa zhuan*, T. 2125), also contain many valuable observations on Buddhist medical and hygienic practice he witnessed during his travels.

Bodhiruci

Bodhiruci (d. 727), written "Putiliuzhi" in Chinese, was a South Indian Brahman who is also said to have trained in the Five Sciences and is reputed to have lived for 155 years.[18] He was recruited to come to China by Emperor Gaozong (r. 649–83) of the Tang. Eventually arriving in the Chinese capital in 692 or 693, he became a major translator under Empress Wu. While his output included many titles that were dedicated to upholding the legitimacy of his patroness, he also produced several medical translations, including the *Sutra Spoken to Ānanda on Abiding in the Womb* (*Fo wei Anan shuo chutai hui*, T. 310.13) and the *Sutra on the Dhāraṇī for the Protection of All Children* (*Foshuo hu zhu tongzi tuoluoni jing*, T. 1028A).

Amoghavajra

Amoghavajra (705–74), whose name was translated into Chinese as "Bukong Jin'gang" (or "Bukong" for short), was born either in Samarkand or in Ceylon.[19] He arrived in China at age ten and went on to become one of the most famous promulgators of Tantric Buddhism in East Asia. In the last decades of his life, he worked for the Chinese government as a ritual specialist, organizing rites for the defense of the state. Amoghavajra is mentioned later in this book as the promoter of highly foreignizing methods of transliterating

Sanskrit. He is also important to our story for his many translations relevant to medicine. These include texts devoted to healing deities, such as the *Ritual Procedure for Recitation to the Master of Healing Tathāgata* (*Yaoshi rulai niansong yigui*, T. 924A–B) and the *Sutra on Samantabhadra's Adamantine and Superlative Dhāraṇī for Prolonging the Life Span, a Radiant Blessing Bestowed from the Hearts of All the Buddhas* (*Foshuo yiqie zhu rulai xin guangming jiachi Puxian pusa yanming jin'gang zuisheng tuoluoni jing*, T. 1136). He also translated two texts containing healing incantations, the *Sutra on the Dhāraṇī to Eliminate All Illnesses* (*Chu yiqie jibing tuoluoni jing*, T. 1323) and the *Sutra on the Dhāraṇī That Can Clear Up All Eye Ailments* (*Nengjing yiqie yan jibing tuoluoni jing*, T. 1324). Finally, Amoghavajra also translated a number of texts describing Tantric healing rituals mentioned in Chapter 3.

*   *   *

Many other translators, figuring somewhat less prominently in Chinese Buddhist historiography more generally but still significant in the translation of Buddhist medicine, are introduced in the pages below. In addition to those individuals engaged in translation proper, a number of commentators and synthesizers also made significant contributions to the reception of Buddhist medicine. These include such paragons of Chinese Buddhism as Zhiyi (538–97), Daoxuan (596–667), and Daoshi (d. 683), all of whom will be discussed in further detail below.

Translation Assemblies

While the named individuals introduced here loom large in both traditional and scholarly accounts of the Buddhist translation project, target texts were most often produced by the efforts of a group rather than a single translator. Initially ad hoc affairs, over the course of the early medieval period, organized "translation assemblies" (*yichang*) developed in both northern and southern China. These assemblies were headed by a "presiding translator" (*zhuyi₂*)$ who in many cases was a foreign monk with only a limited grasp of Chinese.[20] Though his was the name featured as "the translator" in the byline of the completed text, he was often only responsible for reciting the sutra aloud to the assembly in the source language. The presiding translator was assisted by a team, the makeup of which varied on a case-by-case basis. Assemblies typically included one or more bilingual interpreters ("word transmitters," *duyu* or *chuanyu*) who helped orally render and explain his words in Chinese. Members of the audience, who could number well into the hundreds, took notes on these explanations. One or more scribes (*bishou*₁) then collated notes from the various participants and finalized the translation.

Even if they were more directly responsible for the act of transfer than the more famous presiding translators, only rarely do those who assisted in interpreting, sculpting, and polishing the target text appear in the historical record. Nonetheless, from the statements by and about interpreters and recorders that have been handed down to us, some details can be sketched in.[21] The first point to note is that these people were a highly diverse group. Dharmarakṣa's colleagues, for example, are known to have included people of Parthian, Kuchean, Sogdian, Tocharian, Khotanese, Kashmiri, Indian, Yuezhi, and Chinese heritage.[22] While the majority of participants were Buddhist clerics and lay disciples, Chinese scholars and sometimes even Daoists also participated in the translation efforts.[23]

Second, the shape of the translation assemblies and the division of labor changed over time. In the earliest phase, presiding translators depended heavily on interpreters (although some translators appear to have become more proficient in the Chinese language over time and were able to take on increasing responsibilities).[24] By the early fifth century, however, translation assemblies began to be led by polyglot individuals who were themselves learned in both Chinese and the relevant Indic language(s) and therefore did not need to rely as much on interpreters. Kumārajīva, for example, provided an oral translation of the text himself, which would be committed to writing directly by the recorder. Later, in the Sui-Tang period, translation assemblies began to comprise smaller, more exclusive groups of scholar-monks with a higher degree of linguistic and doctrinal expertise.

Third, we note the increase in state patronage of the assemblies in the sixth to eighth centuries. Emperor Wu of the Liang dynasty was a generous patron of translation, as were many emperors of the later Sui and Tang dynasties. One of the most influential translation teams of the Tang, for example, was established by Xuanzang (602–64), a native of Chang'an who had traveled to India between 627 and 645.[25] Upon returning to China, he received official support for his translation activities from Emperors Taizong (r. 626–49) and Gaozong. Empress Wu was also an enthusiastic supporter of a number of translators and participated materially in the process of translation.[26] Such support did not come without strings attached, however. Government officials were increasingly involved with the translation effort, even assuming official positions on the assemblies from which they could oversee the procedures and influence the output.

Given the international and multiethnic background of this cast of characters, the collaborative nature of their work, and the complexity of their institutions, we should not imagine that the texts such men translated were composed in a vacuum by individuals who were limited to a strictly local worldview. On the contrary, they were written by cosmopolitan men who were aware of the world around them, and who were educated about not only domestic Chinese traditions but also the leading cross-cultural currents of thought of their time. These individuals thought deeply about the processes of translation necessary to interface between different languages and cultures and developed specific strategies to bridge those gaps.

Translation Strategies

One scholar has said of translation that it "may very probably be the most complex type of event yet produced in the evolution of the cosmos."[27] While this is surely an exaggeration, there is no doubt that translation involves much more than a straightforward lexical transfer from one language to another. If translation is complicated when a single text is taken up by a single individual, the multiparty Chinese Buddhist translation project involved a number of particularly complex challenges. First and foremost of these was the matter of the distance between the languages. Though, as a matter of convenience, scholars often refer to the source language as "Sanskrit," in fact Buddhist texts were more often written in various Sanskrit-like regional dialects or Prakrits (including Gāndhārī and Buddhist Hybrid Sanskrit among others) rather than the classical language.[28] Belonging to the Indo-European family, these languages were highly inflected, grammatically intricate, and utterly unrelated to the Sino-Tibetan tongues of China proper. Only a minuscule number of Chinese people in the medieval period ever learned any of these Indian languages.

Not only was there a wide linguistic gulf, but Buddhist translators also perceived a steep hierarchical differential between the languages of China and those of India.[29] Sanskrit itself was held to have been a divine gift to humanity from the deva-king Brahmā. Many Buddhist texts were brought to

China in written form, and the most common alphabets in which they were written, *brāhmī* and *kharoṣṭhī*, were considered to be "celestial scripts" (*tianshu*) invented by the Buddha, Brahmā, or other deities. The translation downward into Chinese of the Buddha's holy utterances written in these sacred scripts was never a casual affair. Capturing the authentic meaning of the Buddhist scripture was of paramount importance for the propagation of the true Dharma. It was an event of high religious and social significance, rife with the opportunity for error.

Despite such high stakes, there were also significant practical hurdles to be crossed when translating—or, as contemporaries said, "bringing forth" (*chu₁*)[30]—Buddhist texts into Chinese. Buddhist translators, like all translators, had to deal with losses and gains in meaning, untranslatable turns of phrase, and a whole host of other syntactical, lexical, and semantic considerations. The assemblies' teams of international collaborators worked out through a process of oral negotiation the meanings of the originals and how to express these in the target language.[31] Since these deliberations were not recorded in writing, they are now lost to us. The target texts that were the outputs of these complex multiparty translation procedures, however, contain evidence of the struggles and compromises that accompanied their production. These translations are written in a dialect the sinologist Victor Mair has called "Buddhist Hybrid Chinese." This new dialect incorporated new characters and thousands of neologisms, infused preexisting Chinese characters with new meanings, was written with new grammatical structures reflecting foreign syntactical patterns, and blended vernacular and classical vocabulary and syntax.[32]

There is every indication that Buddhist translators were well cognizant of the challenges they faced. Far from being careless or haphazard, they reflected upon their work, and the methods and goals of translation remained topics of continual debate and discussion throughout the medieval period. Spilling across a variety of prefaces, postscripts, and biographies, their conversation centered on how best to ensure fidelity to the source text (*ben*), the all-important benchmark of authenticity. The debate hinged on the tension between what were known as "unhewn" (*zhi₂*) and "refined" (*wen*) translation styles, a distinction reminiscent of "word for word" versus "sense for sense" translation, or of "formal" versus "dynamic" equivalence, as discussed in the introduction.[33]

Throughout the medieval period, leading Buddhist authorities occasionally attempted to establish guidelines for translators. For example, one of the first Chinese monks to offer a lucid explanation of the challenges of Buddhist translation, Dao'an (312–85), argued in favor of prioritizing closely literal (i.e., formally equivalent) translation.[34] He rejected the use of "categorizing concepts" (*geyi*), which involved correlating Buddhist lists with indigenous analogues.[35] He also warned against five types of losses in translation, which he called "losing the source" (*shiben*): (1) when the original word order is changed to fit Chinese syntax, (2) when unhewn source texts are translated in refined language to suit the Chinese audience, (3) when repetitive parts of sutras are abridged, (4) when large sections of repetitive content are excised altogether, and (5) when digressions are omitted.[36] Dao'an also noted three inescapable difficulties that plagued translators: (1) the changing norms in the target language, (2) the gap between the subtle words of the Dharma and the unenlightened audience for whom the translations were made, and (3) the translator's temporal distance from the time of the Buddha and the temptation to reinterpret the text in contemporary terms. Dao'an critiqued earlier translators for being too clever in their work, with the result that the scriptures were distorted, and he advised translators to overcome these difficulties by cleaving closely to their source texts.

As a respected scholar and head of a translation assembly himself, Dao'an's words carried weight—especially in the north of China.[37] The famous Chinese pilgrim Xuanzang, who lived several centuries later in the reunified empire, was an even more influential advocate of fidelity to the source text. He echoed Dao'an in condemning categorizing concepts, and also rejected analogy (*lianlei*). Questioning the wisdom of translating some Buddhist terminology at all, Xuanzang was a strong advocate of the use of transliteration. According to his well-known five recommendations, a foreign word should be transliterated rather than translated (1) if it was esoteric, (2) if it was multivalent in meaning, (3) if it referred to an object that did not exist in China, (4) if the word was already well known in transliteration, or (5) if by translation a word would lose its positive associations, sense of authority, or gravitas.[38]

Though Dao'an's and Xuanzang's rules of thumb may have sounded attractive in the abstract, individual translators were not always able to freely decide how they would approach their work. Translation choices were in no small part constrained by the makeup and proficiency of the team. The presence of imperial authorities in the assemblies and the influence the state could assert on the translation process were already mentioned above. In addition, the linguistic strengths and experience of the rest of the team were also significant factors. Scholars have noticed that assemblies headed by foreign monks who had a weaker grasp of the Chinese language tended to fall back on the safety of formal equivalence and transliteration, while those who were more fluent could confidently produce texts in a more literary style.[39] It has also been suggested that translators would closely follow the Sanskrit syntax in places where they failed to fully understand the source text, while those who were more sure of their interpretations could write more freely in Chinese.[40]

On the other hand, translation decisions could also be purposeful and strategic. As the medieval commentators well knew, seemingly small lexical choices could have a striking effect on the reader's experience when confronting the target text, and on the ways in which the target texts could be used socially or politically. By employing a more natural language within the text, translators could make their work seem familiar and accessible. By using refined or learned writing styles, they could give their finished product an air of authority. By emphasizing the features of the source language and culture, it could be clearly marked as an authentic rendering of a foreign text. By using an abundance of transliterations, the text could be shrouded in what one scholar of Buddhism has called "a strangeness, a feel that perhaps charged it with an aura of exotica."[41]

Over the long term, certain trends can be seen in the use of such strategies. Generally speaking, the initial attempts to translate Indian texts into Chinese in the second and third centuries were idiosyncratic in their lexical choices. Some translators, such as Lokakṣema (fl. ca. 179–85), employed a great deal of foreign terminology and transliteration while also using many Chinese vernacularisms from the spoken language. Others, such as Kang Senghui (fl. ca. 252), favored a more classical style and readily employed indigenous vocabularies. Scholars have argued that these patterns are indicative of discrete "rhetorical communities"—groups of foreign immigrants and Chinese literati that preferred different styles of translations.[42] Many translators in the early phase followed the syntax of their sources so closely that their target texts would have appeared to the contemporary educated reader as "strangely hybrid, semiliterary productions."[43] In all cases, copious use of unstandardized translation terms and neologisms make the vocabulary employed difficult to fathom. These difficulties have led more than one scholar to complain that these writings are "no more than free paraphrases or extracts of the original texts . . . coated in a language which is chaotic to the extreme and not seldom quite unintelligible."[44] But, of course, this seeming chaos is simply a sign that translation norms had yet to emerge.

While translators operated independently across China in the Period of Division, texts could circulate rapidly and the strategies employed by one group could greatly influence the translational activity of their successors.[45] Soon, decisions made independently and in dialogue among translators coalesced into more consistent norms. After the fourth century, many domesticating translation terms and stylistic choices utilized by Kumārajīva were widely emulated and eventually became conventional. In the reunified empire, the structure of translation assemblies became more consistent, which also meant a more consistent quality in their output. From the seventh century onward, increasing familiarity with Indian thought and culture shifted norms toward nuanced translations that employed complex foreign technical terminology.

Translation Tactics

Understanding the tactical choices made by the translation assemblies on a word-by-word basis is never easy, but this task is especially problematic with medical terminology. Unlike many other types of Indian knowledge, the lexicon for translating Indian medical ideas into Chinese was never fully standardized. Translators frequently used divergent Chinese characters for even the most fundamental medical doctrines.[46] While evolving norms certainly had an impact on the practice of translation overall, when it came to medical terminology, translators throughout the medieval period utilized an entire spectrum of translation approaches—from close adherence to the Indian originals, to freely rendered approximations that captured the spirit but not the letter of the originals, to complete disregard for the source syntax, and everything in between. Most translators were quite willing to utilize multiple translation tactics within the same text, for example, using different characters with similar meanings in translating successive iterations of the same phrase or, conversely, using the same Chinese graph for a variety of source words.[47]

Some historians of medicine have interpreted these inconsistencies as evidence that translators were "clumsy" or "superficial" and have blamed them for the failure of Buddhist medicine to thrive in China.[48] Scholars who regularly work with Buddhist texts are well aware that translation assemblies did in fact make errors, and no one would deny that there are times when we simply cannot figure out what the translators were thinking.[49] However, those who would forward a wholly negative assessment of the handling of Indian medical doctrine seem to be basing their opinion on the assumption that translators must adhere to only the most narrow and literal translation of Indian medical terminology if their efforts are to be judged successful.

In contrast, linguists and translation theorists have long taken for granted that perfect one-to-one equivalence between terms in two languages is impossible.[50] As discussed in the introduction, most scholars of translation approach target texts as evidence of a translator's active attempt to negotiate between two different cultural-linguistic systems. They also understand this process to be inseparable from the specific social context and concrete historical moment in which the translational acts take place, and they are interested in understanding how these environmental factors interconnect with translation decisions. Applying this approach to the Buddhist translations necessitates switching from prescriptive to descriptive language. That is to say, moving away from judging the accuracy of Chinese translators' output according to some imagined standard of perfect equivalence and instead investigating the cultural and social logics that influenced how and why translators dealt with Indian doctrines in particular ways.

To greatly simplify a complex subject, we can identify four basic tactics translators could choose from to render any given Indian medical idea in Chinese, depending on their strategic aims. Moving along the spectrum from formal to dynamic equivalence, a foreign term could in the first place be transliterated. This tactic, advocated most famously by Xuanzang, consisted of approximating Sanskrit pronunciation with a nonsense string of Chinese syllables. It was employed, for example, by Bodhiruci in his translation of an eighth-century obstetric text I will discuss in more detail in Chapter 3. Here, the Sanskrit words for the five stages of embryonic development—*kalala, arbuda, peśi, ghana,* and *praśākha*—are rendered in Chinese characters as *ge-luoluo, anfutuo, bishou₂, jia'na,* and *boluoshequ.*[51] Because most of the Chinese characters used in these terms are specialized graphs frequently used in transliteration, it is clear to any reader even passingly familiar with Chinese Buddhist texts that they are being used here for their phonetic rather than semantic value. It is also clear that the terms in question are to be understood as foreign concepts.

Second, the translator could choose to translate a specific Indian idea with a calque, an accurate root-for-root reconstruction of the original term using existing Chinese characters. An example of this tactic is found in the same embryological text mentioned above when we encounter the words *sheng-zang* and *shuzang.*[52] Literally meaning "receptacle of the raw" and "receptacle of the cooked," these are calques of the Sanskrit terms *āmāśaya* (*āma* = raw; *āśaya* = receptacle) and *pakvāśaya* (*pakva* = cooked; *āśaya* = receptacle). They refer to the stomach and intestines where, according to Indian physiology, the food is stored before and after being "cooked" by the digestive fires. While representing the etymology and structure of Sanskrit words fairly accurately, these sorts of neologisms are, in the choice words of one scholar, "glaring eyesores."[53] The decision to introduce these neologisms instead of simply using the ordinary Chinese characters for stomach and intestines (*wei* and *chang*) was unnecessary if the goal was simply to transfer the meaning of the Sanskrit. Translators used calques to purposefully introduce into the target text terminology that smacked of foreignness and was difficult to comprehend without adequate contextualization (such as comes from wide reading experience, commentarial interpretation, or at least a good dictionary).[54]

Moving toward more domesticating translation options, a third tactic consists of utilizing existing Chinese words to render foreign terms. This approach results in a target text that appears more familiar and reads more naturally, but because words in two languages are never perfect correlates of one another, it typically involves either shifting or extending the semantic fields of the Chinese terms in order to bend them to new usages, or else losses of meaning from the source. In yet another example taken from the same embryological treatise as the above two, "karma" is translated throughout the sutra with the Chinese word *ye*.[55] Though it does not capture the full range of meanings and implications of the Sanskrit term, the use of *ye* as an equivalent for "karma" makes a certain amount of sense since both the Sanskrit and the Chinese words have the core meaning of "action." Choosing a common word such as *ye* as a translation term helps the foreign concept retain a familiar feel; however, the surrounding text and context have to nudge the semantic field of the Chinese term in a new direction in order to fully reflect the meaning of the Sanskrit.

The Buddhist translation project introduced many transliterations and neologisms, and expanded the meaning of many preexisting words. It is these three types of translation equivalents that scholars have had in mind when speaking of the "influence" or the "impact" of Buddhism on the Chinese language. However, there is also a fourth approach to translation, one that is usually characterized as the "sinicization" of Buddhist terminology. This fully domesticating tactic involves translating Buddhist terms with perceived equivalents from the existing Chinese religiomedical vocabulary. To take two examples from the embryological treatise we have been discussing, the various tubes, ducts, and other channels of the body known to Indian medicine—which might be written in Sanskrit as *nāḍī*, *sirā*, *dhamanī*, or *srotas*—are expressed in this text with the character *mai*, a term that in Chinese medical and self-cultivation texts refers to the vessels that circulate qi.[56] Elsewhere, the 101 vital points (Skt. *marman*) of the body are translated as *xue*, the term commonly used to refer to acupuncture points.[57] These attempts to map Indian anatomical and physiological ideas onto the indigenous vocabulary are examples of what some scholars have called "metaphorical equivalence."[58] By using translation terms with known indigenous resonances, translators traded fidelity to the Indian source context for the ability to tap into native cultural and linguistic repertoires.

It is worth underscoring at this point that these four translation tactics are not mutually exclusive approaches. The above examples of each tactic are drawn from the same embryological text, so clearly translators could mix multiple approaches together in the same composition. Moreover, the foreignizing or domesticating effect of each of these approaches would have constantly been shifting as words that initially may have seemed foreign were integrated into the Chinese lexicon and became more familiar over time. For example, transliterations such as *fo* (buddha), *pusa* (bodhisattva), and *bore* (Skt. *prajñā*; i.e., wisdom) probably struck the readers of early translations as bizarre foreign terms. However, they soon became so common in Buddhist discourses that they eventually ceased to have any foreignizing effect whatsoever. Though it might be hard to pin down exactly when a term lost its foreign associations at our historical remove, this process of integration means that what started out as an exotic flair might eventually have become so familiar that it could serve as a domesticating translation for an even newer idea.[59] The point is that in order to understand the strategies behind these translation choices, we must focus not just on what type of equivalence was used, but also on the meanings and connotations of those equivalents in specific settings. By approaching target texts as records of choices made by translators for certain rhetorical effects, we can move beyond whether or not the translators got it right and gain a greater appreciation for the performative nature of their work in historical context.

To provide a few examples of how this approach changes our thinking, let's look at the translation of two common Indian medical doctrines, the Four Elements and the *tridoṣa*. Like most Indian medical terms, the Four Elements are translated into Chinese differently in different cases. The most common translation is "Four Great Ones" (*sida*), though other terms can also be used such as "Four Realms" (*sijie*), the "Four Seeds" (*sizhong*), or the "Four Illnesses" (*sibing*). Likewise, the *tridoṣa*, the pathological Bile, Wind, and Phlegm that constitute core concepts in Indian nosology, can be rendered alternately as the "Three Major Imperfections" (*san dabing*), "Three Internal Calamities" (*san neizai*), or "Three Poisons" (*sandu*).[60]

If we are exclusively concerned with accuracy, we may feel that this range of translation terms is indicative of slippages in medical logic. To refer to the Elements as "Great Ones," "Realms," or "Seeds" is to recognize their role in Indian thought as the all-pervading constituents of the material universe and the building blocks of the human body. It is quite another thing to say that the Elements are "Illnesses." Similarly, there is a significant difference between saying that the *tridoṣa* are "Poisons" that cause illness, and that they are "Imperfections" or "Calamities" in and of themselves. Indeed, some scholars have pointed to these very discrepancies as evidence translators failed to understand Indian medicine.[61]

However, when the translation tactics introduced in the preceding pages are taken into consideration, these seemingly erroneous translations can be seen in a different light. The terms "Great Ones" and "Three Major Imperfections" are simply calques of the Sanskrit *mahābhūta* (*mahā* = "great"; *bhūta* = "existing, present") and *tridoṣa* (*tri* = prefix meaning "three"; *doṣa* = "imperfection" or "defect") respectively. The term "Realms" is using a common Chinese word to translate *dhātu* ("constituent part" or "essential ingredient"), also routinely used in Indian literature to refer to the Earth, Water, Fire, and Wind that compose the body.[62] The translation terms "Seeds" and "Poisons" are ordinary and immediately comprehensible Chinese terms that more or less capture the respective roles of the Elements and *tridoṣa* in Indian medical thought. "Internal Calamity," on the other hand, is a metaphorical equivalent most likely preferred by some translators because it is a term for illness commonly found in texts about classical Chinese medicine and other indigenous writings.

When such inconsistencies in translation are understood as differences in translation tactics rather than as errors, our perspective shifts from the normative to the descriptive. Rather than judging the translations as failures, we now can appreciate how translators actively attempted to build conceptual bridges between Indian and Chinese medical knowledge in order to enhance their readers' understanding of foreign doctrines. Rather than writing off these texts as irrelevant to the history of medicine, we can now begin to explore the evidence they provide that Buddhist writers consciously retooled

Indian medicine in China, and to understand how they pursued their broader strategic goals even at the level of the individual Chinese character.

Negotiating the Religiomedical Marketplace

Having discussed the translators, their assemblies, their debates, their strategic approaches, and their options for rendering Indian terms in Chinese, we now must turn our attention to what it was about the contemporary intellectual climate, cultural context, and social milieu that encouraged or demanded certain translation decisions be made. While ideas about equivalence and other cultural-linguistic concerns always guided the work of translators, where they stood on important tactical decisions varied according to individual tastes and social contexts, and according to the goals individual translators might have for specific translations. This section focuses on the relationship between those translation decisions and translator's attempts to position Buddhism in the religiomedical marketplace of medieval China.[63]

From all available evidence, Chinese patients—whether commoners, members of the elite, or the emperor himself—have at all times in history patronized healers of many different persuasions. The range of competitors in the marketplace (including physicians, Daoists, spirit healers, sages, pharmacists, and other adepts in addition to members of the Buddhist sangha) was introduced in Chapter 1. However, we did not discuss the social dynamics among these groups or between them and their patients. In fact, a medical system is never a completely unified "free market" in the sense that any given patient is willing and able to patronize any given practitioner. In all societies, social networks, economic hierarchies, political machinations, and other forces play important roles in shaping the distribution of and access to different types of healers. In fact, rather than a single unified field, the overall health-care sector typically consists of numerous marketplaces—sometimes overlapping, sometimes fractured—in configurations that are unique to each historical time and place. In medieval China, many factors encouraged, shaped, and constrained the interactions between buyers and sellers of medicine. Official patronage could have a stimulative effect upon certain groups, such as when Empress Wu lavished support upon monastic hospitals in the early eighth century. Periods of political disunity, dynastic transition, or repressive policies, on the other hand, could have an opposite effect, disrupting the distribution or restricting the supply of Buddhist medical institutions and practitioners.

As fundamental as these external factors in influencing patient choices was the perceived legitimacy of different types of practitioners. The immediate struggles between religious healers revealed in medieval texts, in fact, seem more often to have been over cultural capital rather than economic resources. Patients would never have seen all of the practitioners and therapies available to them as an undifferentiated muddle. In seeking out a healer in the religio-medical marketplace, they made choices between practitioners who were socially distinguishable from one another regardless of the syncretic overlaps in their healing practice or ideology. Such distinctions could have been collective (i.e., pertaining to the group to which the healer was perceived as belonging) or individual (i.e., concerning the qualities the healer was perceived as possessing personally). In either case, such distinctions would always have been based on socially agreed-upon cues.

Though they only represented a small fraction of the total number of practitioners in the marketplace, physicians associated with classical Chinese medicine certainly occupied the most authoritative position during the Han dynasty due to the cultural legitimacy they achieved by association with the imperial ideology. The crumbling of the empire and the subsequent social and political disunity dealt a blow to the established order, however, providing an opening for new ideas to gain more social acceptance and official patronage than might have been possible otherwise. Into this gap stepped Buddhist and Daoist authors, who busily got to work renegotiating the social hierarchy to their own advantage.[64]

The primary ear toward which their sectarian arguments and self-promotional pronouncements were directed was the state. While the state was ever fluctuating in the medieval era, the reigning ruler or rulers always represented the greatest source of financial support and prestige. The state was also the most significant patient. In order to win official patronage—the crown jewel of cultural capital—the various competing religious groups had to provide concrete means of intervening in the medical matters of most interest to the state: the health of the ruler and the protection of the realm against epidemics.

Given the structural homology between the body, state, and cosmos in Chinese thought, for any group to write about illness or healing was to engage in political discourse. Since high antiquity, Chinese political thinking had held that the prosperity of the state and its people hinged on the benevolence and moral propriety of the ruler.[65] His role as mediator between the divine and worldly realms was already established as early as the first historical dynasty: when disaster struck the people of the Shang, it was the king who consulted the oracle and performed the necessary ritual remedies. From the Zhou through the Han, calamities of all sorts were interpreted as signs of the ruler's own moral transgressions. Epidemic disease was not a separate category in this thinking; it was one of many natural disasters, celestial phenomena, and other ominous occurrences that were read as political auguries and as signs of the possible loss of the ruler's Heavenly Mandate (*tianming*).[66] The early medieval period was an era in which multiple dynasties competed in the political vacuum left by the dissolution of the Han. It also was a time when epidemics frequently and violently erupted onto the Chinese stage. The anxiety that this combination caused rulers in search of legitimacy cannot be overstated.

If epidemics were the result of the ruler's shortcomings, however, rulers could mobilize a range of rituals of purification, propitiation, and sacrifice to right the cosmos, renew the imperial mandate, and maintain or increase their grip on power. As they began making inroads into Chinese political discourse, some Buddhist authors began to take advantage of the sense of crisis and despair—and even to fan the fire—by promulgating millenarian literature announcing the arrival of the apocalypse (*moshi* or *famie*).[67] Simultaneously, however, they also offered a range of solutions drawn from Indian kingship practices for preserving and restoring the ruler's legitimacy in such dire times.

The first documented example of a Buddhist monk exorcizing an evil portent on behalf of a ruler comes from 372 C.E.[68] By the sixth century, such events were commonplace. Moreover, by that time, several key texts had become available that enabled beneficent rulers to employ a range of Buddhist rites to protect their kingdoms against epidemics, natural disasters, and calamities of all kinds. One example, the early fifth-century *Sutra of Golden Light,* offered the righteous king who even just listened to its sacred words an increase in his own physical strength and power.[69] It also taught the ruler how to protect his realm from epidemics through invocation, incantation, and other ritual means. Likewise, the *Sutra on the Perfection of Wisdom for Benevolent Kings* (*Foshuo renwang boreboluomi jing*, T. 245), a pseudotranslation of the late fifth century attributed to Kumārajīva that became one of the most important texts for the ritual protection of the state, also promised that Buddhist deities would intervene to relieve epidemics and other calamities in response to the meritorious actions of a Dharma-king.[70] The fact that both were retranslated during the Tang is evidence of the continuing importance of these texts, and the rituals they describe, in the reunified period as well.[71]

The sangha's ability to compete successfully for cultural capital and official patronage hinged on the language it mobilized in such texts. Words were the battlegrounds upon which religiomedical practitioners fought for recognition and legitimacy. The various rivals hurled the same invectives and defended the same lexical turf. Each called the others "transgressive" (*xie*), "confused" (*diandao*), "deluded" (*wang*), "sinister" (*zuo*), and "perverse" (*yin*), while laying exclusive claim to knowledge of the "Law" (*fa*) or the "Way" (*dao*) that was "upright" (*zheng*) and "true" (*zhen*). They painted their competition as "sorcerers" (xi_1) and "evildoers" (*e'ren*), while using such titles as "King of Physicians" and "King of Medicine" for heroes from their own ranks. Such labels were of critical importance in jockeying for position in the marketplace of ideas, as the cultural capital earned through such contests could be converted into increasing patronage across ever-widening swaths of society.

As disparate Daoist sects began to coalesce into a viable competitor in the early fifth century, they began to target their opprobrium at Buddhism in a more systematic fashion. The production of polemics and apologia on both sides hardened these fault lines as the medieval period progressed, and imperially sponsored debates between representatives of both groups raised the stakes to new levels of urgency.[72] Sometimes, competitive exchanges between Buddhists and Daoists specifically centered on questions of translation. A 570 Buddhist apologetic called *Laughing at the Dao* (*Xiaodao lun*, T. 2103: 143c–152c), for example, belittles Daoists for misunderstanding Buddhist translation terms.[73] Daoists, the text tells us, erroneously read the phrase *namo fo* as "south-no-Buddha," not realizing that it was a transliteration of a Sanskrit phrase paying homage to the Buddha. Daoists also took the terms *youpose* and *youpoyi* literally as "frightened on the [mountain] pass" and "frightened of the Kapilavastu [people]," rather than understanding they were transliterations of *upāsaka* and *upāsikā*, meaning "layman" and "laywoman." The Buddhist apology characterizes these errors as "disgraceful and foolish," and as signs of Daoism's unsophistication. However, it is clear from these passages that these Daoist readings were not unintentional. The literal interpretations of these transliterations were shrewd intentional misreadings designed to undercut Buddhist legitimacy by feeding into the *huahu* ("converting the barbarians") controversy. This nativist position, forwarded by Daoists throughout the medieval period, held that the Buddha was actually Laozi, who had made the long journey to the South in order to convert the barbarians of India from their frightful and violent nature to a more civilized way of life.[74]

If some Daoist attacks on Buddhism concerned translation, many specifically focused on healing practices. One Daoist scripture, for example, denounced Buddhists for "eating impurities"—that is, taking urine as medicine.[75] Another tract complained that Buddhist monks "anxiously scheme and strive without a moment's rest" and that they "presume on their medical skill and recklessly fabricate cold and warm (drugs)."[76] Popular tales from the period reveled in pitting practitioners of various sectarian persuasions against one another. A well-known story in the fifth-century compilation *A New Account of Tales of the World* (*Shishuo xinyu*), for example, involves the healer-monk Yu Fakai's victory over Daoist healers.[77] We are told that his patient, an ardent Daoist, had had much difficulty obtaining a cure for a condition of the bowels. Fakai takes his pulse and at once apprehends the cause of his ailment being his "excessive zeal." Upon taking one dose of Fakai's prescription, the patient defecates "several wads of paper, each as big as a fist." These are inspected and turn out to be the Daoist talismans he had piously swallowed in vain.

In a less humorous vein, a narrative from *Records of Signs from the Unseen Realm* (*Mingxiang ji*), completed around 490 by the lay devotee Wang Yan (b. ca. 454), revolves around the illness of He Danzhi.[78] When he is afflicted by a demonic illness, He has a Daoist priest perform a number of ritual remedies. These are ineffective, we are told, and since the patient steadfastly refused to practice Buddhism he consequently died. Another story from the same source tells of a female patient, the wife of Zhang Ying, who beseeches her husband to stop making useless sacrifices to the "profane gods" and perform Buddhist rituals instead.[79] This patient acquiesces. Zhang seeks the services of a monk, who is able to help drive away the disease-causing demon as the layman dreams. In a third story, a Daoist supporter is convinced by a friend to stop disrespecting Buddhist images and to make an image of Guanyin himself. He does so, and his acute illness is cured.[80] Such stories are clearly indicative of the competitive environment in which religious healers operated.

In negotiating these struggles for cultural capital, the authors and translators of Buddhist treatises had to emphasize the novelty of their healing approaches while simultaneously expressing their compatibility with Chinese ways. They needed to claim that Buddhism was new and superior, while still conforming to established cultural expectations and expressing themselves in socially acceptable language.[81] In this rhetorical tightrope walk of conformity and subversion, Buddhism's perceived Indianness was simultaneously a limitation and an asset that translators worked both to overcome and to capital-ize upon. When faced with the task of explaining Buddhist medicine to their contemporaries, Buddhist translators and writers frequently employed the terminology of their rivals. They often framed foreign medical knowledge in terms of the normative religiomedical language of sympathetic resonance, divine retribution, spirits, and qi. They appropriated longevity practices, self-cultivation techniques, and demon lore from the competition and used them as metaphorical equivalents for Buddhist practices. When they employed these strategies, they did so precisely in order to demonstrate their legitimacy and relevance in culturally acceptable language. But, in the very next breath, the same Buddhist authors also were quick to capitalize on long-standing Chinese stereotypes that arcane and powerful wisdom was to be found in faraway places, and they loaded their translations with foreignizing formal equivalents that showcased the exotic origins of Buddhist wisdom.[82]

Meanwhile, despite all of their objections to the "barbarian" culture of India, Daoist authors appropriated Buddhist techniques of healing, astrology, demonology, and ritual protection into their own compositions, and they mimicked Buddhist textual and paratextual conventions.[83] Physicians, too, were eager to exploit their connections with Buddhism. Official dynastic his-tories recount the medical feats of the physician Hua Tuo, for example, in narrative sequences modeled after Indian prototypes.[84] The famed physician Sun Simiao, who is said to have had personal associations with the Buddhist master Daoxuan, was posthumously deified and given the title "Medicine King" (yaowang), a term that in the medieval period was in common use for Buddhist deities.[85] The increasing appearance of Buddhist tropes in the self-representations of physicians indicates the increasing impact of Buddhism on medieval Chinese medical culture and frames of authority quite aside from matters of doctrine and practice.

Such examples of appropriation and exchange between competing groups are obvious examples of syncretism and hybridity, and Buddhism's interac-tions in the religiomedical marketplace can indeed be described in terms of influence and sinicization. But, while such terms helpfully highlight the permeability of the boundaries between the different religiomedical systems competing in medieval China, they tend to lead us to overlook the fact that these interactions were also efforts at strategic positioning by specific groups and individuals. The extent to which Buddhist medical texts relied on indig-enous idioms to justify or explain Indian medical ideas is a measure of how much pressure Buddhists were under to conform to the established conventions

of Chinese religiomedical discourse. The extent to which Buddhist medicine
was appropriated and mobilized by practitioners of other traditions, on the
other hand, is a measure of how much the sangha began to enjoy increasing
legitimacy in medieval China and to set the standards to which other groups
had to conform. Similarities in vocabularies, ideologies, and representations
are thus evidence not of homogenization, but of struggles on the part of authors to dominate the religiomedical discourse and to dictate the terms on
which such discussions would be had.[86]

*   *   *

Traduttore traditore. The Italian proverb famous among translators and translation scholars alike implies that translators are traitors to their source texts.
But, could a translator ever be otherwise? Each instance where a translator
builds bridges between the source and target contexts requires him to com-
promise the literal meaning of his text. Relying on formally equivalent translation, on the other hand, produces a target text that is potentially confusing,
alienating, or, worse, irrelevant to his readership. In all cases, his decisions
about how to proceed will be inseparable from his attempts to position his
target text—and himself—in the reception environment.

As one scholar of translation put it, every act of translation "walks a fine
line between reconstructing and reinventing the message and meaning to be
conveyed."[87] Buddhist translators walked this line carefully, employing multiple tactics within the same text in pursuit of their strategic goals. Whether
they translated Indian medical terminology into Chinese employing foreignizing or domesticating tactics, conformed to prevailing norms, or employed
their own idiosyncratic preferences, translators were aware that their choices
had far-reaching political and social implications.

Indeed, Buddhism's success in China depended on these decisions. Because of the homology between the cosmos, the state, and the human body in
Chinese thought, in order to compete in China, Buddhism's claim to mastery
over the cosmos had to be manifested in its ability to cure disease. The con-
verse also was true: Buddhist claims of healing power were by extension asser-
tions of the authority of Buddhist institutions and worldviews. All attempts to
position Buddhist medicine as an authoritative, legitimate, and effective healing model in China hinged on how individual writers translated this knowledge and situated it within the Chinese religiomedical landscape.

CHAPTER 3

Translating Medicine in Buddhist Scriptures

This chapter explores in the aggregate the large number of medieval Chinese Buddhist scriptures containing medical knowledge in order to provide a corpus-level analysis of translation norms. As mentioned previously, the translation of Buddhist medical doctrine was never thoroughly standardized at the level of vocabulary. Individual translators rendered medical terms in a variety of ways throughout the many centuries of their activity. At the same time that their lexical choices were highly variable, however, the basic strategic approaches Buddhist translators took to the translation of the medical material in their source texts followed some surprisingly consistent patterns over the long term. This chapter illuminates these patterns and explores what light they might shed on the priorities, goals, and intended audiences of the translators who produced these target texts.

Buddhist Medical Metaphors

Rather than provide an exhaustive transeme-by-transeme analysis of the corpus, this chapter focuses on the Chinese translation of five important metaphors that are pervasive in Buddhist scriptures dealing with medical topics. These five can be understood as "conceptual metaphors," as famously defined by cognitive linguist George Lakoff and philosopher Mark Johnson.[1] Lakoff and Johnson (and a number of scholars following in their footsteps) have taught us that metaphors are much more than mere wordplay. Conceptual metaphors are deeply ingrained patterns that structure our speech and our thought. They are fundamental to human cognition, allowing us to think about and express complex ideas by mapping those abstractions onto more concrete processes and objects.

Though they are central to our speech and thought, conceptual metaphors are unlike conventional metaphors used as rhetorical flourishes in that they often remain invisible to those who use them. To repeat an often-cited example that Lakoff and Johnson discuss extensively: in English, we often say that an argument is something to be "won," that positions taken by one's opponent are to be "attacked" or "shot down," and that particularly valid points are "right on target."[2] Lakoff and Johnson claim that, while few in the English-speaking world may consciously realize the connection, this constellation of ways of speaking points to an underlying conceptual metaphor, ARGUMENT IS WAR. As they point out, this particular metaphor (and many others such as TIME IS MONEY, THE MIND IS A MACHINE, THEORIES ARE BUILDINGS, LOVE IS A JOURNEY, and so on) not only structures the way we speak and think about but also how we experience and perform some of the most basic everyday activities in our lives.

This chapter illuminates five conceptual metaphors that are inherent within Buddhist writings on medicine. While these certainly do not encompass the sum total of all Buddhist references to medical knowledge, each metaphor lies at the foundation of a complex edifice of dependent metaphors, similes, imagery, symbols, and other patterns of language that include many of the most basic and influential Buddhist medical ideas. These five metaphors are: (1) THE BODY IS A COLLECTION OF PARTS, (2) HEALTH AND DISEASE ARE REWARDS AND RETRIBUTIONS, (3) THE DHARMA IS MEDICINE, (4) DEITIES ARE HEALERS, and (5) HEALING IS AN OCCULT POWER. While the local reception and translation of individual medical terms and doctrines could vary greatly from place to place across Asia, these metaphors represent enduring cultural-linguistic structures at the very heart of the pan-Asian Buddhist tradition. These conceptual metaphors are evidenced in the earliest Indian Buddhist texts known to us, and they maintained their explanatory power as they were translated into other languages throughout the first millennium.[3] These five metaphors were highly influential in shaping medical thought in many recipient cultures, where they often continue to form the basis of discourses on health, illness, and the body and to provide the foundation for systems of traditional medicine even in the contemporary period.

More to the point for the present discussion, these metaphors are ubiquitous in medieval Chinese Buddhist literature, transcending all phases of translation in China. Clearly defined "schools" or "lineages" (*zong*) of Chinese Buddhism did not emerge until the Tang and are not reflective of social realities in the earlier period. However, these metaphors are notable for the ways in which they supersede conventional designations such as "Tiantai," "Pure Land," and "Yogācāra," and transcend such megacategories as "Hinayana," "Mahayana," and "Tantric" or "Esoteric" Buddhism.[4] These metaphors also cut cleanly across scholarly categories of analysis extrinsic to the tradition, such as "early Mahayanic," "proto-Tantric," and so forth, and even across the basic distinctions between authentic translations from Indic languages versus pseudotranslations authored domestically (i.e., "apocrypha"). Below, I will illustrate these metaphors with a selection of passages drawn from across this wide range of Buddhist scripture. (In the interests of space, I will not attempt to provide a comprehensive accounting of all possible texts of relevance. Rather, the discussion below concentrates on representative examples of the metaphors, supplemented with citations to additional passages. I should also point out that this chapter is focusing on describing norms. By definition, norms have exceptions, although I will not be able to focus on those to any great extent.)

Interwoven individually and in combination throughout the Chinese Buddhist corpus, the five conceptual metaphors discussed here can be held up by scholars as obvious examples of the influence of Indian cultural-linguistic structures on the Chinese system. However, at the same time as they may be deemed influential, how these metaphors of Indian origin were dealt with by Chinese translators was always highly contingent on their intended audiences and their goals for their texts. While we do not have exact copies of their source texts, and thus cannot perform a word-for-word correlation of sources and targets, we can make some general observations about the strategies and tactics involved in the production of the Chinese translations. These strategies and tactics, rather than the metaphors per se, are the focus of the present chapter. As I will show below, the ways in which these medical metaphors were rendered in Chinese could have a major impact on how these ideas—and by implication, Buddhism itself—were received domestically. Translators could adjust the language they used to express these metaphors in order to build bridges between foreign and indigenous medical doctrines, or conversely to make Buddhist ideas seem exotic and highly specialized to their readers. They knew that the right combination of translation tactics could further the sangha's claim to knowledge that was effective and specialized and help them consolidate their position in the contemporary religiomedical marketplace. These metaphors therefore provide compelling examples of how the translation of imported cultural-linguistic systems could be manipulated locally for local purposes. They also illustrate how the study of translation can shed light on the multiple meanings of medical discourse in a specific historical time and place.

The Body Is a Collection of Parts

Mainstream Buddhist thought holds that "the body" is merely a conventional label for a collection of more subtle parts that can be separated out for further analysis. In Buddhist traditions across Asia, this way of thinking is closely related to ascetic discourses that speak of the body as a constant source of disappointment and entrapment.[5] The ordinary physical body is continually in need of maintenance and attention, frequently experiences pain and suffering, and constantly falls ill. As stated in the highly influential *Mahāparinirvāṇa-sūtra* (*Da banniepan jing*, T. 375), it should be seen as a wound that must be dressed, oozing "pus from the nine orifices in proportion to the food and drink that is supplied."[6] Always in need of attention, the body demands lodging to protect it from the natural world and medication for its constant sickness. It is a fleshly prison that one must struggle to transcend if one is to be liberated. But at the same time, merely having a body is also one of the greatest impediments to spiritual progress. The clinging attachment to the physical form arising from misunderstanding its contingent and constructed nature is seen as one of the main sources of humankind's self-induced suffering and dissatisfaction (Ch. *ku*; Skt. *duḥkha*).

These great disadvantages notwithstanding, a human body is also an indispensable tool for generating the kind of insight that leads to enlightenment. Because of the pivotal role played by the corporeal form in mankind's entrapment in suffering, ascetic practices often center on analyzing and understanding its constituent parts as an essential ingredient in the process of liberation. Analysis of the body thus represents one of the most basic pillars of Buddhist meditation practice. Such exercises typically are said to lead to the realization that self-identification with the body is misguided and, from there, to the transcendence of the individual self and release from all suffering.

The body is deconstructed, subdivided, and subjected to analysis in any number of different ways in Chinese translations of Buddhist treatises on meditation, asceticism, and philosophy.[7] Many texts encourage reflection on the Impurity or Loathsomeness of the physical body (Ch. *bujing guan*; Skt. *aśubhabhāvanā*), characterizing it as a collection of repulsive anatomical substances.[8] Some passages instruct the meditator to contemplate the stages in the decomposition of the physical body after death, when it breaks down into pieces. Another way of stressing the disgusting nature of the physical form is to describe each body part as a home for parasites that slowly eat away one's strength and vitality.

One shared feature of these different descriptions of the body is that they are organized around lists of body parts. Although Chinese texts have preserved many variations upon these lists, these formulaic enumerations of anatomical structures are closely related to discourses in the wider Indian religious and medical literature. Similar in both tone and content to certain passages of the Āyurvedic treatises as well as the much more ancient Vedas, these lists are probably indicative of widespread Indian oral traditions.[9] However, in Buddhist texts, as opposed to the Vedic or Āyurvedic, the reader's focus is normally directed toward the ascetic goal of detachment from the physical form, and it is within this doctrinal context that such lists of body parts should be read.

Another conventional Buddhist way of speaking of the body that echoes the broader Indian medical, religious, and philosophical tradition is to view it as an inherently unstable collection of the Elements. While this figure of speech can be found in many places across the Chinese Buddhist corpus, one of the most lucid explanations of the idea is a sutra preserved in section 16 of the *Mahāratnakūṭa* (*Da baoji jing*, T. 310.16). A product of the translation assembly of Narendrayaśas (517–89), a monk from northern India, this sutra repeats the conventional Indian wisdom that the Earth Element (*tujie*) makes up the solids in the body, Water (*shuijie*) the liquids, Fire (*huojie*) the body's heat and digestion, and Wind (*fengjie*) the mobility of the body and the circulation of substances within it.[10] The text further explains the Space Element (*xukongjie*) as the empty cavities within the body, and the Element of Consciousness (*shijie*) as that which allows the person to experience sensual perception and mental processes.

It is typical for Buddhist texts to stress that the Elements constituting the physical body are mutually conflicted because of their inherently antagonistic qualities. Because the Elements are neither stable nor harmonious, the body is always in a state of flux. The "internal" Elements are perpetually unstable because they are in constant interaction with their "external" counterparts in the world outside. Pathological states can occur as the result of shifts in the weather or seasons; the influence of environmental factors on the body; the excessive, irregular, or unwise consumption of foods; the violation of other aspects of proper regimen; baleful astrological configurations; or the predominance of negative mental and emotional states. When the Elements can be managed successfully, one may experience a period of tenuous balance, peace, or calm (*tiao, he, an,* and so on). Inevitably, however, a change in the internal or external conditions disturbs them and they fall back out of equilibrium. The Elements then become excessive or depleted (often written *zeng* and *sun* respectively), imbalanced (*butiao*), or "coarse" (Ch. *cuse*; Skt. *karkaśa*). Such fluctuations of the Elements are among the main explanations of illness in Buddhist texts, and the expression "404 illnesses of the Four Elements" (i.e., 101 each for Earth, Water, Fire, and Wind) is a conventional way of saying "all illnesses."

While the other ways of dividing up the body mentioned above focus on the disgusting qualities of the physical form, the Elements usually appear in Chinese Buddhist texts in connection with the doctrine of Emptiness (Ch. *kong*; Skt. *śūnyatā*). This discourse emphasizes that the body is an ephemeral, temporary, and constructed object. From the moment of conception, the Elements are held together in a contentious and tenuous relationship. This lasts as long as the period of time that one is alive. Upon death, they fall apart again and dissolve away. The sutra by Narendrayaśas, for example, repeats for each Element the following formula:

> When the body's internal Wind Element arises, it is Empty; when it is extinguished, it is also Empty. The body's internal Wind Element is of an Empty nature.[11]

The point is that any self-identification with any aspect of the body—or attempt to militate against its continual changes—is misguided.

Having introduced the metaphor of THE BODY IS A COLLECTION OF PARTS and its relationship to the ascetic values of detachment and transcendence, we can now turn to examine how Chinese translators dealt with these ideas in their target texts. In the first place, it is clear that the translators of the texts that showcase this metaphor—though they were different individuals whose work spanned many centuries—consistently prioritized a high degree of fidelity to the source context in their handling of this particular constellation of ideas. When encountering this metaphor, translators typically avoided drawing to any great extent upon metaphorical equivalents from the Chinese repertoire (as we will see authors doing below). Translations of body-part meditations and lists of parasites do not rearrange their presentations to conform to the organizational structure of the yin and yang Viscera, for example, nor to the body parts' relative importance in Chinese medicine. They do not remove items appearing in these lists that had less clinical relevance in China (such as "membranes" or "brain stem"), or interpolate important Chinese anatomical concepts missing from Indian sources (such as the so-called "Triple Burner," *sanjiao*). In fact, there is little if any overlap in these translations of Buddhist anatomy and physiology with Chinese models of the body at all. It is not the case that Indian and Chinese medical ideas were utterly incommensurable: indigenous Chinese discourses describing the body as a composite object were readily available to translators.[12] Nevertheless, the norm was to mobilize native knowledge only in limited ways, relying instead primarily on foreignizing terminology that privileged the source language and context.

The metaphor THE BODY IS A COLLECTION OF PARTS, with its two related discourses of Loathsomeness and Emptiness, is found across a wide spectrum of texts on asceticism, meditation, and philosophy. The consistent handling of this particular metaphor with foreignizing translation tactics across these genres and across centuries of translation activities suggests that medical knowledge that was specifically marked as being foreign had a role to play in supporting the ideals and practices of Buddhist asceticism in China. I will return to the larger significance of these translation decisions in the last section of this chapter. Before coming to that, we should briefly introduce the other four medical metaphors, the translation of which unfolded quite differently from the first.

Health and Disease Are Rewards and Retributions

In Buddhist thinking, one's health is first and foremost a matter of one's karma. It is karma that brings the constituent parts of the body together at the moment of conception and that determines the appearance, strength, and susceptibilities of the physical form. The idea that one's physical body is an outward manifestation of one's karmic status is a ubiquitous topic in Buddhist scripture worldwide. In the words of one scholar, Buddhist literature is replete with descriptions of living beings that "stink with sin, are disfigured by vices, and, conversely, are perfumed or adorned with merit or virtue."[13]

Some of the most medically relevant texts focusing on the physical effects of karma are a series of embryological texts translated into Chinese between the late third or early fourth and the early eighth centuries.[14] Found both embedded within larger composite texts and circulating as separate sutras in their own right, these accounts dramatize conception, fetal development, and birth, while forwarding an ascetic interpretation of the process of reincarnation. In a representative example of the genre, the *Sutra Spoken to Ānanda on Abiding in the Womb,* produced by Bodhiruci's translation assembly in 703–13, the action unfolds over thirty-eight weeks as the fetal body develops from a small cluster of the Four Elements into a newborn baby. Along the way, the text traces the week-by-week emergence of anatomical structures and substances such as the limbs, orifices, organs, joints, *rasa* (nutritive essence), vital points (Skt. *marman*), channels, blood, bones, flesh, skin, hair, body hair, and nails.

This is another conventional way of talking about body parts shared widely among Indian religious and medical traditions.[15] In Buddhist embryological texts, however, it is not the body parts per se, but rather the workings of karma, that take center stage. In Bodhiruci's text, although conception requires the fertility of the mother, the sexual act, and the presence of a being awaiting reincarnation, it is karma that unites these factors at the opportune moment.[16] When the karmic conditions align and conception occurs, forces described as "Karmic Winds" (Ch. *yefeng*) begin to blow through the womb, driving the subsequent development of the fetus's body. Some of these winds directly influence the attractiveness, completeness, and health of the developing body depending on the merits and faults accrued in previous lives.[17] Karma also determines whether the birth will go well, how much pain there will be, and whether the newborn lives or dies.[18]

Buddhist embryological treatises, like the texts on body parts discussed in the previous section, are ascetically minded. There is no role for medical intervention in the processes they describe, and there is no avoiding the effects of the karma generated in previous lives. Even in the best of circumstances, these accounts hold, the process of coming into the world is unfortunate and unpleasant. In Bodhiruci's translation, for example, the new life begins when a being awaiting reincarnation descends into the womb as a result of generating anger, delusion, and sexual desire upon seeing the act of intercourse between the parents.[19] Though the fetus initially deludes itself into thinking otherwise, the uterus is described as a site of impurity, stench, imprisonment, darkness, and Loathsomeness.[20] The eventual birth is a process of unspeakable pain and suffering, comparable to being flogged, being skinned alive, and other tortures.[21] Finally, in the week immediately following birth, the newborn baby's body is infested with eighty thousand parasites and begins a life full of suffering.[22]

Taken as a whole, the embryological genre seems chiefly intended as an opportunity for authors to dwell on the pollution of sexual relations, the ignorant nature of ordinary human beings, and the unsatisfactoriness of the corporeal body.[23] The ultimate purpose of this excursion into Indian gynecological and obstetric doctrines is to encourage ascetic practice and to inspire the individual to seek liberation from the cycle of rebirth (Ch. *lunhui*; Skt. *saṃsāra*). The Buddha admonishes the audience that allowing oneself to be born into a new human life through such a grotesque and painful process is calamity of monumental proportions that should be avoided at all costs. In one passage of Bodhiruci's translation the Buddha unequivocally denounces rebirth, saying:

> The instant the Five Aggregates of mind and body [i.e., the various parts that make up an individual] form a person, there already are all kinds of suffering. How much more deplorable is continual repeated rebirth in *saṃsāra*! Even a small turd is foul; how much worse when there is a great amount! The Five Aggregates of the fetal body being such as they are, who could take pleasure in it?[24]

The only way to avoid the unfortunate and highly unpleasant fate of repeated rebirth into a repulsive, ephemeral, turd-like body, according to the Buddha, is to generate disillusionment with the world, to strive toward achieving complete enlightenment, and to escape permanently from the cycle.

Embryological texts, like other ascetic discourses discussed in the previous section, feature many foreignizing translation tactics. The names of the phases of fetal development and the Winds that drive the process are typically rendered in transliterations and calques.[25] Likewise, the terms for the body parts taking form each week are usually derived from specialized Indian medical terminology and transliterated or calqued rather than mapped onto Chinese analogues (the two exceptions in Bodhiruci's text, *mai* and *xue*, were discussed in Chapter 2). Equally notable is the copious use of patently Indian similes and imagery. In the first place, the characterization of the forces of karma as winds blowing inside the uterus is quite foreign to Chinese embryological thinking.[26] The texts also use Indian tropes when they speak of the fetus being "cooked" by the mother's Fire Element, compare certain anatomical structures to lotus plants, and equate the development of the fetus to the curdling of milk. The translators likewise chiefly employ Indian models of anatomy and physiology when describing the processes taking shape in the uterus—the growth of the Elements, the development of the eighty thousand channels of the body, and the mother's nutritive essence (Ch. *ziwei*; Skt. *rasa*) entering through the fetus's navel chakra (Ch. *qilun*; Skt. *nābhicakra*), for example—rather than replacing these with Chinese anatomical or physiological models.

In contrast to these embryological treatises, when other types of texts written for nonascetic audiences discuss the effects of karma on health, they employ a different translation strategy. While ascetic texts emphasize the futility of seeking medical care for the ailing body and the acceptance of pain and illness as inescapable consequences of human embodiment, texts on medical karma geared toward wider audiences focus mainly on the possibility of ameliorating this unpleasantness through the cultivation of merit. These texts stress that those who accumulate negative karma will suffer the retributions of disease, disfigurement, and physical discomfort; however, they also promise that freedom from illness, beautiful bodies, and corporeal comfort in future lives will flow from devotional practices such as following the precepts, venerating and recopying sutra texts, and cultivating Buddhist virtues.[27]

Rather than prioritizing formal equivalents as the embryological treatises do, translators of texts meant for broader consumption tend to prefer a domesticating lexicon that expresses the medical ramifications of karma in terms that medieval Chinese readers would have found familiar and accessible. This is not a black-and-white distinction, but rather a matter of emphasis. Terms such as "resonant responses" (*ying*), "retribution" (*bao*), and "auspiciousness" (*fu*) are used in many types of Buddhist treatises (including sporadically in the embryological sutras just mentioned); however, highlighting the connections between Buddhist merit-making practice and indigenous beliefs and practices concerning sympathetic resonance and divine retribution allowed translators of other works to infuse their texts with a wellspring of indigenous cultural resonances in order to boost their appeal.

One of the most significant merit-making practices mentioned in Buddhist texts as a source of corporeal well-being is performing acts of medical or hygienic charity. The *Sutra on Bathing the Sangha in the Bathhouse* is one text that specifically correlates the type of charitable gift given with the type of karmic merit that is thereby earned. Traditionally attributed to An Shigao, this text is most likely to have been translated by Dharmarakṣa in the third or early fourth century.²⁸ The framing narrative of the text tells a story about Jīvaka, the King of Physicians, who invites the Buddha and his assembly to use his bathhouse.²⁹

According to this sutra, donating the use of the bathhouse involves giving the sangha seven gifts: a hot fire, clean water, soap, ointment, pure ash, willow twigs used for cleaning the teeth, and monastic undergarments used to preserve modesty.³⁰ The text links each item that Jīvaka has donated with the particular medical benefit each will bring to the monks: the fire promotes the equilibrium of the Four Elements, the water promotes the cure of Wind Illness (*fengbing*), soap eliminates Damp Paralysis (*shibi*), ointments counter Cold Frost (*hanbing*), pure ash cures Feverish Qi (*reqi*), the willow twig removes pollution, and the undergarments promote the comfort of the body and the lucidity of the eyesight.³¹ It is worth noting that Wind Illness, Damp Paralysis, and Feverish Qi are all familiar disease names found in indigenous Chinese medicine, and that, aside from the conventional references to the Four Elements, there are no technical Indian medical terms in the text.³² The use of these metaphorical equivalents indicates that expressing the benefits of bathing in the normative language of Chinese medicine was more important to this translator than preserving the literal meaning of the source text.

Karma enters into this text when the Buddha explains that, because Jīvaka's generosity will relieve the sangha of these pernicious ailments, he himself will accrue seven auspicious rewards (which in various places the text calls *fu*, *bao*, and the combination *fubao*) related to health and hygiene.³³ Though it is not stated explicitly, it is clear that each reward correlates with one of the gifts given. Because of his gift of fire (i.e., one of the Four Elements), to the sangha, Jīvaka will in future lives enjoy balance of his own Elements. Because of the gift of pure water, he will be pure, clean, and dignified. Because he gave soap, his own body will become fragrant and his clothing clean. Because he gave a lubricant for the skin, his own skin will be lustrous and radiant. Because he gave ash, he is ensured that he will have attendants to sweep away dust (from his person or his living quarters is not made clear). By virtue of his gift of the implements for oral hygiene, his own teeth and mouth will be healthy and attractive. Finally, because he donated the undergarment, his own needs for clothing and adornments will be fulfilled.

The text stresses that because he will be able-bodied, healthy, clean, fragrant, lustrous, and well-dressed in future lives, Jīvaka will be respected and revered and will bring joy to those who see him.[34] Lest we wonder whether gifts to the sangha can only lead to physical benefits, the Buddha also promises that all of the abovementioned rewards from Jīvaka's donation to the sangha will result in his rebirth in ever-higher realms of human and superhuman existence.[35] However, the most notable part of this sutra for our purposes is not the potential for otherworldly rebirths but the connection made between merit making of a medical or hygienic nature and the health-related merits Jīvaka stands to earn. The sympathetic and retributive nature of these rewards is underscored by the parallelism between each gift and its effects, and by the familiar vocabulary of reward and retribution used throughout the sutra.

The two texts discussed in this section are intended only as representative examples. Many additional scriptures proclaiming the medical benefits of merit making and warning of the physical dangers of sinful acts could be mentioned. The important point to highlight is that the same core metaphor of medical karma might be translated in different ways depending on the genre of the text in which it appears and the intended audience. A comparison of the translation tactics employed in an embryological treatise emphasizing asceticism versus an appeal to the laity for patronage of monastic infrastructure demonstrates that translation choices could diverge when dealing with a single doctrine, and that translators could strategically mobilize distinct vocabularies when writing for different ideological purposes.

The Dharma Is Medicine

As mentioned previously, Buddhist texts conventionally count birth, old age, illness, and death as the four principal afflictions of humanity. The power of the Dharma to cure illness thus is a common synecdoche for its ability to improve the human condition as a whole.[36] The Dharma is frequently compared to a wonder drug (Skt. *agada*; Ch. *ajiatuo*), or is called the "King of Medicines." The Four Noble Truths (Skt. *catur-āryasatya*; Ch. *sidi*), ostensibly the foundational doctrines of the Dharma, were even interpreted as representing the medical logics of diagnosis, etiology, therapeutics, and cure.[37]

Beyond similes and comparisons, this metaphor is also taken quite literally in Buddhist scriptures that claim for themselves the power to vanquish physical disease. The fifth-century translation of the *Lotus Sutra* by Kumārajīva, for example, proclaims itself an "excellent medicine" (*liangyao*) for the illnesses of the world.[38] If a sick person merely listens to the text, it promises, all his or her illnesses will disappear. The *Sutra on the Contemplation of the Two Bodhisattvas King of Medicine and Supreme Medicine* (*Foshuo guan Yaowang Yaoshang er pusa jing*, T. 1161), the principal scripture on the two healing bodhisattvas translated by the Central Asian monk Kālayaśas (fl. 424–42), also calls its teaching an "excellent medicine," and bestows upon itself the title "Wondrous Medicine of Ambrosia That Cures Afflictions and Illnesses."[39]

This metaphor is also the force behind passages that stress that illness is a trifling matter for one who has mastered Buddhism—or, conversely, that mastery over illness is a sure sign of enlightenment. The locus classicus for this formulation is the fifth chapter of the *Vimalakīrti Sutra,* entitled "Mañjuśrī Inquires About the Illness," also translated by Kumārajīva.[40] When asked about the illness that presently afflicts him, the enlightened Vimalakīrti answers with complete nonchalance. Since it is only a false sense of self that causes one to identify with the physical body, he says, the whole idea of being ill is ultimately "unreal and illusory" (*feizhen feiyou*).[41] It arises from "delusion" (*wangxiang*), "confusion" (*diandao*), and "mental agitation" (*fannao*). If one realizes the Emptiness of all things, then one can simply "curtail" (*duan*) the suffering of sickness.

Not only does the enlightened person possess perfect knowledge about the Empty nature of the body, but he also enjoys total control over how this illusory form manifests. According to Vimalakīrti, such a person can transform himself endlessly—taking on any form, becoming a deity, or becoming one of the Four Elements.[42] If there is an epidemic, he can transform himself into medicinal herbs that can be taken by the populace to eradicate illness. He may also choose to manifest sickness, old age, or death if he compassionately deems that doing so will in some way assist other beings.[43] (This, incidentally, is precisely what Vimalakīrti is doing in the sutra: he has manifested his own illness so that others will visit him and receive his teachings.)

While total power over health and illness remains the prerogative of the fully enlightened, the DHARMA IS MEDICINE metaphor extends the opportunity to improve health and vanquish disease to all devotees—not through the deferred mechanism of karma as described in the previous section, but in this very lifetime as a direct result of the proper practice of the Dharma. Many sutras stress the protective, strengthening, and curative benefits of fasting, repentance, chanting, adhering to the precepts, listening to the sutras, and other virtuous Buddhist deeds.[44] In addition, the tranquillity, purity of mind, and insight achieved through meditation, contemplation, or understanding the Dharma are frequently named as primary factors in maintaining health.[45] Refraining from sexual excess and from eating meat, while advocated primarily on moral grounds, are also connected with promoting health in some instances, as is the moderation in diet and daily regimen that result from taming craving and aversion through meditation and self-discipline.[46] (Like karma, however, the power of the Dharma cuts both ways: disparaging the Dharma, insulting Buddhist deities, or desecrating its sacred implements results in all manners of severe disease; likewise, eating meat, immoderate regimen, or failing to keep the precepts can bring illness and even death.)[47]

Translators of the metaphor THE DHARMA IS MEDICINE frequently borrow language from indigenous Chinese medicine and cosmology when expressing the benefits of the practice of Buddhism. They do frequently employ the stock phrase "404 illnesses of the Elements" when explaining what ailments the Dharma cures, but, just as often, the translation of such passages explicitly establishes associations between Buddhist knowledge and indigenous models.

One place where this tactic is persistent is in the Chinese translation of the Indian doctrine of *tridoṣa*.[48] References to these "three defects" appear frequently in a wide range of Buddhist texts, often specifically in order to draw a parallel between the ease with which a good doctor can cure illnesses of Wind (Skt. *vāta*), Bile (Skt. *pitta*), and Phlegm (Skt. *śleṣman* or *kapha*), and the efficacy with which the Buddha's teachings can alleviate the mental impurities of greed, anger, and delusion. When encountering such passages, translators often rendered the three defects in characters that evoked basic Chinese medical categories. The translation for the Wind defect was virtually always *feng*, a term that also meant "wind" in Chinese, and that had been recognized as one of the major pathogenic factors in China since the beginning of recorded history.[49] "Bile," on the other hand, was routinely translated with characters evocative of yang disorders, such as *re* ("Heat) and *huang* ("Yellow"). "Phlegm" from the sixth century onward was most often translated as *tan* ("Phlegm") or *tanyin* ("Phlegm Congestion"), but prior to that time was rendered with yin words such as *han* or *leng* ("Cold"), *shui* ("Water"), *feibing* ("Lung Illness"), and *xiantuo* ("Saliva"). The intent of making such connections was clearly not to explicate the subtleties of Indian medical doctrine, but rather to evoke indigenous medical resonances while still conveying the central message that Buddhist practices can vanquish all mental and spiritual anguish. By establishing these metaphorical equivalences between the Indian defects and the native ideas of Wind, yin, and yang, translators made the foreign doctrine of *tridoṣa* and the benefits of Buddhist practice more accessible and meaningful to a Chinese audience.

Beyond passing references to the *tridoṣa*, integrating indigenous Chinese knowledge also was a central concern for the translators of the *Sutra on the Buddha as Physician* (*Foshuo foyi jing*, T. 793), one of the most influential treatises on Buddhist medicine in Chinese.[50] This text, ascribed to the translation efforts of Zhu Lüyan (fl. ca. 224–30) and Zhiyue (fl. ca. 230), purports to present the Buddha's advice on diet and regimen. It includes long sections on how the practice of basic aspects of the Dharma—such as moral restraint, self-regulation, and vegetarianism—can benefit one's health. The advice given is similar in tone to the guidelines found in monastic disciplinary codes. This connection is especially striking in the lists of faulty regimen appearing throughout the text, such as the ten causes of illness, nine causes of premature death, four immoderate cravings, and five results of overeating (similar lists are found in the medical sections of the monastic codes).[51] While much of the form and content may have derived from Indian literature, however, what is most interesting for our present purposes is the text's tendency to interweave indigenous Chinese medical and cosmological terminology in an attempt to mold Buddhist medical wisdom to conform with Chinese cultural expectations.

In striking contrast to the descriptions of body parts discussed in an earlier section, the translators of this sutra begin establishing connections between Indian and Chinese anatomical and physiological models from the outset. The sutra's opening lines read:

> Human bodies from the beginning consist of Four Elements: Earth, Water, Fire, and Wind. When Wind increases, qi rises. When Fire increases, Heat rises. When Water increases, Cold rises. When Earth increases, one's strength will flourish. From these original Four Elements, there arise the 404 ailments.[52]

The passage starts by using the translation *sibing* ("Four Illnesses") for the Four Elements rather than the usual calque *sida* ("Four Great Ones"), which as already discussed would make more intuitive sense to a Chinese reader unfamiliar with Buddhist terminology than the latter. The translators then invoke native Chinese models in the description of each Element's medical significance by deploying terms with obvious indigenous medical resonances such as "qi," "Heat" (*re*), "Cold" (*han*), and "flourishing" (*sheng$_2$*).[53]

After these opening lines, the *Sutra on the Buddha as Physician* launches into a discussion of the relationship between the seasons and the balance of the Four Elements in terms of the creation, flourishing, and decay of the Myriad Things (*wanwu*) and changes in yin and yang—important concepts from indigenous Chinese cosmology.[54] The text then goes on to explain the appropriate activities and foods for each season in passages that incorporate the seasonal fluctuations of yin and yang and that echo in both tone and terminology the seasonal advice given in indigenous Chinese medical and self-cultivation literature.[55]

We do not have access to the sutra's source text, and therefore do not know for certain whether it represents a translation of a lost Indic treatise, a pseudotranslation composed anew in China, or a sort of "transcreation" that combines aspects of both.[56] While the core ideas of the text may indeed have originated in Indian tradition, however, it is clear that during the translation or compilation of this sutra in China in the third century, Buddhist knowledge was strategically interpreted using indigenous frameworks. The integration of Chinese medical and cosmological models into the text's medical advice is a sure sign of efforts to rework standard Buddhist dietetics and regimen in order to fit better with Chinese prototypes. Certainly, a third-century Chinese person encountering this text would have found the indigenous models of cosmic energies more accessible than the newly arrived Indian medical doctrines of the Elements and the *tridoṣa*. In all likelihood, the translators also reasoned that adding references to these Chinese medical and cosmological doctrines would reflect well on the Buddha and would be a more convincing display of medical wisdom in the eyes of a domestic audience.

Deities Are Healers

If THE DHARMA IS MEDICINE, it follows that DEITIES ARE HEALERS. The comparison is as routine in Chinese Buddhist texts as it is in Buddhist discourses across Asia. Representations of the Buddha as a healer are ubiquitous: he is the physician who administers the superlative medicine unknown to other doctors; he is the surgeon who extracts the poisoned arrows of suffering; he is the ophthalmologist who clears away the cataracts of ignorance.[57] Other deities are also frequently represented as healers, including the Master of Medicines Buddha, the Buddha of Infinite Life, and the bodhisattvas Guanyin,

King of Medicine, Supreme Medicine, and Samantabhadra, plus a whole collection of devas, spirits, and enlightened beings who grant boons of health. Such figures are routinely spoken of in terms that emphasize their medical omnipotence: they are given titles such as "King of Physicians," "Great Physician" (Ch. *dayi*), and "Bestower of Medicines" (Ch. *shiyao*). These same monikers are also regularly applied to medical heroes from the sangha or the laity, notably Jīvaka.[58] Beyond mere rhetorical flourishes, as in the case of THE DHARMA IS MEDICINE, this metaphor also could be interpreted quite literally: many Buddhist texts promise that beneficent Buddhist healers will intervene personally on behalf of devotees who perform specific ritual actions.

While there are important divergences between the rituals associated with various categories of beings, as well as shifts in their practice over time, healing rites in sources as diverse as the *Sutra on the Master of Medicines Buddha*, the *Sutra of Golden Light*, ritual manuals associated with various bodhisattvas, spell texts, and Tantric writings all tend to hinge on a common logic.[59] The rites usually begin with preparatory measures to purify the supplicant (for example, confession, fasting, bathing, and washing the clothes) and to consecrate the ritual space (which can be an altar, a ring of cow dung, or simply a "ritual perimeter" [*jiejie*]). Once these preliminaries are completed, the crucial act in the healing rite is the performance of *gongyang* (Skt. *pūjā*). Meaning "supplying and supporting" in ordinary Chinese, *gongyang* in Buddhist contexts takes on the meanings of "to worship," "to venerate," and "to make offerings." *Gongyang* usually involves the presentation of material objects in a symbolic gesture of devotion. Gifts to be offered in the course of healing rites include typical votive items such as lamps, incense, food, vessels, seats, canopies, Buddha images, and banners. Donations of money, perfume, musical instruments, mirrors, weapons, and medicines are also mentioned. In addition to making these material offerings, bodily and mental gestures of devotion are also considered *gongyang*, including the performance of prostrations and other ritual behaviors. A common action called for in healing rites is ritual speech. Conventionally, this involves the recitation of the name of the deity in rites for buddhas, or *dhāraṇīs* (incantations or spells) when calling upon lesser beings. In some cases, the supplicant may additionally write out a *dhāraṇī* or a sutra, or draw images of the entity being invoked.

The premise of all such ritual actions is that, in return for performing *gongyang* with sincerity, the devotee may receive a response from the deity to whom the offerings are directed. Among the many boons promised if the performance is successful, the supplicant may be rewarded with the spontaneous cure of a particular ailment, the exorcism of demons, the eradication of the 404 illnesses of the Four Elements, or relief from "all illness whatsoever" (*yiqie bing*).

Oftentimes, such beneficial outcomes are simply said to be "caused" or "granted" (*ling*) from afar. Other texts are more specific. Visualization treatises, for example, often suggest that through meditation one may invoke a deity's actual presence in order to be healed in the flesh.[60] On the other hand, the *Sutra of the Samādhi of the Five Attendants of the Buddha* (*Wufoding sanmei tuoluoni jing*, T. 952), translated by Bodhiruci, encourages supplicants to sleep on the altar platform before an image of a particular deity in order to receive him in a dream.[61] A series of texts appearing from the seventh century onward describes a range of other methods for invoking apparitions of Guanyin's multiple manifestations (especially the eleven-headed, thousand-armed, and horse-headed forms) for healing purposes.[62] Beginning in the eighth century, Tantric texts began to detail the practice of *āveśa* (*aweishe*), or spirit possession, in which the invoked deity descends into the body of a medium (often a child) in order to be consulted directly, often offering medical diagnosis or prognosis.[63] Invoked deities could also be called forth to inhabit a finger, mirror, blade, flame, jewel, pearl, piece of flint, vessel of water, or statue in order to become present within the ritual space.[64]

In healing rituals focusing on invocation, the beneficial intervention of superhuman beings in everyday affairs is conventionally spoken of using terms such as "added support" (*jiachi*), "added protection" (*jiahu*), "added assistance" (*jiabei*), "added consideration" (*jianian*), and other similar phrases. These are all translations that render the Indian term *adhiṣṭhāna*—literally meaning "basis" or "position," but in the Buddhist context connoting something like "divine empowerment," "divine assistance," or "divine blessings"—in phrases that were readily accessible to a Chinese audience.[65] In addition to these domesticating translations, many texts also explicitly employ metaphorical equivalents from the indigenous vocabulary of cosmic resonance. Buddhas are said to respond to ritual acts by manifesting "transformation bodies" (*huashen*, *bianhuashen*), "response bodies" (*yingshen*), or "dream responses" (*menggan*).[66] Such vocabulary explicitly connected Buddhist healing rituals with indigenous Chinese models, reframing the invocation of deities with *gongyang* as yet another example of how the stimulus-response principle operates in the resonant cosmos.

In addition to describing the means of ritually invoking them, texts that engage with the metaphor of DEITIES ARE HEALERS often portray buddhas, bodhisattvas, and other divine beings as masters of particular medical disciplines or specific therapeutic interventions. Deities wield numinous medicines, emanate healing lights from their bodies, perform surgeries, and administer all sorts of other therapies. The details of such descriptions are frequently drawn from foreign medical traditions; however, these texts also often feature indigenous Chinese healing techniques. For example, the *Secret Essential Methods for Treating the Maladies of Meditation* (*Zhi chanbing miyao fa*, T. 620) mentions a great range of healing deities and techniques. This is said to be a 455 translation by the layman Juqu Jingsheng (d. 464), who studied in Khotan and who is credited with the translation of several Central Asian visualization texts. Scholars, however, believe it to be a pseudotranslation.[67] The sutra relates the Buddha's teachings on the cure of various maladies that may arise during the practice of meditation. It contains advice for dealing with mental conditions such as madness, loss of concentration, excessive sexual arousal, and temptation to break discipline, as well as a range of physical disorders resulting from the imbalance of the Four Elements. Though it includes several meditations on the Loathsomeness of the body as well as spells for driving away demons, the majority of the text focuses on the visualization of deities, devas, spirits, departed masters, and other beings, and on the therapeutic actions these powerful allies perform on the meditator's body within the virtual world of the visualization.

Secret Essential Methods is unusual in the sheer number and diversity of beings it introduces as healers. The meditator is instructed to visualize all sorts of "transformation buddhas" (*huafo*), bodhisattvas of various levels, devas and demigods, sagely disciples of the Buddha from the Āgamas, other ascetics and enlightened people, snakelike *naga* spirits, eagle-like *garuḍa* spirits, and an array of other fantastical figures.[68] Within the visualization, this cast of characters takes turns healing the meditator with their Dharmic teachings, flashes of light, numinous gemstones, visionary surgery, and all sorts of other procedures.

Indigenous and imported knowledge are liberally intermixed in *Secret Essential Methods*. For example, in one meditation to cure the imbalance of the Four Elements, the reader is instructed to visualize a series of multicolored celestial youths (*tiantongzi*) that each administer a different therapy.[69] Throughout this sequence, the meditator's head is cut open and medicated ghee is poured into the opened skull, medicine is applied topically to the skin and hair, acupuncture and massage are performed in various ways, an anthelmintic enema is administered, the channels are flushed with both ghee and rosewater, the body is pierced with a diamond and rubbed with a "Wish-Fulfilling Jewel" (Ch. *ruyi zhu*; Skt. *cintāmaṇi*), the orifices are irrigated with medicines, and so on and so forth through visitations by all nine celestial youths. Though many of these are recognizable as Indian and Central Asian medical procedures, indigenous religiomedical knowledge has also been purposefully incorporated. Of course, the mention of acupuncture is of Chinese provenance, and the language utilized in that particular passage (which mentions several acupuncture channels) is clearly invoking Chinese models of the body.[70] The interpolation of indigenous material is not limited to incidental details, however, but is integrated into the very structure of the passage: the multicolored celestial youths that provide the framework for this section themselves are thinly veiled adaptations of the body gods found in numerous Daoist texts.[71]

While perhaps especially kaleidoscopic in its presentation, *Secret Essential Methods* is not unique in its strategic embedding of indigenous knowledge within a Buddhist primer on intercessory medicine. Chinese Buddhist literature is filled with similar representations of Indian heroes wielding Chinese medical knowledge and technologies. In all likelihood, one goal of such an approach was to make the healing acts of the Buddhist deities more compelling in the eyes of a Chinese reader. Adding to the deities' competence as well as lending a localized patina of medical legitimacy, such representations contributed to these figures' omniscience and omnipotence in matters of healing (and by extension in all other matters as well). Undoubtedly, another strategic aim for such an approach was to co-opt the therapeutic tools of the competition into the Buddhist healing repertoire.

Healing Is an Occult Power

Scriptures that deal with this fifth and final conceptual metaphor focus on the use of objects (such as texts, relics, icons, and talismans) as well as actions (such as body postures, *mudrās*, and speech) that have the apotropaic power to protect from disease or the exorcistic power to eliminate it once it has taken root. Knowledge of such things is routinely characterized in Buddhist texts as occult—that is to say, it is enveloped in language that heightens its mysteriousness and inscrutability. These healing objects and actions are characterized as lying beyond the scope of ordinary human knowledge; they are frequently also characterized as as transgressing social norms, and thus needing to be hidden from ordinary uninitiated people. Such occult therapies were usually heavily exoticized through the purposeful manipulation of translation tactics.

While some scholars of religion have drawn a strong distinction between "magical" and "religious" ritual techniques, the healing powers discussed in this section are in fact inseparable from the ideas presented in the previous one.[72] It is their explicit and implicit connections with the protective powers of buddhas, bodhisattvas, devas, demons, enlightened people, and other supernormal beings that give occult practices the ability to transform illness into health. When Buddhist texts ascribe occult therapies to the teachings of deities well known for their beneficence (such as the Buddha, Amitābha, Guanyin, or Brahmā), these practices can stand on their own merits. When revealed to humankind by more ambiguous beings (such as devas, demons, sorcerers, and the like) their use usually needs to be explicitly sanctioned by the Buddha or another higher authority in order to make clear that it is authorized and effective.[73] Examples of the latter class of beings include the Demon General Āṭavika (lit., "Forest-Dweller"; Ch. Azhapoju), the Deva-King of the North Vaiśravaṇa (Pishamen Tianwang), the "Poison Woman" Jāṅgulī (Rangwuli or Changjuli), and even the Hindu god Śiva (Ch. Moxishouluotian; Skt. Maheśvara).[74]

Buddhist occult practices can be used to achieve a whole range of religious and secular goals. A single talisman or incantation, for example, may confer political power, divine protection, supernormal abilities, and total enlightenment in addition to freedom from illness. At the same time, there is also a wide variety of texts that present specific instructions for the deployment of occult healing. These simple ritual instructions for vanquishing illness, dissipating poison, assisting with obstetric and pediatric crises, and so forth are often found alongside those for rainmaking, protecting the crops in the field, ridding grain of pests, raising silkworms, and keeping one's possessions from falling into the hands of thieves. While they draw upon the transcendent power of deities, then, these techniques are intended for the practical management of the vicissitudes of everyday life.

Translators dealing with the Buddhist occult often went to great lengths to shroud these techniques in cabalistic language. While most Chinese scriptures contain examples of foreignizing language and imagery, translations of occult therapeutics generally represent the extreme end of the spectrum. At the same time that they heavily exoticized their material, however, writers of this type of literature also needed to be sure to advertise the efficacy of occult therapies to their readers in accessible terms in order to ensure their broad appeal and relevance. Each act of translation thus represented a careful balancing act between the impulse to heavily foreignize and the need to domesticate at least some aspects of the text.

The most common occult therapy in our medieval sources on healing—and the one that most obviously showcases foreignizing translation tactics—is the *dhāraṇī,* a short spell or incantation intended to counter demonic entities, maleficent forces, and misfortune of all kinds. As briefly mentioned in the previous section, *dhāraṇīs* are often listed among the types of *gongyang* performed during healing rites. In addition to being incorporated into these larger rituals, however, they were also frequently presented as a stand-alone healing technique.

Dhāraṇīs appeared in China as early as the late second century.[75] Over the course of the subsequent centuries—assisted by their incorporation into influential texts such as the *Lotus Sutra*—their popularity exploded, and hundreds of incantations were added to the Chinese Buddhist arsenal.[76] Healing spells make up a voluminous portion of the extant *dhāraṇī* literature from the medieval period. Early catalogs indicate that independent spell texts for enhancing medicines, dissipating poisons, and treating various disorders (such as seasonal afflictions of qi, childhood illnesses, toothache, and eye pain) had come into circulation by the sixth century.[77] A number of additional spell texts appeared in the reunified period, including remedies for pediatric illnesses, ophthalmological problems, skin disorders, and "all illnesses."[78]

In addition to these independent texts, dozens of additional incantations appear within large compendia compiled in the medieval period. Three such collections are extant from the Period of Division: the *Sutra on the Consecration of 72,000 Devas for Protection of the Sangha* (known simply as the "Consecration Sutra," *Guanding jing,* T. 1331), the *Sutra of the Great Dhāraṇī Spirit Spells Spoken by the Seven Buddhas and Eight Bodhisattvas (Qifo bapusa suoshuo da tuoluoni shenzhou jing,* T. 1332), and the *Collection of Miscellaneous Dhāraṇī (Tuoluoni zaji,* T. 1336).[79] Subsequent compilations from the Tang include the *Dhāraṇī Compilation (Tuoluoni ji jing,* T. 901) and the *Forest of Pearls in the Garden of the Dharma (Fayuan zhulin,* T. 2122.60), both composed in the mid-seventh century. Collectively, these compilations include dozens of simple *dhāraṇīs* that mention healing in their titles, or that include healing among their primary benefits. The diseases they claim to be able to cure provide an overview of the ordinary complaints of the time, from toothache to malaria, childhood illnesses, diarrhea, poisoning, snake and insect bites, and even malodorous armpits.

The methods for using *dhāraṇīs* to heal were varied. Spells could be written out in order to create healing talismans that could be hung or worn on the body to resolve illness or offer protection.[80] Most often, however, *dhāraṇīs* were to be recited aloud. Often the text prescribes a specific number of times the spell should be recited, and sometimes gives instructions on how to amplify the curative effect with ritually significant gestures or objects.

The "active ingredient" of a *dhāraṇī* spell text—the incantation itself—could derive from various sources. It might be translated from Sanskrit, composed anew in China, or appropriated from indigenous traditions, and the boundaries between translation proper and pseudotranslation were especially fluid in this arena. Perhaps the simplest example of an incantation found in multiple medieval texts is the Homage to the Triple Gem: *namo fo, namo fa, namo biqiuseng* ("Homage to the Buddha, homage to the Dharma, homage to the sangha").[81] In most cases, however, incantations consist not of well-known phrases such as these, but of strings of specialized transliteration characters used for their phonetic value. When recited, these syllables were said to harness the mantic power inherent in the Buddhist scriptures and in the celestial language of Sanskrit. Whether the utterances preserved in medieval *dhāraṇī* texts actually represent transliterated Sanskrit, though, or if they are pseudo-Sanskrit invented by Chinese authors instead, cannot be known in most cases. Neither can we always ascertain what other secret meanings or mnemonic significance specialists believed these utterances to hold.[82]

Whatever their ultimate source or meaning for the initiate, however, one undeniably important social function of these mysterious foreign syllables written with specialized graphs was to convey the message that Buddhist practitioners had access to unique and mysterious occult techniques of foreign provenance. By the eighth century, some translators began to further draw attention to the non-Chinese origin of *dhāraṇīs* by devising even more foreignizing translation strategies for presenting them. The Tantric master Amoghavajra was a leading proponent of a new method of transcribing Buddhist incantations.[83] His method involved inserting into the text special characters notating the pronunciation of individual Sanskrit phonemes, a somewhat more accurate—though certainly much more byzantine—way of specifying the sounds of the source language. Amoghavajra and his students also began advocating writing *dhāraṇīs* in a variant of the *brāhmī* script known as *siddhaṃ* (*xitan*).[84] The enthusiasm for such methods may indeed have been grounded in a pious concern to preserve the integrity and divine nature of the original Sanskrit sounds and scripts. At the same time, we must not forget their performative value: these techniques, which some contemporaries called "nontranslation," were strategic choices that heightened the perceived foreignness, and hence both the authenticity and specialized nature, of translated knowledge.

Who was the audience for these performances of esotericism? The intended audience for *dhāraṇī* texts included the sangha, of course; however, occult healing apparently was first and foremost pitched toward the laity. The location of healing *dhāraṇīs* among other spells for the vicissitudes of everyday agrarian life suggests that they were intended primarily for the benefit of ordinary people, and the large proportion of ritual therapies for problem pregnancies and children's illnesses can only have been meant for non-monastics. Thus, unlike the ascetic treatises and manuals discussed earlier in this chapter that employed foreignizing translation tactics mainly in order to appeal to the sangha's own notions of authenticity, texts on occult healing techniques were, at least in part, designed to promote the services of Buddhist clerics as healers. The use of difficult-to-read transliteration systems and foreign scripts ensured that precious few could read the incantations or fathom their hidden meanings, but the same tactics also boldly announced their arcane and secretive nature.[85] *Dhāraṇīs* written in such extremely foreignizing ways exuded an unquestionable aura of mystery, highlighted Buddhism's difference from its domestic competitors, and made clear the fact that the sangha offered something novel in the religiomedical marketplace.

While Buddhist texts on occult healing are more loaded with foreignizing translation terms than any other genre, however, it is telling that such exoticisms are used chiefly in the syllables to be incanted, the proper names of deities and demons, and incidental details about ritual objects or procedures, but not in discussing the effectiveness of the therapies or the problems they overcome. In these texts, healing is seldom explained in terms of Indian anatomical and physiological models. They do not belabor how the corporeal body parts are to be enumerated or in what season the *tridoṣa* are to be pacified. Nor do they engage in any sustained way with indigenous Chinese medical models.[86] On the contrary, illnesses are simply said to be instantaneously "treated" (*zhi₃*), "healed" (*liao*), "cured" (*yu*), "purified" (*jing₂*), "expelled" (*chu₂*), "cast out" (*tuo*), or "removed" (*li₁*). The names of the illnesses that can be treated are also typically drawn from indigenous vocabularies—Seasonal

Qi (*shiqi*), malaria (*nüe*), carbuncles (*yongzhong*), and other common disorders that are readily found in contemporary medical treatises as well.

The terminology used to refer to the *dhāraṇīs* themselves also served to establish connections between Buddhist occult techniques and indigenous precedents. The Sanskrit word *dhāraṇī* is often transliterated as *tuoluoni* or calqued as *zongchi* (literally "encompassing grasp," a combination of characters that captures the original's meaning of "to hold" or "to grasp").[87] However, in the texts under discussion here, the term is often also translated as *zhou,* an indigenous word in widespread use in early and medieval China for the spells, curses, and incantations of Daoists and other ritual specialists.[88] Often, within the healing *dhāraṇī* texts or in their titles, both the transliteration and the metaphorical equivalent are found alongside one another, a strategy that simultaneously asserts the foreign status of Buddhist incantations and establishes connections with native practices.

Aside from *dhāraṇīs*, other Buddhist occult therapies such as talismans and *mudrās* were also typically referred to with terms that were long in use by the indigenous traditions (*fuzhou* and *fuyin*).[89] By far the most common word used to describe the whole gamut of Buddhist occult healing practices, however, is *shen*. This character had a wide semantic range as early as the Zhou dynasty, by which time it already could refer to spirits (deities, ancestors, and others), marvelous or clairvoyant powers, penetrating intelligence, and mystical realization. By the medieval period, in addition to these meanings, the term was also in common usage as an adjective roughly analogous in scope and fuzziness to the English words "paranormal," "magical," and "divine." In texts on occult therapies, *shen* is often used in conjunction with other characters, such as in the common translation of *dharaṇi* as *shenzhou* (lit., "numinous spell" or "spirit spell") or of consecrated water as *shenshui* (lit., "numinous water"). When deployed in Buddhist texts, such indigenous terminology brought to the compositions a thick web of connotations and expectations derived from the autochthonous context. The vocabulary suggests that Buddhist incantations can manifest spontaneous transformations by stimulating changes in the resonant cosmos, by transforming qi, and by communicating with spirits.[90]

The use of such metaphorical equivalents created or magnified points of connection with the techniques of Daoists and other indigenous groups. This increased their appeal, but also allowed Buddhist writers both to absorb specific techniques from their rivals as well as to tap into the conceptual systems and cultural resources that undergirded them. Meanwhile, however, on the other side of the ideological fence, Daoist texts began to be composed that employed pseudo-Sanskrit and mimicked Buddhist *dhāraṇīs*. Many texts on occult healing and protection were written by practitioners of one group with the specific aim of appropriating incantations, rituals, talismans, and other therapies from the competition.[91] In turn, both Buddhist and Daoist occult techniques found their way into the writings of prominent physicians such as Sun Simiao and came to be officially taught at the imperial medical bureau. The resulting integration of foreign and indigenous traditions of therapeutic magic was so thorough that it is now impossible to draw clear-cut distinctions between the practices of one group of practitioners or another, or between pseudotranslation and translation proper. This synthesis of such markedly foreignized Buddhist practices into the Chinese religio-medical world was only possible because of the simultaneous efforts to explain these techniques using the tools of the indigenous cultural-linguistic system.

The Social Logic of Buddhist Medical Translation

The five conceptual metaphors discussed in this chapter played critical roles in structuring the presentation of medical knowledge in Buddhist texts. These metaphors undergird five interrelated clusters of doctrines, practices, and ways of speaking that predominate across a wide range of literature introduced to China and composed domestically. If we accept Lakoff and Johnson's argument about the nature of conceptual metaphors, these not only profoundly shaped the way Chinese Buddhists wrote about but also how they thought about health, illness, and their bodies. The translation of the medical ideas expressed through these metaphors was apparently guided by a different logic than the translation of other types of Buddhist knowledge. While the specific translation equivalents used are highly variable across the corpus of scriptures discussed here, the consistency of the broader strategic approaches to these metaphors is striking. The crucial variable that seems to have been guiding these norms is not geography, temporal era, or sectarian affiliation, but rather the rhetorical value of translation and of foreign origin in specific types of discourse.

As discussed above, medical content in texts advocating ascetic perspectives was typically translated in language that prioritized fidelity to Indian source texts and discouraged the integration of Chinese models. Such an approach made sense in terms of these translators' purposes, social contexts, and goals. After all, these were for the most part meditation manuals, philosophical treatises, and other aids to asceticism primarily intended for the internal consumption of the sangha. It is not surprising that translators appealing to this interpretive community prioritized translation tactics that made the foreign origin of their ideas clear. For this audience, foreignizing vocabulary and unfamiliar imagery could serve to explicitly mark the texts as a product of translation—and therefore make it seem more authentic. A foreignizing flavor also could underscore Buddhism's break with Chinese religiomedical traditions. These texts inscribe foreign ideas like detachment, Emptiness, karma, and *saṃsāra* onto the body, turning the flesh into a heuristic tool for a specifically Buddhist model of insight and liberation. They make clear that undertaking Buddhist forms of ascetic practice involved steeping oneself in a new body culture, a new vision of health and illness, and a new experience of embodiment that was distinct from indigenous precedents.

In contrast, translators with a mind to reach broader audiences followed a different strategy. While ascetic texts tend to forward few if any marketable medical therapies and frequently argue that pain and suffering are the natural condition of the corporeal body, scriptures targeted more broadly work to demonstrate the power of Buddhist therapeutic interventions and the importance of Buddhist clerics as brokers of the beneficial forces in the cosmos. Buddhist scriptures composed outside of China had long been expounding on the healing effects of Buddhist practice, describing Buddhist deities as healers, and touting the power of Buddhist therapeutic thaumaturgy. When translating such ideas for Chinese audiences beyond a narrow circle of ascetics and philosophers, translators did so in ways that expressed these discourses in appealing and accessible ways—even if it meant distorting Indian doctrines in the process. Capitalizing on real and perceived points of similarity between foreign and indigenous knowledge, Buddhist writers reached for indigenous Chinese doctrines, therapies, and terminology whenever advantageous. They borrowed concepts, symbols, and idioms from native cosmological models, placing this appropriated knowledge in the mouths and in the hands of their Buddhist heroes. However, they simultaneously also peppered their translations with foreignizing words whenever they wished to create an aura of novelty or exoticism.

The norms discussed in this chapter do not only speak to us about the whims of Buddhist translators. Because translators were always embedded in the target economic, political, and ideological contexts, they also tell us a great deal about the nexus of religion and medicine as a site of social contestation in medieval China. For example, they bring into focus the role of medical knowledge as a legitimating factor in the marketplace of religious ideologies. Any religious group worth its salt was expected to promulgate a model of healing. In that environment, it was unthinkable that the sangha would not also promote its own ideas about illness, health, and the body—or that its medical ideas would not be one of the criteria upon which judgments of its value would be based. In order to forward Buddhism's position in China most effectively, it was essential that the translators, authors, and editors of Buddhist texts demonstrate the compatibility of their knowledge and practices with the indigenous ideas of recompensatory rewards and sympathetic resonance. However, they also had to be clear that they were offering novel therapeutic interventions. With the right combination of translation tactics, Buddhist translators could have their cake and eat it too: incorporating indigenous medical material into their texts could bolster Buddhism's appeal in the eyes of the medieval Chinese populace, while a foreign mystique could signal to the uninitiated that this was a difficult field best handled by clerical specialists, who should be sought out and given patronage in exchange for their healing services.

*   *   *

The fact that different translation norms prevailed in different social and ideological contexts has important implications for how we think about the reception of Buddhist medicine in China. The medical contents embedded in these texts clearly had important ideological functions in the medieval era—including supporting the practices of Buddhist asceticism, lending an aura of legitimacy, facilitating the appropriation of rival knowledge, increasing Buddhism's relevance among the laity, and bolstering the sangha's attempts to win patronage. The use of particular blends of foreignizing and domesticating language in large part determined how well such goals could be realized. The choice to translate a Buddhist medical doctrine with metaphorical equivalents drawn from the texts of rival groups—or, conversely, to use transliteration and calques that emphasized the foreignness of the source text—was a strategic decision that had to be made each time a translational act was performed. Over the course of the medieval period, it was precisely those aspects of Buddhist medicine that were captured with the right mix of the familiar and the novel that succeeded in attracting official patronage, integrated well into the state cult, and spread throughout all layers of society. The widespread acceptance of these foreign ideas and practices in popular Chinese culture and within the official ritual repertoire thus was not due to some kind of structural affinity between Indian and Chinese ideas.[92] Nor is it fully captured by speaking of India's pan-Asian influence or the hybridization of cultures. Rather, it was the cumulative result of the decisions of the many individual translators who worked to resituate Buddhist knowledge strategically within the Chinese religiomedical world.

CHAPTER 4

Rewriting Buddhist Medicine

This chapter shifts gears from the broad analysis of norms to look more closely at how a handful of individual authors tailored their presentation of various aspects of Buddhist medicine in specific compositions. The texts under consideration in this chapter include commentaries, manuals, reference materials, and other writings that can be thought of as "Buddhist secondary sources" in the sense that they describe, reconcile, systematize, and codify the scriptural knowledge discussed in the previous chapter. Although they were not necessarily engaged in translation proper, these commentators, anthologizers, and other rewriters of Buddhist medicine were intimately involved in intralingual translation. Like those who engage in translation of any kind, they employed divergent strategies in response to shifts in patronage patterns, sociopolitical context, changing perceptions of the source culture, and other factors beyond questions of language and equivalence.

Each of the authors introduced here responded as an individual to the perceived needs of his time. Nevertheless, a general historical trend emerges. In contrast to the relative stability of the translation norms for scriptures discussed in the previous chapter, a close reading of these secondary sources suggests that a shift took place between the sixth and eighth centuries in how Chinese writers approached the Indian medical knowledge that was being made available to them by the translation assemblies. Authors in the earlier period tended to try to explain Buddhist medical doctrines in terms that were more compatible with indigenous repertoires. They liberally employed metaphorical equivalents and other domesticating translation strategies and emphasized the compatibility of Indian medical thought with Chinese ideas. Following the broader trend in post-reunification China, however, discussions of Buddhist medicine from the mid-seventh century onward became increasingly concerned with fidelity to the source context. Secondary sources on Buddhist medicine composed in this period exhibit a marked increase in familiarity with Indian medical terminology and contain technical language rarely seen in the earlier era. This chapter investigates these historical developments, focusing on how such choices dovetailed with translators' strategies and goals as individual actors in their own social and political worlds.

Early Commentaries on the *Sutra of Golden Light*

Chinese Buddhist exegetes in the early medieval period struggled to make sense of the sheer volume of the Buddhist scriptures that were being introduced to China. In the earliest period of textual transmission, Chinese Buddhists were often unable to discriminate among the doctrinal positions of the various competing Indian schools or to reconcile their conflicting messages. As familiarity with Buddhist thought increased, making sense of these differences became a central focus. In the sixth century, exegetes such as Paramārtha (Ch. Zhendi, 499–569), Zhiyi (538–97), and Jizang (549–623) began to posit elaborate hierarchical systems that purported to show definitively how all Buddhist doctrines fit together. Departing from Indian commentarial tradition, these "taxonomies of teachings" (*panjiao*) placed the diversity of the Tripitaka within a hierarchy of truths that made sense in the Chinese context.[1] Taxonomies based on the "three turns of the [Dharma] Wheel" (*sanlun*) proposed by Paramārtha and Jizang organized all scriptures into three discrete temporal phases supposedly correlating to chronological periods of the Buddha's teaching career. In Zhiyi's system, on the other hand, he enshrined the *Flower Ornament Sutra* (*Huayan jing*, T. 278–279, T. 293) and *Lotus Sutra* as the undisputed paragons of truth, with other texts arrayed below these.

During an era of political transition, such rationalizing systems attempting to unify Buddhist teachings closely mirrored initiatives to reunite the cultural and social diversity of the Chinese subcontinent under a single emperor. This connection was not lost on ambitious rulers, who frequently supported the systematizing efforts. Emperor Wu of the Liang, for example, invited Paramārtha, a Tripitaka master from western India living in Southeast Asia, to Jiankang as part of his attempt to use Buddhism to bring peace to the realm.[2] Zhiyi, a native of Anhui, received patronage from the upper strata of the Chen dynasty before the reunification and was specifically sought out by the rulers of the Sui as part of their efforts to consolidate their reabsorption of the South into the reconstituted empire.[3] Likewise, Jizang, who was born in China but was of Parthian heritage, received patronage and was given multiple abbotships by the rulers of the Sui as well as by the founder of the Tang.[4]

It is not surprising that these commentators writing in the Period of Division and the early reunification era returned again and again to the *Sutra of Golden Light*. The first translation of this text is credited to the Indian monk Dharmakṣema (Ch. Tanmochen; 385–433), shortly after his translation career at the capital of the Northern Liang began in 420.[5] The sutra deals primarily with Buddhist ideals of kingship and the power of Buddhist ritual to provide for the protection of the state, and thus was a natural focus of attention for exegetes with royal or imperial patronage. However, a chapter of this sutra also happens to contain one of the most coherent explanations of Indian medical doctrine in the Chinese Tripitaka. Thus, as they worked to interpret the sutra's content, commentators necessarily also grappled with how to present foreign medical ideas to their audiences. Forging a compatible relationship between Buddhist and Chinese medical terminology was not their central concern, but was nonetheless instrumental to these writers' broader goals, for showing that Buddhist texts contained relevant medical wisdom meant that the texts could also be trusted on other matters such as statecraft.

Part of the task facing these authors was simply to make the foreign medical ideas in the *Sutra of Golden Light* comprehensible in the Chinese context. However, Indian medical ideas could not simply be accepted at face value. The metaphor of the body as an assemblage of impermanent, disgusting, and essentially incompatible Elements, for example, might have dangerous political implications. In a cosmos where bodies and states were thought to have a homologous relationship, such a view of the physical body could have implied that any efforts at reunifying the realm were contrary to nature and doomed to eventually fail. On the other hand, reinterpreting Indian medical doctrines in terms of Chinese equivalents could reinforce Buddhism's compatibility with doctrines such as yin-yang and Five Phases that underpinned the classical political models and worldview, and thus could neutralize any potentially subversive political message.

The bulk of the medical content in the *Sutra of Golden Light* appears in chapter 15 of Dharmakṣema's text, where a doctor's son (who is in fact the Buddha in a previous life) is inspired to relieve the suffering caused by an epidemic and asks his father to teach him the art of medicine.[6] The father replies to his son in verse with a summary of the basic principles, concentrating primarily on the relationship between the seasons, the arising of the *tridoṣa*, and the medicinal Flavors (*rasa*, i.e., the therapeutic effects of food and drink by which the *tridoṣa* can be ameliorated). Though this passage may have struck a reader of the Sanskrit source text as a fairly straightforward précis of Indian medical doctrine, it was clear to the Chinese systematizers that these laconic verses filled with foreign medical terms and concepts required further clarification. All three of the sixth-century exegetes wrote commentaries that purported to explain this chapter. (Only the later commentaries by Zhiyi and Jizang are now extant, but both authors quote extensively from a lost original attributed to Paramārtha.)[7]

Although Paramārtha was from western India, Zhiyi was Chinese, and Jizang was Parthian, these commentators all explained Indian medicine in terms of indigenous Chinese doctrines. For example, where the sutra discusses how illnesses arise according to the Indian calendrical divisions of Six Seasons (Ch. *liushi*; Skt. *ṛtu*), the commentators adduce lengthy explications on how to calculate the periods of the year based on the logic of yin and yang and the Five Phases.[8] These computations take up an inordinate amount of space (over forty lines of dense prose) given the brevity of the mention in the original sutra text (only five lines of verses [Skt. *gāthās*]), indicating that the incorporation into the commentaries of detailed Chinese calendrical knowledge was a principal goal of the authors' presentation of the material.

In order to elucidate the connections between food and illness mentioned in the sutra's verses, the commentators discuss six ways that improper consumption of food and drink can cause illness. These include (1) eating too much, (2) eating too little, (3) waiting too long to eat, (4) eating when one is not yet hungry, (5) eating "forbidden foods," and (6) eating "unfamiliar or strong foods."[9] The first four items on this list are generic sorts of recommendations on regimen similar to those found in the *Sutra on the Buddha as Physician* mentioned in Chapter 3 and many other Buddhist texts.[10] But, in order to explain what is meant by "forbidden" and "unfamiliar or strong" foods, the commentators provide examples of indigenous Chinese food taboos. The two extant commentaries differ slightly in these passages, but they both mention the prohibition against eating meat and drinking milk at the same meal.[11] They both also advise that southern people should not drink *jiang* (a type of broth); that northern people should not drink milk or take honey; that eating bitter vegetables together with honey will prevent the

conception of a male child; that certain flavors will exacerbate a cold; and
that ingesting alcohol, wheat, or raw meat when one has a Fire Illness results
in blindness, bloody vomit, and bloody diarrhea. Zhiyi additionally mentions that eating white heron meat fried in lard will cause leprosy (*lai*), while
Jizang adds that eating Cold and Moist flavors when one has a Wind Illness
can be lethal.

Continuing in this domesticating vein, the commentators explain the
sutra's passages on the arising of the *tridoṣa* by invoking a doctrine on the
opening and closing of the hair follicles that is drawn from Chinese etiological theory:

> [When the sutra says that] in summertime, the Wind [i.e., the Wind
> *doṣa*] is aroused, this means that in summertime the hair follicles
> (*maokong*) open up. Winds from outside get in and arouse the inter-
> nal Wind.

> [When the sutra says that] Heat Illness [i.e., the Bile *doṣa*] is aroused
> in the autumn, this means that the hair follicles are closed tightly
> and the Heat trapped inside cannot circulate, resulting in illness.[12]

The commentators also employ this same doctrine to explain the efficacy
of the Oily Flavor (Ch. *ni*; Skt. *snigdha*) in treating illness. When the hair
follicles open up, they state, foods of this category can be used to stop them
up and prevent external Wind from entering. Likewise, in cases of disorders
caused by the Phlegm *doṣa*, the Oily Flavor can stop up the hair follicles and
prevent Water from entering.[13]

The commentary by Zhiyi, who as we will see below was quite familiar
with indigenous medical models, goes even further than the other two in his
domesticating explanations. In making sense of the sutra's connections between the seasons and the onset of illness, Zhiyi wholly departs from Indian
models and instead introduces a Chinese system based on the Viscera:

> Liver illnesses arising in spring can be cured. Spleen illnesses arising
> in spring are difficult to cure. Heart illnesses arising in summer can
> be cured. Lung illnesses arising in summer are difficult to cure. Lung
> illnesses arising at the end of summer, at the beginning of winter, or
> in mid-autumn can be cured, but if Liver illness arises [at that time],

this will be difficult to cure. Kidney illnesses arising in winter can be cured, but if a Heart illness arises, this will be difficult to cure.[14]

This section echoes passages in the *Inner Canon,* which also associate illness of the Liver with springtime, of the Heart with summer, of the Lungs with autumn, and of the Kidneys with winter. The passage quoted above could just have easily come from Daoist or self-cultivation literature.

Let us be clear: these examples of indigenous medical ideas introduced into the commentaries to explain Indian medicine are not indications of confusion or error. Given their multicultural origins and their deep knowledge of Buddhist scriptures, there is no chance that these translators were not aware of the distinctions between Indian and Chinese medical models. Rather, these are examples of the commentators' conscious and strategic deployment of indigenous metaphorical equivalents. They were able to engage in this kind of bridge building due in no small part to the metaphorical equivalence already established by Dharmakṣema's choices in his initial translation of the sutra. For example, in translating the *tridoṣa* he gives the Wind *doṣa* as Wind (*feng*), Bile as Heat (*re*), and Phlegm as alternately Water (*shui*), Lung Illness (*feibing*), or Water Entering the Lungs (*shuiguofei*)—all of which, as discussed in the previous chapter, are double entendres connoting both Indian and Chinese doctrine.

Given their penchant for reinforcing and elaborating on such metaphorical equivalencies, it is fair to say that unpacking the meaning of Indian medical doctrine was not these three commentators' top priority. Indeed, we might point out that some of their correlations are made in only the most desultory way, if we were concerned only with formal equivalence. For example, they equate the Buddhist Six Elements with the Chinese Six Viscera (*liufu*), but since these two doctrines have virtually no common ground, and the commentators do not support their position in any detail, they most likely are being equated here based only on their numerical correspondence.[15] Instead of exploring Indian medicine in any detail, what the commentators seem to prioritize most in these passages is the demonstration of indigenous Chinese medical and scientific expertise. They mobilize a whole gamut of Chinese doctrines that would have been recognized as a performance of erudition by any contemporary reader. If we were to investigate further the authorship of these texts, we might be able to conclusively link their writing to specific bids for patronage. In any case, it is clear that these authors were more interested in showcasing for their politically ambitious patrons Buddhism's compatibility with a whole range of indigenous Chinese medical, scientific, and culinary knowledge—and their own ability to make these connections—than in explaining the meaning of foreign medical doctrines with reference to the source context.

Zhiyi's Meditation Manual

The close connection between a translator's audience, his goals, and the interpretive strategies he employs is epitomized by the fact that, while Zhiyi glossed Indian knowledge with Chinese equivalents in his commentary on the *Sutra of Golden Light*, he pursued a different strategy when writing meditation manuals intended for the sangha. Zhiyi is famous for his creation of taxonomies of Buddhist knowledge and is also credited with the founding of the Tiantai School (*tiantai zong*). In the annals of Buddhist medicine, however, he is most well known for being the first Chinese author to systematically integrate Indian and Chinese medicine.[16] One of his earliest compositions to take such a stand, written while in retreat on Mount Tiantai between 575 and 585, is a short but influential meditation manual commonly known as *The Shorter [Treatise on] Śamatha and Vipaśyanā Meditation* (*Xiao zhiguan*).[17] Part and parcel of his lifelong project of systematizing Buddhist knowledge more generally, this manual was intended to unite various styles of meditation into a single coherent system. The ninth chapter of this text, entitled "Treating Illness" (*zhibing*), provides a concise overview of Zhiyi's thoughts on how to treat illness with meditation.

The chapter begins with a discussion of two separate approaches to the diagnosis of illness. The first method involves an analysis of the excess and depletion of the Four Elements, in which Zhiyi delineates various symptoms and signs according to the usual Buddhist division of 101 illnesses each for Earth, Water, Fire, and Wind.[18] A close reading of this passage reveals that Zhiyi has employed few terms drawn from indigenous medical vocabularies. Instead—and in contrast to his commentary on the *Sutra of Golden Light* discussed in the previous section—he presents the Indian doctrine of the Four Elements on its own terms. Immediately following this passage, however, Zhiyi presents a second method of diagnosis that is based entirely on indigenous categories. Here, he provides a list of symptoms and syndromes based on the logic of the Five Viscera (*wuzang*). The correlations he gives between symptoms, organs, and bodily functions in this section have no connections with Indian medicine, but rather draw exclusively on indigenous models and vocabularies.[19]

Zhiyi continues this strategy of juxtaposing foreign and domestic medical models as he introduces various methods of treating illness with meditation. The first category of therapies he presents is drawn from the Buddhist context. He considers these to be types of *śamatha*, or meditations that involve single-minded concentration on a particular object. In the first place, the meditator has only to fix his attention on the location of the illness and he will be able to cure it.[20] This is because, says Zhiyi, the mind can control the karmic retributions (*guobao*) of the present life. The second method involves fixing the mind just below the navel, a location that the text names in both Chinese (*dantian*, lit. "field of cinnabar") and Sanskrit (*udāna*, here transliterated as *youtuona*). He does not explain this technique any further than to say that if one is able to fix one's mind there without wavering for a length of time, one will be healed.[21] A third practice involves concentrating on the soles of the feet. This is effective because the mind usually focuses on the upper parts of the body, which can cause the imbalance of the Four Elements. By training the mind on the soles of the feet, Zhiyi states, the "Four Elements will naturally come into balance and illnesses will disappear."[22] Finally, citing the *Vimalakīrti Sutra*, he states that realizing the Empty nature of the body and quiescently abiding in calmness is sufficient to cure all illnesses.[23]

These healing meditations centering on concentration practices are typical of advice on the management of illness found in the broader Buddhist tradition and would be familiar to Buddhists across Asia. In his second category, *vipaśyanā* meditations, however, Zhiyi again introduces indigenous Chinese practices. While Zhiyi uses little by way of domesticating terminology in the preceding section, speaking in terms of karma and scriptural precedents, he here shifts his idiom strongly in favor of indigenous models. The meditation he presents in this section is the Six Breaths (*liuzhong qi*), an indigenous Chinese breathing practice with a long history in domestic religiomedical literature that involved the recitation of six syllables as a means of both regulating the Viscera and repelling demons.[24] In Zhiyi's description of the practice, the therapeutic logic hinges on the Chinese Viscera, and there is no hint of the Buddhist language employed in the *śamatha* section above.

The language changes back again when discussing a second therapeutic practice called the Twelve Breaths (*shi'er xi*). Rather than being named for syllables, these techniques are named the Upward (*shangxi*), Downward (*xiaxi*),

Full (*manxi*), Scorching (*jiaoxi*), Lengthening (*zengchangxi*), Dissipating (*miehuaixi*), Warming (*nuanxi*), Cooling (*lengxi*), Forceful (*chongxi*), Retained (*chixi*), Harmonizing (*hexi*), and Nourishing Breaths (*buxi*).[25] Here, Zhiyi is referring to Indian techniques of breath control (Skt. *prāṇāyāma*), and he distinguishes the Indian exercises from the aforementioned Chinese ones by using the term xi_2 instead of qi for the breath. Predictably, when he correlates each of these Indian breathing exercises with the symptoms it cures, he draws on the therapeutic logic of the Four Elements instead of indigenous Chinese doctrines.[26]

While the bulk of the *vipaśyanā* section consists of the two practices of breath control, Zhiyi does briefly mention a third healing meditation in this category. He states that if one suffers from Cold, he can visualize within his body "a Fiery Qi arising" and thereby cure himself.[27] While only mentioning Fire, this is in all likelihood a domesticating translation of the Four Element absorption (*samādhi*) meditations, mental exercises that are said to be able to transform the physical body.[28] He then mentions again the power of the realization of Emptiness to spontaneously resolve illness.[29] Next, Zhiyi explains that if an illness is of demonic origin, the incantation of *dhāraṇī* will help with its treatment, and if it is of karmic origin, one should repent and practice merit making.[30] In conclusion, he insists that there is no illness that is impervious to the curative effects of *śamatha* and *vipaśyanā* meditation, so long as they are practiced by one who is consummate in Buddhist virtue. For such a person, learning the meditations well will benefit both himself and others and will enable him to practice the "correct Dharma" (*zhengfa*).[31]

There is no question that Zhiyi understood the Indian and Chinese medical systems he presents to be distinct. Unlike in his commentary discussed in the previous section, where he interprets the medical doctrines in the *Sutra of Golden Light* in terms of Chinese models, in this text, Zhiyi characterizes Buddhist and Chinese medicine as compatible but separate bodies of knowledge. Though he does not utilize much Sanskrit, throughout his chapter he maintains a high degree of separation between the two models he discusses by using different lexicons—one foreignizing, one domesticating—to talk about them. That Zhiyi uses different translation tactics in this composition suggests his strategic goals are different. By absorbing the widely known practices of Visceral diagnosis and the Six Breaths into the framework of his manual on *śamatha* and *vipaśyanā*, he addressed the need to systematize or reconcile Buddhist and Chinese models of diagnostics and therapy.

Zhiyi's chapter provides a rationale for the use of indigenous medical knowledge by Buddhists, but not everyone believed that all indigenous practices were compatible. In the closing section of the *Taishō Tripitaka* version of Zhiyi's essay, an interpolated passage by an unknown author explicitly draws boundaries that exclude certain techniques advocated by Buddhism's rivals. The passage reads:

> Nowadays people have only superficial spiritual attainments and use *śamatha* and *vipaśyanā* without any result, and therefore in our time these are not transmitted. Because [these orthodox teachings] are unattainable, people practice the arts of qi and grain avoidance, and I fear they have given rise to heterodox views. Medicines of metal, stone, herbs, and wood can be taken when appropriate for the symptoms of an illness.[32]

The unknown author of this rebuke apparently saw no irony in criticizing practitioners of the arts of qi (*qishu*) and grain avoidance (*xiuliang*), while at the same time approving of Zhiyi's appropriation of indigenous diagnostics and breathing exercises as well as allowing for indigenous pharmacological therapies. Although all of these practices had associations with rival groups, for this unnamed editor, the latter were legitimate methods that could be safely incorporated into Buddhist practice, while the former were "heterodox views" that were misleading and did not belong in this synthesis of truths. Thus, within the very same text, Buddhist medicine could be a location both for absorbing the competition and for policing the boundaries of orthodoxy.

Daoxuan's Vinaya Commentary and the New Reception Environment in the Tang

The view that Chinese and Indian medical systems were compatible or even interchangeable as forwarded by Zhiyi and other systematizers in the sixth century became problematic in the seventh. Social realities had changed, and the boundaries of what constituted acceptable medical approaches for Buddhists were open for renegotiation. With the empire now united and the political situation stabilized, Buddhist medical doctrines may have seemed less subversive. With Buddhism flourishing and cross-cultural exchange with India intensifying (no fewer than fifty embassies to India would be mounted by the Tang rulers between 619 and 753 for a range of economic, political, military, and religious purposes), Chinese authors were becoming more acquainted with Indian culture. Chinese markets and materia medica literature were making room for Indian medicinals, and elite physicians at the government medical bureaus were incorporating Indian doctrines into their treatises. Indian longevity and rejuvenation practices were becoming fashionable in Tang society.[33] Seventh-century rulers were bringing Buddhist relics into the imperial palace during times of grave illness in the hope of stimulating a cure.[34] Emperor Taizong developed an interest in Indian medicine and sent emissaries to the subcontinent to the court of King Harṣa (r. 606–47) to acquire, among other things, medicines to treat his ailments and a doctor specializing in longevity.[35] Taizong's successors, Gaozong and Empress Wu, each would enjoy the ministrations of several such specialists.[36] The translation norms promulgated by Xuanzang (602–64), the famed pilgrim and easily the most respected translator of his day, prioritized the Indian language and cultural context. And many well-known exegetes of the period stressed the need to look to the Buddhist holy land as a model in order to reinvigorate monastic practice and to maintain the purity of the Dharma in China.

As explained in the previous chapter, such social shifts played a surprisingly minor role in influencing the strategic approaches to the translation of the medical content in Buddhist scriptures. In that literature, choices between domesticating and foreignizing translation tactics continued to be made primarily on the basis of the intended audience. However, changes in the reception environment greatly influenced how Buddhist authors framed and explained Buddhist medical doctrines in their secondary literature. Engaging with Buddhist medical ideas now became an opportunity to bring to the fore the particulars of Indian culture, as well as to demonstrate an author's personal commitment to and knowledge of Indian precedents. It presented the opportunity both to enrich the Chinese language and also to address perceived shortcomings in the Chinese culture. Some of the signs representative of this shift were that authors now began to codify Buddhist medicine and to downplay the role of Chinese medical doctrine in their treatises.

The seventh and eighth centuries saw the rise of new classes of indigenous Chinese Buddhist literature. Reference materials such as catalogs, dictionaries, encyclopedias (*leishu*, lit. "category books"), and monastic disciplinary handbooks (*qinggui*, lit. "rules of purity") began to be composed in large numbers. Such texts were deeply implicated in social functions such as defining schools of thought, constructing lineages, and inventing origin stories.[37] They were also devoted to the codification of Buddhist knowledge of all types and were instrumental in bolstering Buddhism's image as a legitimate body of wisdom about human affairs, the natural world, and the cosmos as a whole. As part of this general trend, some authors began collecting, organizing, and codifying Buddhist medical knowledge from across the scriptures.

Daoxuan (596–667), a towering figure in Chinese Buddhist history who has already been mentioned several times in this book, is traditionally recognized as the founder of the Nanshan Vinaya School (*Nanshan lü zong*) and is widely known as an important reformer of monastic discipline.[38] Several of his most notable writings were distillations of rules from the Indian monastic disciplinary codes, in which he attempted to develop a consistent monastic disciplinary system for the Chinese sangha. In such tracts, Daoxuan sometimes explicitly commented on the proper handling of medical substances, tools, and literature. His guidelines were largely designed to limit the private control of medical knowledge by individual members of the sangha and were particularly concerned with curtailing the practice of non-Buddhist medical traditions.[39] At the same time as he established limitations on indigenous medical knowledge and practice, Daoxuan not only allowed but encouraged the sangha to care for one another according to principles set out in the Tripitaka. He elaborated this position most influentially in the sixteenth chapter of his *Emended Commentary on Monastic Practices from the Dharmaguptaka Vinaya* (*Sifenlü shanfan buque xingshi chao*, T. 1804.16), compiled in 626–30. Titled "Nursing the Sick and Sending Off the Dying" (*zhanbing songzhong*), this chapter purported to outline the proper way to administer nursing and hospice care within the monastic order.[40]

Despite its name and Daoxuan's preference for the Vinaya of the Dharmaguptaka sect, the commentary is not entirely based on that source. Rather, it weaves together relevant passages from the Dharmaguptaka Vinaya with materials drawn from across a wide range of monastic disciplinary literature available in Chinese translation in Daoxuan's lifetime.[41] These sources— including the Vinayas of the Mahāsāṃghika, Sarvāstivāda, and Mahīśāsaka sects in addition to a number of imported and domestically produced commentaries—were originally composed in different historical eras and geographic areas and in fact represented the views of competing Buddhist orders. Daoxuan's chapter also integrates several examples of other genres, including sutras from both the Āgama and Mahayana literature, as well as metaphysical texts of the Abhidharma variety. As he brought passages from all of these disparate sources together, he ignored or glossed over the many differences between them in order to construct a unified synthesis for his readers.

One of the principal concerns of Daoxuan's chapter is to provide a strong doctrinal justification for the practice of caring for the sick within the monastic community. At the beginning of the chapter, he refers to a narrative from the Dharmaguptaka Vinaya in which the Buddha instructs the monastic community to care for one another when sick.[42] In the original narrative (which Daoxuan does not repeat in full but clearly expected his audience to know), the Buddha comes across a sick monk who is lying in his own urine and excrement within the monastic quarters. The Buddha approaches the monk and asks why he is in this condition. The monk replies that in the past he had failed to care for sick monks within the community, and now that he had fallen ill no one is caring for him. Upon hearing this, the Buddha helps the monk to rise and cleans his body. He washes his clothing, cleans out his dwelling, makes a new bed for him out of grass, and lays out fresh bedding. Later, the Buddha informs the sangha of his actions, giving them the following admonition: "*ruo you yu gongyang wo zhe, ying gongyang bingren.*"[43]

The interpretation of this line spoken by the Buddha hinges on the double meaning of the term *gongyang*, which as discussed in Chapter 3 means both "to give care" and "to make offerings." The Buddha's instruction can be read as saying "If you would care for me, then you should care for the sick," but it could just as well be understood as saying "If you desire to make offerings to me, then you should care for the sick." When he interprets this line in his commentary, Daoxuan capitalizes on the ambiguity of the term in order to argue that to care for the sick is both to emulate the Buddha and to make offerings to him.[44]

With the rationale for providing assistance to the sick thus established, the chapter continues by presenting a long list of quotes from Buddhist literature illustrating the proper methods of doing so. These include, for example, instructions from the Mahāsāṃghika Vinaya on what a member of the sangha should do if a monk or nun falls sick while traveling,[45] a passage from the same source enumerating nine deviations from proper regimen that can cause premature death,[46] a reference to the Dharmaguptaka Vinaya's list of five virtues of the sick nurse that facilitate the cure of the patient,[47] and other short passages from assorted Vinayas and disciplinary commentaries on the proper means of caring for and supplying the needs of the sick.[48]

After covering these medical topics, Daoxuan's chapter turns to hospice facilities, the importance of the moment of death, funeral arrangements, and disposal of the corpse, which were all matters of great concern for the reformer.[49] These sections focus a great deal of attention on the importance of the patient's state of mind at the moment of death for ensuring his or her salvation. They also stress that an attendant should assist the dying to control their thoughts and preach the Dharma to them in order to ensure auspicious rebirth. In this part of the commentary, Daoxuan includes an idealized description of a hospice facility at the Jetavana monastery in India (which he ascribes to "a Chinese tradition" [*Zhongguo benchuan*]).[50] He also invokes a number of scriptural authorities, including the *Vimalakīrti Sutra*, the *Mahāprajñāpāramitā-śāstra* (Ch. *Dazhi du lun*, T. 1509), the *Flower Ornament Sutra*, *Biographies of Eminent Monks,* several Āgama texts, the Vinayas, and a number of other disciplinary texts.[51] Though they mostly deal with death rather than curing, some of these citations are relevant to us in that they give us glimpses into what Daoxuan thought were the important nursing practices to promote within the monastic community.

Daoxuan's commentary was written with specific goals in mind. Reacting against what he perceived to be the chaotic heterogeneity of the Chinese sangha's disciplinary practice, he wished to consolidate the most important principles from the various strands of literature available to him in a new monastic guide that was customized for the Chinese sangha. While it was intended to serve contemporary purposes, however, by producing this treatise Daoxuan began the process of fashioning an enduring template for subsequent writings on Buddhist medicine. The texts he chose to cite, the doctrines he decided to include, and his justification for the practice of medicine by the devout all would continue to lie at the heart of writings about Buddhist medicine for centuries to come.

Daoshi's Encyclopedia Entry

One author who rapidly adopted Daoxuan's synthesis was Daoshi (?–683), a contemporary who sometimes collaborated with him on the composition of disciplinary texts and collections of short narratives.[52] Daoshi had previously worked on a translation team headed by Xuanzang and surely was intimately acquainted with the developing norms that advocated stricter adherence to Indian sources. In addition to texts on merit making and other facets of lay practice, Daoshi compiled two important encyclopedias that dealt with all manners of historical and literary topics, contemporary politics, material culture, daily life, ritual practices, philosophical doctrines, and other matters of interest to monastics.[53] Daoshi's magnum opus was the one-hundred-fascicle *Forest of Pearls in the Garden of the Dharma*, which he completed in 668 after many years of labor. The ninety-fifth chapter of this work, called "On the Suffering of Sickness" (*bingku pian*), reinscribed many of the choices made in the compilation of Daoxuan's Vinaya commentary, while expanding the scope to include an even wider range of scriptural material.[54]

The chapter opens with a preface in which Daoshi adapts and expands upon an essay from another of Daoxuan's famous compilations, the *Expanded Hongming ji* (*Guang hongming ji*, T. 2013).[55] The piece revolves around core Buddhist medical perspectives, such as the impermanent and mutually antagonistic nature of the Four Elements, the disgusting and dissatisfactory nature of the physical body, and the inevitability of illness as a part of human embodiment.

Five sections then follow that focus on basic doctrine, nursing, therapy, hospice, and death practices. Each of the chapter's sections contains a few opening lines of commentary that, like the introduction to the chapter as a whole, are pastiches made up of Daoshi's own words and passages from the *Expanded Hongming ji* (and possibly other contemporary sources as well). Following these introductory lines, Daoshi presents a series of quotes drawn from a wide range of Buddhist canonical literature. These include many passages previously quoted in Daoxuan's Vinaya commentary, interspersed with fundamental statements of doctrine from the *Sutra on the Buddha as Physician* and the *Sutra of Golden Light*; bits of doctrine and inspirational narratives from early Āgama texts, *jataka* tales, and the *Dharmapāda*; passages from major Mahayana texts such as the *Vimalakīrti Sutra,* the *Flower Ornament Sutra*, and the *Mahāprajñāpāramitā-śāstra*; quotes from a number of sutras of varying importance on Maitreya Buddha and the Pure Lands; and monastic disciplinary strictures from the Dharmaguptaka, Mahāsāṃghika, and Sarvāstivāda Vinayas as well as from disciplinary texts for both the sangha and the laity. In the final section of the encyclopedia chapter, Daoshi includes a selection of fourteen narratives culled from hagiographies of monks and from secular collections of strange tales that were circulating widely in the medieval period (these will be discussed further in Chapter 5).[56]

Doctrines introduced within the encyclopedia entry include practically all of the main principles of Buddhist medicine mentioned previously in this book: the connections between the Four Elements, the seasons, and the Flavors; the causes of illness due to inappropriate regimen; the basic division of 404 illnesses; the importance of caring for the sick as meritorious practice; guidelines regarding proper and improper nursing; the *tridoṣa* and their treatment; the idealized hospice facility that supposedly operated at Jetavana; the invocation of deities through the practice of chanting and meditation; the importance of the moment of death; and the use of occult practices to assist in preserving and regaining health.

Like Daoxuan before him, Daoshi surely was interested in using his writing to speak to a range of issues in contemporary society as well as to pursue his own personal advancement. He no doubt wished to demonstrate the richness of the Buddhist medical tradition, but also to showcase his own status as an authoritative and well-read scholar. For our purposes, Daoshi's approach to his compilation is most notable for the relative lack of interest he exhibits in building explicit bridges between Indian and Chinese medical doctrine. The tales appended to the end of the chapter do, in fact, domesticate Buddhist healing by suggesting its connection with indigenous notions of retribution, resonance, and the spirit world. This suggests the continuing importance of domesticating translations in arguments for the efficacy of Buddhist healing—a topic I will return to in the next chapter. However, in the sections where he is discussing what Buddhist approaches to healing actually consist of, the author relies on the available literature in the Tripitaka. Granted, some of the passages he quotes, such as the introduction of the *Sutra on the Buddha as Physician*, use metaphorical equivalents to suggest that foreign and domestic medical knowledge are compatible. However, Daoshi does not explicitly engage with Chinese medical doctrines in an attempt to explain or justify Buddhist ideas, as did Zhiyi and other sixth-century authors.[57]

These choices of how to present Buddhist medicine are of a piece with the changing norms in the seventh century. Daoshi's treatment of scriptural passages in the encyclopedia entry continued the process of systematization begun by Daoxuan. Although he only rarely cites Daoxuan explicitly, he clearly relied on the latter as a source of inspiration and material.[58] Both authors cherry-picked diverse items from across the Tripitaka and organized them under topical headings to create a unified Chinese tradition of Buddhist medicine where one had not existed before. Daoshi's chapter encompasses a much greater diversity of source texts and medical doctrines than did its predecessor, and it represents a further development of the codification of knowledge begun by his predecessor. It also shows us that Buddhist medicine was increasingly being recognized as a legitimate body of knowledge that need not be compared or explained with Chinese categories.

Yijing's Travelogue

If Daoxuan and Daoshi were relative purists in their approach to what constituted Buddhist medicine, Yijing (635–713) was even more so. A native of Shandong, Yijing embarked on one of the most celebrated pilgrimages in world history aboard a Persian ship in 671. Stopping in Śrīvijaya (present-day Sumatra) for training in Sanskrit, he eventually made his way to the east coast of India and on to the Buddhist university at Nālandā, where he remained translating Buddhist texts and studying the Indian monastic curriculum for nine years. He set sail back to Śrīvijaya in 687, settling there for a time until eventually returning home in 695. In 691, while still abroad, Yijing completed his travelogue, *Records of Buddhist Practices Sent Home from the Southern Seas*, which he dispatched back to China along with new translations of Buddhist texts.

During his time in India, Yijing studied medicine. Although he eventually abandoned this pursuit, feeling it was not a proper vocation for a monk, he nevertheless paid close attention in his travelogue to the medical and hygienic practices of the monks in Indian monasteries. Amid much reportage on aspects of monastic life such as ordination, master-disciple relationships, and clerical clothing, Yijing's travelogue contains valuable observations on daily ablutions, regimen, healing, and the maintenance of health.

Yijing was not a purely disinterested reporter.[59] One of his stated goals in writing his travelogue was to provide an account of monastic life in India as a guide for Chinese monks and as an encouragement for them to follow Indian monastic discipline more closely. He particularly emphasized the need for the Chinese sangha to learn Sanskrit and advocated that monks study and follow the Mūlasarvāstivāda Vinaya. On the topics of medicine and hygiene in particular, he held Indian practice to be the unquestioned standard of authenticity. Yijing forwarded his antisyncretist position by repeatedly criticizing Chinese deviation from Indian norms in his travelogue. He had little tolerance for any Chinese modifications, which he considered to be misunderstandings. All admixtures and adaptations were backward, dangerous, and contrary to the Buddha's teachings, and the Chinese sangha needed to clearly understand and more closely adhere to Indian ways.

On occasion, Yijing is conciliatory in his travelogue toward certain types of indigenous medical knowledge not overtly associated with Buddhism, such as when he praises Chinese innovations in acupuncture, pulse taking, longevity drugs, and herbs. These contribute to China's fame in India and around the world, says Yijing: "In all the five parts of India, who does not esteem China, and who within the four seas does not hold her in respect?"[60] However, although some of China's medical traditions are worthy of respect, the pilgrim argues that Chinese knowledge is lacking in certain key areas, most particularly in etiology and therapeutics, and it is here that China must learn from India.[61]

Yijing takes many opportunities to highlight India's superior knowledge of medicine. Of particular interest is his chapter titled "Rules for Taking Medicine" (*jinyao fangfa*).[62] Chief among the Indian therapies he praises in this section is fasting, which he says may cure an imbalance of the Elements in a matter of days. One should also massage the abdomen or practice self-induced vomiting in order to clear out undigested food. Using these therapies, he says, one need not trouble with medicines or a physician: "each person is then a King of Physicians, and every person becomes a Jīvaka." If medicines are necessary, Yijing recommends a number of herbal simples, ointments, and compound remedies. This medical knowledge, he says, echoing a common Indian legend about the origins of medicine, was handed down by Indra and was now commonly practiced all over India.

Elsewhere in the travelogue, the pilgrim takes up the topic of hygiene.[63] He describes in glowing terms the daily practice of bathing and applying ointments among the Indian sangha. The monastics bathe in an "open-air pool with bricks" and take medicinal baths for illness, as taught by the Buddha. These ablutions prevent problems with the eyesight and afflictions of Cold, says Yijing. It is also particularly beneficial if one bathes on an empty stomach, as one thus partakes of food when the body is "pure and empty" and one's appetite is increased. Additionally, bathing relieves Phlegm and mental depression.

Yijing also reports at length on oral hygiene.[64] The teeth are to be cleaned, he says, by chewing on a length of "dental wood" (Ch. *chimu*; Skt. *dantakāṣṭha*), which are twigs of a Bitter, Astringent, or Pungent flavor. In addition to the usual willow tree, these could be cultivated from quercus, pine, ampelopsis, mulberry, peach, locust, or from xanthium root. The latter is preferable as it "hardens the teeth, and makes the mouth good smelling, and also helps the digestion" as well as curing illnesses of the Heart. It can also cure toothache and other dental problems. The tongue is scraped with the same twig, or one can fashion a tongue scraper from metal. Bamboo should be used to make a toothpick. Yijing also describes the practice of nasal irrigation with water, which he calls "Nāgārjuna's art of longevity" (Ch. *Longshu changnian zhi shu*, known today as *jala-neti*). Cleansing oneself is especially important after eating a meal, says Yijing.[65] The monk must wash his hands, cleanse his teeth, pick his teeth, scrape his tongue, and use "bean dregs" (*douxie*) or mud to wipe his lips. Then, he should clean the vessel and his hands with bean dregs, dry earth, and cow dung.

Yijing is quick to point to differences between Indian and Chinese practice in such matters of personal cleanliness and is unreservedly critical of what he saw as the Chinese misunderstanding of Indian wisdom. He notes, for example, that the practices of oral hygiene have been grossly misinterpreted in China.[66] In the first place, the type of wood has been incorrectly identified. Second, rather than using a single stick with which to brush the teeth, members of the Chinese sangha use many sticks, chewing all of them in their mouth without rinsing. Others even swallow the juice "thinking it will cure their ailments." Such practices, says Yijing, are not only wrong, they are dangerous: "They try to be clean, but contrarily they become filthy, and though they hope to get rid of disease, they incur more serious illness." Adding what must have been a grave insult to his fellow Chinese monastics, he states that in India "even a child of three" is taught to do it properly.

Also a target of Yijing's criticism is the lack of attention to personal hygiene on the part of the Chinese sangha when answering the call of nature.[67] The proper rules were unknown in China, he says, and even if they had been introduced, they would not have been followed scrupulously. Consequently, Chinese monastics have been continually committing disciplinary infractions by not maintaining their own purity. If a monk behaved in such a way in the holy land, "the people of the five parts of India will laugh at him and he will be sneered at wherever he goes." Yijing also contrasts Indian and Chinese practices when discussing the cleanliness of Indian methods of food preparation, the careful attention to distinctions between "pure" and "impure" foods and drinks, the proper technique to maintain clean drinking water, and the beneficial effects of exercise on one's health.[68]

Yijing's most stinging barbs, however, are reserved for the Chinese sangha's "despicable" and "vulgar" practice of using "dragon decoctions" (*longtang*), medicines he says are made from the excrement of pigs and cats. Yijing's personal anxiety about this particular allegation, and the chance that it may reflect poorly on him as a member of the Chinese sangha, is almost palpable: chief among the reasons he gives for shunning the use of dragon decoctions is that "if foreigners were to hear about it, it would be detrimental to the good name of our morals and manners."[69] He explains that, while the Vinaya does prescribe the use of dung and urine as medicine, this refers strictly to the dung of a calf and the urine of a cow.[70] Even with this allowance, however, he stresses there is in fact no need for such unpalatable medicines. "We have plenty of fragrant medicinal herbs," he says, "and why should we not use them?" In utter condemnation of those who choose to use dragon decoctions, he declares that "although they have some small benefit in mind, they are not aware that it is a great offense against the holy teaching."

All of the abovementioned critiques of Chinese adaptation of Indian medical and hygienic practices were part and parcel of Yijing's strategy to bill himself as the indisputable authority on authentic monastic discipline. He rested his claim to being a privileged cross-cultural translator on the fact that he had seen Indian practices with his own eyes while studying in the holy land over many years—in marked contrast to the vast majority of Chinese exegetes who had never set foot on the subcontinent.[71] Most accounts of Indian monasteries prior to Yijing's had relied largely on a combination of speculation and divine inspiration. For example, in the decades prior to Yijing's voyage, Daoxuan had written his utopian description of the famous Jetavana monastery, already mentioned above.[72] In this text, Daoxuan had described Jetavana's hospice facility, or "Hall of Impermanence" (*wuchang yuan*), as a wondrous place where magnificent silver and crystal bells made by Indra and the moon deity Candradeva (Ch. Yue Tianzi) rang by themselves, chiming with the sound of the Dharma. In the "Buddha's Infirmary" (*fo bingfang*), eight sets of musical instruments given by Brahmā spontaneously played music that cured the Buddha of any illness he might choose to manifest. Daoxuan also described the monastery's "Infirmary of the Saints" (*shengren bingfang yuan*) where the enlightened disciples were healed, the bathing quarter (*yufang*), and the running-water toilet (*liuce*). In his preface to the text, Daoxuan claimed that his image of Jetavana was culled from the monastic disciplinary literature and the work of previous writers, and that it was confirmed and supplemented in a vision revealed to him by a divinity.[73] Yijing, on the other hand, summarily dismissed Daoxuan's description as "entirely baseless."[74]

Despite their differences, Yijing and Daoxuan both engaged in the idealized representation of Indian Buddhism and thus were both contributors to a Chinese discourse that glorified "Heavenly India." However, Yijing's portrayal of Indian magnificence was not based on fantastical monastic trappings such as automated bells, self-playing musical instruments, and self-cleaning toilets. Rather, the pilgrim ascribed a great deal of importance to the Indian sangha's attention to monastic discipline and to their meticulous hygienic practice in particular. To hear Yijing speak of it, the stakes in accurately managing the loathsome nature of the physical body could not be any higher. He repeatedly insists that properly managing its inputs and outputs is critical not only to ensure physical health, but also to maintain ritual purity. By committing infractions in even minor points of discipline concerning the body, he suggests, one becomes polluted and thus incapable of performing the basic tasks of the sangha, or of receiving any of the benefits. Such a position is, of course, an example of the equation between cleanliness and holiness that has been widely discussed by scholars of both religious studies and the history of medicine and that is found in countless traditions worldwide.[75] For Yijing, though, asserting this connection—and forwarding his own antisyncretic vision of Indian hygienic and medical discipline to maximize it—allowed him to promote himself in his role as a uniquely qualified translator of Buddhism in China.

Huizhao Revisits the *Sutra of Golden Light*

In 703, after his return to China, Yijing produced a new translation of the *Sutra of Golden Light*. By this time, the text's précis of Indian medicine discussed at the beginning of this chapter had been significantly augmented.[76] New Indian medical material that had accreted to the passage since the last time it was translated into Chinese included dream interpretation, the analysis of death signs, and other additional Indian medical doctrines. The text now also mentioned familiar Indian medicinals not present in the earlier version. Given Yijing's training in Indian medicine as well as his emphasis on adhering to Indian precedents as a measure of authenticity, it is not surprising that his retranslation of this chapter for the most part emphasized formally equivalent language. But when the exegete Huizhao (648–714) undertook the task of writing a commentary on Yijing's translation, he abandoned his predecessors' strategy of explaining unfamiliar Indian terms and doctrines in the sutra with Chinese metaphorical equivalents. A native of Henan transplanted to the Tang capital in Chang'an, Huizhao had been a student of Xuanzang, and in his commentary he followed his teacher's dictum to prioritize close fidelity to Indian language and culture.

By Huizhao's time, China's interest in India was at its zenith. Under Empress Wu, for the first time in centuries, the reigning ruler was an unshakable supporter of the Dharma and was highly interested in Buddhist institution building. She constructed Buddhist temples and monuments, employed Indian scientists and clerics at court, sponsored translations of scriptures, and even famously had pseudotranslations written proclaiming herself to be the reincarnation of the bodhisattva Maitreya.[77] This passion for Indian culture and knowledge at the highest levels of society was reflected in a heightened attention to the Indian cultural context and language across a wide gamut of Buddhist commentarial literature.

The change in approach was greatly facilitated by the increasing availability of the very kinds of reference materials discussed in this chapter. In addition to commentaries, manuals, encyclopedias, and travelogues, by Huizhao's time a welter of writings were available that were specifically intended as translation aids. Sanskrit studies had become increasingly well established among Buddhist exegetes over the medieval period.[78] In Huizhao's lifetime, great scholar-translators such as Xuanzang, Yijing, Fazang (643–712), Yixing (684–727), and their students were writing treatises expounding upon Sanskrit grammar and admonishing translators to be more precise in their work. This trend would continue to intensify after Huizhao passed away. In the latter half of the eighth century, Amoghavajra and his student Huiguo (746–806) would introduce their complex method of transliterating Sanskrit phonemes, and the definitive textbook of the *siddhaṃ* script, *An Explanation of Siddhaṃ Letters* (*Xitan zi ji*, T. 2132), would be composed by the turn of the century.[79] This flurry of activity in the mid-seventh to early ninth centuries would represent the peak of China's engagement with Indian scripts and languages. Huizhao's commentary was written in the earlier part of this period but already exhibits a markedly heavier use of Sanskrit than the other texts discussed in this chapter.

In a discussion of the relationship between the *tridoṣa* and the seasons, Huizhao allows that in order to understand Indian doctrine, one might "use the Five Phases as a reference."[80] In a variation on the familiar tactic of metaphorically equating the *tridoṣa* with Chinese medical categories, he suggests that one can understand their seasonal arising and passing by thinking of Phlegm as Water, Wind as Wood, and Bile as Fire. These brief lines aside, however, Chinese medical terms do not feature prominently in Huizhao's explanation of Buddhist medical doctrine. Nor does he engage in a performance of expertise in other Chinese arts and sciences as did the sixth-century commentators on the earlier version of the *Sutra of Golden Light* discussed at the beginning of this chapter. He makes no mention of Chinese food prohibitions, nor of native cosmological models. Although Paramārtha, Zhiyi, and Jizang each took up dozens of lines discussing the interactions of yin and yang in order to explain the six seasons of the Indian year, Huizhao summarizes the foreign calendrical method in a few sentences without even mentioning the Chinese doctrines.[81]

Instead of dwelling on indigenous parallels, Huizhao elucidates the medical terms encountered in the sutra by appealing to the source context and language. Where the sutra text mentions the Seven Constituents (Ch. *qijie*; Skt. *saptadhātu*), the Eight Arts of Medicine (Ch. *bashu*; Skt. *aṣṭāṇgāyurveda*), and the Six Flavors (Ch. *liuwei*; Skt. *ṣaḍrasa*), Huizhao lists out these items individually in a matter-of-fact way that leaves little room for domesticating associations.[82] Where the sutra mentions the Indian doctrine of *rasa* (the nutritive essence of digested food), he gives an explanation of how food is separated out into *rasa* and waste products that is drawn wholly from Indian tradition and that revolves around transliterated technical terms.[83] Even more striking, in several instances, Huizhao clarifies terms that Yijing had translated into Chinese in the sutra text by back-translating them into Sanskrit. For example, Yijing had calqued the common Indian remedy *triphalā* by using ordinary Chinese words meaning "Three Fruits" (Ch. *sanguo*). Huizhao, in turn, glosses this term by naming the three fruits in transliterated Sanskrit: *helilejia* (Skt. *harītakī*; i.e., *Terminalia chebula*), *amoluojia* or *awuluojia* (Skt. *āmalaka*; i.e., *Emblica officinalis*), and *pipidejia* (Skt. *vibhītaka*; i.e., *Terminalia bellirica*).[84] Here, he helpfully warns against an erroneous interpretation of the second term as referring to mango (Skt. *āmra*; Ch. *anmoluo*). The author also employs transliteration when explaining that the "Three Spices" (Skt. *trikaṭuka*; Ch. *sanxin*) consist of dried ginger, black pepper, and *bibo* (Skt., *pippalī*; i.e., *Piper longum*).

Huizhao's practice of using transliterated Sanskrit to clarify unfamiliar Chinese terms and his limited use of indigenous metaphorical equivalents is a notable reversal of earlier commentarial practice when explaining this sutra. His approaches are indicative of the new norms that were developing among interpreters of Buddhist medicine, with strong preference for illuminating the source context over establishing connections with Chinese models. They are also exemplary of the deepening engagement with the specific details of Indian medical knowledge by Chinese exegetes more generally, not to mention an unmistakable performance of Huizhao's personal expertise in Sanskrit terminology.

*   *   *

The authors of the texts discussed in this chapter exhibited different attitudes toward Indian medical knowledge, forwarded divergent interpretations of its core doctrines, and took distinct stances on how it should be represented in the Chinese cultural context. These examples demonstrate that how medieval Chinese rewriters approached the task of translating Buddhist medical doctrines could vary widely—even on the part of a single author when writing for different audiences. They also show how closely translation strategies were connected with the historical contexts, intellectual milieus, and social goals of the translators.

This chapter has described the deepening engagement of Chinese Buddhist authors with Indian medicine between the sixth and eighth centuries, which I have suggested is related to the contemporaneous consolidation and stabilization of the reunified empire and the strengthening of Indo-Sinitic economic and political contacts. Ironically, however, the turn away from the use of metaphorical equivalence and domesticating translations is likely to have contributed in the long term to a decline in the importance of Indian medical doctrines in Chinese thought. Buddhist authors' increasing engagement with the source context would have greatly enhanced the specialized reader's familiarity with a range of Indian doctrines; however, as discussed in the foregoing chapters, the appeal of Buddhist medical models in broader society was directly related to the accessibility of the texts explaining them and their compatibility with indigenous linguistic and cultural repertoires. An increasingly foreignizing presentation of Buddhist medical knowledge by Tang-era exegetes meant that such doctrines were increasingly bring marked as specialized, non-Chinese knowledge. Over time, learned discussions of Buddhist medicine consequently became accessible to fewer and fewer outside of the most educated among the sangha.

In fact, however, almost all of the texts discussed in this book thus far would have been difficult for ordinary medieval people to understand.

Compositions like Huizhao's would have seemed especially abstruse and un-approachable, but all Buddhist texts strewn with transliterations and other foreignizing terms would have presented interpretive problems. In the next chapter, we will leave aside scriptures written in Buddhist Hybrid Chinese and the theoretical musings of exegetes, sectarians, and philosophers, and turn instead to popular genres of literature. These more accurately reflect the common understandings of Buddhism among everyday people, and provide us the opportunity to explore how aspects of Buddhist medicine were, in time, able to become enduring and vibrant parts of Chinese popular culture.

CHAPTER 5

Popularizing Buddhist Medicine

This chapter explores one of the primary avenues for the popularization of Buddhist medicine in medieval China: narratives. Through the refashioning, resituating, and recirculating of stories about healing, many aspects of Buddhist medicine discussed in previous chapters were freed from the confines of abstruse scriptural language and narrow doctrinal contexts and were integrated into the vernacular culture. Out of the many cultural-linguistic elements of Chinese and Indian provenance available to them, authors of narratives pieced together appealing combinations of the familiar and the novel to express their visions of the utility of Buddhist healing for their contemporary society. Of course, this is not simply a case of syncretism: these narratives were also carefully crafted for specific strategic purposes. More than any other type of literature discussed elsewhere in this book, healing narratives provide a vantage point from which we can see the spread of Indian ideas about illness and healing throughout all layers of Chinese society, while also witnessing the adaptation and domestication of foreign knowledge in order to appeal to domestic audiences and forward the sangha's position in the Chinese religiomedical marketplace.

Buddhist Healing Narratives

In Buddhist literature from virtually all times and places (extending back to parables supposedly told by the Buddha himself, if we believe he was a historical figure) the narrativization of complex themes and ideas has always been one of the chief ways that the Dharma has been introduced to and explained by ordinary people.[1] Such was also the case in medieval China. Buddhist notions of compassion and selflessness, for example, were often expressed through stories of bodhisattvas or monks sacrificing their bodies in the name of the Dharma or for the sake of suffering beings.[2] The beneficence and accessibility of buddhas and bodhisattvas were frequently illustrated with narratives about devotees being saved at the eleventh hour from death, disaster, and misfortune by apparitions of the deities, or by relics, icons, or other proxies.[3] Ideals of asceticism, scholarship, and magical potency were captured in tales about the exploits of exceptional monks.[4] Stories of nuns, on the other hand, modeled piety, chastity, and faith.[5] Though the topic has not been studied as extensively as these other examples, Buddhist ideas about illness and healing also ranked high among the most important themes that inspired the composition of narratives in medieval China.

This chapter focuses on this latter category of narratives. There probably was a virtually infinite supply of such tales circulating orally in medieval China. Many of the earliest translators and missionaries in China are traditionally said to have been involved in healing activities, and it is highly probable that stories about their exploits were being told from the very earliest phase of the arrival of Buddhism in China.[6] Unlike in parts of South Asia where oral transmission was preferred, however, Chinese cultural expectations demanded that knowledge be written down if it was to be considered legitimate and authoritative by the elite.[7] It is perhaps predictable, then, that when Buddhism began making inroads into higher social circles, narratives about Buddhist healing began to appear in the written record in significant quantities.

By the fifth century, a number of collections of written narratives were being produced. Though recorded in the literary language, these short and entertaining stories were fashioned from material culled from a variety of oral and textual sources.[8] Once written down, such stories had enormous appeal and circulated widely as sources of enjoyment, wonder, education, and moral suasion. A large proportion of the authors and rewriters of these tales were Buddhist clerics or lay devotees, who wrote or rewrote them as acts of piety and proselytism, but they were just as avidly authored, copied, and circulated by scholars, officials, and other literate segments of medieval society.[9] While they originally may have appeared in collections of religious hagiographies or secular wonder tales, or circulated as independent texts of whatever genre, a significant number of these healing narratives subsequently were canonized—that is to say, incorporated individually or in bulk into the officially sponsored Buddhist Tripitakas and catalogs. Over the course of the medieval period, these very narratives became some of the most important tools in Buddhism's proselytizing efforts in China.

How are Buddhist healing and healers represented in such tales? Analysis of the choice of language and the presentation of content reveals a persistent pattern of domesticating, adapting, and refracting foreign ideas through indigenous cultural and literary lenses. These narratives intensively draw upon the metaphors of HEALTH AND DISEASE ARE REWARDS AND RETRIBUTIONS, THE DHARMA IS MEDICINE, DEITIES ARE HEALERS, and HEALING IS AN OCCULT POWER. As established in Chapter 3, these metaphors were already being rendered in highly compatible and appealing ways by the translation assemblies, and narrativists were keen to capitalize upon and deepen these connections. Authors of healing narratives also liberally wove elements of indigenous Chinese religiomedical lore into their compositions, including symbols, plotlines, tropes, motifs, textual conventions, and specific details drawn from all sorts of native literature. In yet another sign of competition among groups of religiomedical practitioners for cultural and social capital, they especially favored borrowing material from stories about Daoist healers, wonder-working physicians (*shenyi₁*), ritual technicians, popular spirit healers, and other figures who were being portrayed as effective healers in rival writings.[10]

Because of the widespread practice of borrowing and repackaging literary material, most medieval Buddhist narratives strike the modern reader as highly syncretic mosaics of Indian and indigenous elements. At the same time, however, these writings cannot be considered only in terms of the hybridity of their content. Each act of authorship (and by authorship, here I expressly mean to include compiling, editing, adapting, and even oral retelling) represents the attempt by a historical individual to position himself and his tradition within a particular social landscape. Even if we lack details about a particular author's motivations—indeed, even if an author's identity is completely unknown—by analyzing translation strategies we can plainly see that, as a group, the writers of healing narratives were intent upon negotiating the similarity and difference between the sangha and their competition and concerned with arguing that Buddhist therapeutic knowledge was an effective and even superior alternative.

Adaptations of Indian Healers

The first aspect of Buddhist medical narratives that will receive our attention is the refashioning and repurposing of material introduced in imported Indian texts. One major source of material for Chinese adaptations was the monastic disciplinary literature. Though for the initial period of Buddhism's development in China no full translation of the Vinaya existed, five separate monastic codes became available between the early fifth and early eighth centuries.[11] Narratives form an important layer of this literature, as short stories often are attached to certain rules and regulations in order to illustrate the rationale behind them. In India, these explanatory narratives were memorized by the sangha and used as templates for preaching and storytelling.[12] In China, too, the dramatic and persuasive value of Vinaya narratives was quickly recognized.

As Chinese storytellers picked up and disseminated Vinaya narratives, however, they amended their content and manipulated the literary frames surrounding them in order to better appeal to Chinese audiences. Sometimes, these cross-cultural translators reframed individual narratives by extracting them from the disciplinary codes and establishing them as independent sutras, or by using them as prototypes for the composition of new adaptations. Here, I will introduce an example of each of these processes. Both healing tales I discuss were extracted from the Vinaya, modified to fit Chinese expectations, and subsequently reabsorbed back into the Tripitaka in their newly rewritten versions.

Among the many tales in the monastic disciplinary literature that caught the fancy of Chinese audiences were those that featured the Buddha caring for the sick. In a particularly influential episode from the Dharmaguptaka Vinaya already discussed in the previous chapter, the Buddha comes across a sick monk lying in his own excrement within the monastic living quarters. As mentioned previously, the Buddha learns from the patient that the monks are not caring for one another when they fall ill, helps the ailing monk with his own hands, and instructs the assembly to care for one another. It was also already mentioned that this Vinaya narrative was held up by Daoxuan as one of the most important passages authorizing medical charity as a compassionate practice for Buddhist devotees and that it is cited widely for the same purpose in other Chinese Buddhist literature. However, we are revisiting the story in this chapter because it also became the prototype for adaptations written in China featuring exemplary Chinese monks.

One example of this kind of reformulation is the story of Kang Falang. This episode appeared in several places, including in the collection of wonder tales *Records of Signs from the Unseen Realm*. Though this compilation is no longer extant as a separate text, significant portions of it were preserved by virtue of their inclusion in Daoshi's seventh-century encyclopedia *Forest of Pearls in the Garden of Dharma* and other texts.[13] In this narrative, Falang is traveling with another monk westward across the desert toward India. At a desolate location along the way they come across another pair of monks. One is gravely ill with dysentery (*li₂*) and lying in his own filth, while the other is seemingly indifferent to his sick companion and interested only in chanting scripture. Taking pity on the sick monk, Falang and his travel partner stop to take care of him, for many days making his rice gruel and cleaning up after him. Though they think the patient will not live through the seventh night, at daybreak his appearance suddenly changes for the better and the filth that has hitherto filled the room transforms into flowers. At this point, Falang and his travel partner realize that their new acquaintances are in fact enlightened and that they were merely being tested. As a result of passing this test, Falang and his partner receive the blessing of the enlightened monks and are allowed to stay on with them. The text ends by telling us that Falang later went on to become a "great Dharma master" (*da fashi*) at Zhongshan.

The storyline is, of course, modeled on the episode about the Buddha from the Vinaya, complete with the seemingly indifferent monk who does nothing to help his comrade. However, in this retelling, the time and place have been adjusted, and the protagonist has been reimagined as a local Chinese hero. The literary frame of the story has changed as well: the narrative is no longer part of the monastic disciplinary code but now appears in a collection of popular tales appended to an encyclopedia entry on the essentials of Buddhist medicine. These shifts in content and genre indicate that both the narrative's audience and its core meaning have changed. Like the original story in the Vinaya, this tale still models Buddhist ideals of compassion and selflessness. The willingness to deal generously with the sick and to encounter the human body's foulest substances with equanimity is still an important measure of a monk's moral cultivation. However, in its new adaptation, this narrative is no longer an admonishment of the sangha for failing to care for the unfortunate among their ranks. Rather, it now showcases the sangha's moral virtue and lofty spiritual attainments. All of the monks depicted within the story turn out to be exemplars of virtue. It also perpetuates the promise of great rewards for devotion to individual members of the sangha, suggesting that monks are above reproach and are always worthy of devotion: though their behavior may seem immoral or inappropriate to the unenlightened, a monk may merely be testing you to determine if you are worthy of receiving his higher teachings.

While stories involving the sangha's compassionate care of the sick played an important role in modeling Buddhist ideals, the biography of Jīvaka, the

King of Physicians, is an even more significant example of the crosscultural translation of an idealized Indian healer. This protagonist, mentioned several times already throughout this book, appears in numerous Buddhist texts as an interlocutor of the Buddha, an important patron and devotee of the sangha, and physician to the monastic order. In Buddhist traditions outside of China, the biography of Jīvaka appears within the chapter of the Vinaya devoted to the rules regarding monastic clothing.[14] In Chinese, a version of the story is found in that section of the Dharmaguptaka Vinaya.[15] Like most monastic disciplinary material, this version of the biography was meant primarily for the internal consumption of the sangha and therefore exhibits fewer domesticating translation tactics and adaptations. However, over the course of the fifth century, a second recension of the biography began circulating as a separate sutra that was significantly reworked in order to appeal to a wider target audience.

This adapted narrative is today extant in two editions called the *Āmrapālī and Jīvaka Avadāna Sutra* and the *Āmrapālī and Jīvaka Sutra*.[16] The two are erroneously attributed by tradition to the late Han translator An Shigao—an attribution that was most likely added by catalogers in order to paper over its anonymous origins.[17] In reality, the contents represent a patchwork of material cherry-picked from various sources, including perhaps a text translated by Dharmarakṣa's team in the third to fourth centuries, but certainly excerpts from Vinaya texts and adaptations of material from biographies of famous Chinese physicians found in the secular dynastic histories. While the Vinaya version of the story did not undergo a sustained program of domestication when it was translated in the early fifth century, the biographical details in the separate sutras were heavily amended in order to incorporate both indigenous medical doctrines and frames of authority. The narrative was also clearly reworked to stake a claim in the religiomedical marketplace, resituating Jīvaka in competition with the legendary wonder-working paragons of classical Chinese medicine, Bian Que and Hua Tuo.[18]

In the popularized version of the narrative, Jīvaka performs a series of Indian medical procedures including the nasal administration of ghee to treat an illness of the head, trephination to remove parasites in the brain, and abdominal surgery to manipulate the liver. Though common in Indian medicine, these practices were new to China, and the narrative likely derived much of its appeal from the inclusion of such exotic details.[19] However, the separate sutras also contain many references to indigenous medical terminology, texts, and procedures. Jīvaka diagnoses on the basis of qi, the Five Viscera, and the pulses. He is said to have mastered early in life "the classics of materia medica, medical formulary, and acupuncture."[20] In one sequence, he acquires X-ray vision that allows him to see inside his patients' bodies, a plotline that is borrowed from the well-known biography of Bian Que in the Han-era *Records of the Grand Historian (Shiji)*.[21] He also is able to bring the dead back to life, a claim he also shares with both Bian Que and Hua Tuo. Significantly for his position vis-à-vis his competition, Jīvaka is said to have been born with acupuncture needles and herbs in his hands, which the texts repeatedly insist is proof that only he—not any of the other wonder-working physicians who also claim the title—is the legitimate King of Physicians (*yiwang*).

While the authors of the popularized version of the Jīvaka biography made many such additions, they also purposely excluded potentially subversive content they found in their source texts. Most of Jīvaka's healing exploits from the Dharmaguptaka Vinaya were incorporated into the longer of the two separate sutras, but a surgery he performs on King Bimbisāra's anal fistula was not, most likely because this portion of the story has degrading implications for the ruler.[22] Likewise, Jīvaka's treatment of the Buddha with a purgative was also omitted, probably because it would not have fit well with the omnipotent and docetic view of the Buddha being promulgated in China.[23]

The repositioning of this Vinaya narrative as an independent sutra text and the careful selection of material to add, revise, or omit in the rewriting of the biography are illustrative of the sort of adaptation and repackaging narratives underwent as they were molded to fit into the medieval Chinese literary and cultural world. As Buddhist writers adapted healing narratives they thought useful for positioning their protagonists against the heroes of contemporary rivals, they are also windows onto the "turf wars" in the competition for cultural and social capital in the religiomedical marketplace.

Once extracted from their original doctrinal and literary frameworks, however, Vinaya narratives could take on surprising new lives. For example, as stories about a wondrous Buddhist healer named Jīvaka were exchanged among the devout, his narrative was remixed and readapted even further. Accounts of an Indian healer-monk named Jīvaka living in China in the second to third centuries are found in both *Records of Signs* (as quoted in *Forest of Pearls*) and in a hagiography of eminent monks from the Liang dynasty I will discuss further below.[24] This Jīvaka performs a number of therapeutic interventions that combine spell casting, consecrated water, and ritual implements. He is not the King of Physicians, but his biography was undoubtedly linked to the other Jīvaka's in the medieval imagination. Like the story of the Buddha

caring for a sick monk morphing into that of Falang, this tale also updated a
remote Buddhist hero from ancient times and reimagined him as a contemporary actor in Chinese society.

Even more interesting, the reputation of the King of Physicians seems to
have circulated well beyond the Buddhist community and to have been put
to various rhetorical purposes by physicians as well. Details from the Buddhist narrative are likely to be the inspiration behind the surgeries mentioned
in the biographies of Hua Tuo in the *Records of the Three Kingdoms* (*Sanguo
zhi*) and the *Records of the Later Han* (*Houhan shu*).[25] Likewise, Jīvaka's name
appears in a medical prescription in Sun Simiao's formulary (*Qipo fang*), and
in the titles of several texts on classical Chinese medicine listed in the Song
dynastic catalog of medical texts.[26] What is Jīvaka's name doing in these settings, attached to therapeutics and compositions that have little or nothing
to do with Indian medical models? As I have been arguing throughout this
book, the answer has more to do with the strategic appropriation of effective
rhetorical devices than with questions of medical influence. Such references
are windows into the recirculation and popularization of Indian cultural-
linguistic elements in medieval Chinese society, and they are also reminders
of the countless numbers of oral and written conversations that were taking
place among competing practitioners that are no longer recoverable by the
historian.

Doctors of the Dreamworld

A second important category of healing narratives involves the representation
of the healing powers of deities. Indeed, one of the most prevalent themes in
Chinese Buddhist narrative literature as a whole is the transcendental power
of buddhas and bodhisattvas to right the world in times of trouble. Such
miracle tales were specifically designed to evoke surprise, wonder, and awe at
their extraordinary power.[27] Buddhist deities are shown to be omniscient and
omnipotent masters over the cosmos who bring assistance and good fortune
to emperors, members of the elite, ordinary devotees, and to the polity as a
whole. Such stories frequently revolve around the themes of protection from
epidemics or recovery from chronic or fatal illness. Tales of savior deities often use themes or tropes from the Indian sutra literature as their point of
departure—particularly those associated with the DEITIES ARE HEALERS
metaphor. But, while many aspects of these narratives are drawn from Indian

precedents, the appearance of deities is routinely expressed in such stories in the indigenous vocabulary of the resonant cosmos. In fact, one of the most common terms used for stories about deities in the medieval period was "stimulus-response tales" (*ganying yuan*).

Among the many ways that deities responded to human stimuli, they could manifest "response bodies" or "transformation bodies" through which they visited devotees in order to grant their blessings. As briefly mentioned in Chapter 3, such visitations often occur in dreams. While introduced previously in the context of ritual manuals, the idea of dream responses also held much dramatic value for the authors of miracle tales. Perhaps the most famous story about a dreamed deity in Chinese Buddhism is the story of how the Dharma was originally introduced during the Han dynasty.[28] According to the legend, which was already circulating at the end of the second century, Emperor Ming (r. 57–75) dreamed of a flying golden figure. Learning from his ministers that this was a foreign deity known as the Buddha, he dispatched envoys to India to bring back more information. From this point onward, dreamed deities remained a significant feature of Chinese Buddhism.

Many medieval narratives tell of the protagonist's spontaneous recovery from grave illness as a result of the ministrations of deities performed in dreams. One story from the *Records of Signs* (quoted in the *Forest of Pearls*), for example, tells of a woman who had been devout since her youth and had chanted the *Lotus Sutra* diligently for many years.[29] When she becomes sick, she has great faith in the text's ability to give her "beneficial protection" (*shanyou*, another domesticating gloss on the Buddhist concept of *adhiṣṭhāna*). Because of her great devotion to the text, she has a dream in which a Buddha's hand reaches through her window and touches her heart. When she awakens she is completely healed. Of course, it turns out that the visitation is not merely a dream: the Buddha has left behind a golden radiance and a fragrance that are witnessed with awe by her servants and other acquaintances.

Dreamed deities in Buddhist narratives might cure with a touch, as in this story, or they may actually perform medical procedures. One dream-manifestation story appearing in a Tang-era hagiographic collection, for example, involves the medical ministrations of a monk named Sengyai.[30] Sengyai had immolated himself in a dramatic display of his devotion and enlightened detachment and in emulation of a popular story about the bodhisattva Medicine King from the *Lotus Sutra*. As the monk Huisheng lay in his sickbed full of regret for having missed the spectacle, Sengyai appears to him in a dream and relieves his illness by fumigating him with sandalwood chips and

incense. In the dream, Sengyai reveals to the monk that he really is a bodhisattva named Brilliant All-Illuminating Treasure Storehouse (Guangming
Bianzhao Baozang). When Huisheng awakens, the biography tells us, he is
twice as strong as before.

The earliest extant narrative concerning the performance of the Master
of Medicines Buddha healing rite, recorded in the *History of the Northern
Dynasties (Beishi)* and repeated in the *Forest of Pearls*, also involves a dreamed
medical procedure.[31] In this story, a young man has the ritual performed
twice with the intent of restoring his grandfather's lost vision. On both occasions, he has seven monks light seven lamps and recite the sutra for seven
days. On the last day of the second cycle, he dreams of an old man healing
his grandfather's eyes with a golden lancet (*pi*).[32] Three days later, the man's
vision is restored. The implication, of course, is that the Master of Medicines
Buddha, in response to the stimulus of the ritual, had descended in a dream
disguised as an old man and had administered the cure.

The blind regaining sight through contact with Buddhist deities, clerics,
or practices is a frequent trope in the miracle literature. As mentioned in
passing in Chapter 3, the removal of a film or dust from one's eyes often
stands in Indian literature as a metaphor for enlightenment. The step from
such metaphorical statements to narratives about deities literally performing
surgery to restore one's eyesight is not a far leap. Stories such as these thus are
narrativizing the DEITIES ARE HEALERS metaphor, but it is critical to note
that they are not intended as mere allegories. Rather, they were crafted to be
compelling testimonials to the veracity of Buddhist claims. In fact, miracle
tales explicitly were spoken of as "proofs" (*yan*), evidence of the truth and
efficacy of Buddhist healing.[33]

While the abovementioned stories feature a range of deities, the most
common protagonist in medieval miracle stories about healing is Guanyin,
who became famous for medical interventions early on in his career in China.
As mentioned in a previous chapter, the most well-known canonical source
discussing Guanyin's beneficence is the *Lotus Sutra*. This text was first translated in China in 286 by Dharmarakṣa, but it is Kumārajīva's translation of
406 that was most influential. The twenty-fifth chapter of that version was
extracted and circulated as an independent sutra in the fifth and sixth centuries.[34] Entitled the *Guanyin Sutra,* it highlighted the deity's abilities to intervene on behalf of all sentient beings in their times of need. Guanyin, the text
promises, will deliver the devout from natural disasters, the perils of sea-
faring, imminent violence, demon attack, imprisonment, banditry, torment

by lusts and cravings, or the unfulfilled desire for a male child. When invoked, Guanyin can appear to the devotee in any number of forms appropriate to the situation, including by manifesting a Buddha body or various other divine bodies, or by becoming a king, wealthy man, householder, minister, Brahman, monastic, male or female lay believer, wife, young boy or girl, or any variety of heavenly, human, or nonhuman beings. Taking this sutra as inspiration, many medieval tales depict Guanyin's interventions in a range of perilous situations.[35]

The fact that healing is not mentioned in the *Lotus Sutra*'s account of Guanyin's powers, but is frequently featured in Chinese stories, indicates the importance of healing powers in the medieval Chinese conceptualization of ideal deities, as well as cross-cultural translators' willingness to cater to those expectations. As he was increasingly domesticated, Guanyin concomitantly became increasingly important as a healing deity. As mentioned in Chapter 3, he would eventually come to be the most common deity to be called upon in therapeutic rites. By the seventh and eighth centuries, a great number of spell texts and ritual manuals were being translated and composed (i.e., pseudo-translated) that described the invocation of multiple manifestations of this deity for a whole spectrum of healing purposes.[36] A great variety of healing narratives featuring Guanyin came into circulation as well.

Among Guanyin's many therapeutic specialties in miracle tales is washing out the intestines of the sick while they sleep. The earliest extant collection of narratives associated with Guanyin, compiled in the fourth to fifth centuries, includes one such story about the monk Zhu Fayi. This tale is briefly retold in a hagiographic collection from the Liang dynasty and in more detail in the *Records of Signs* (as quoted in the *Forest of Pearls*).[37] In the latter version, Fayi is said to have been sick for a long time, and though he had resolutely sought a cure using conventional medicines, he had found no relief. Instead, he dedicatedly placed his faith in Guanyin. The narrative describes the deity's manifestation thus:

> One day, he dreamt of a holy person (*daoren*) who came to examine him in order to cure his illness. He scooped out [Fayi's] intestines and stomach and washed out his organs. [Fayi] could see they were clogged up with a great quantity of putrid stuff. Having finished washing them, [the holy person] put them back inside and announced "Your illness is gone!" When [Fayi] awoke, all of his afflictions had cleared up and he was back to normal.[38]

The apparition, of course, is a manifestation of the deity appearing in response to the stimulus of the devotee's faith. (While I have translated the
term *daoren* as "holy person" in the quote above, the Chinese literally means
"man of the Dao." This was a common term for members of the sangha in
the medieval period, but the domesticating value of this choice of words is
obvious.)

Narratives about dream surgery are intended to showcase the deities' accessibility and the power of accomplished monks to invoke their presence
through their prayers. However, these episodes must always be read against
contemporary narratives about other wonder-working healers that were also
circulating in the medieval period. The washing out of the intestines is, of
course, a well-known component of ancient Indian medicine and yogic practice alike. Entire sections of the most famous Āyurvedic classics are dedicated
to the procedure and the tools for medicated enemas.[39] But, by the time that
the Zhu Fayi story was being written down, the washing of the inner organs
was already a well-known literary device in several strands of Chinese literature as well. The trope appears in the late Han biography of Bian Que, for
example, where the physician is compared to Yu Fu, a great surgeon of ancient times who is said to have "washed and rinsed the stomach and intestines,
washed and rinsed the Five Viscera, and practiced with such perfection that it
transformed the physical form."[40] Likewise, the third-century biography of
Hua Tuo contains a passage in which he washes out the intestines to remove
diseased tissues while his patient is under anesthesia. Intestinal washing also
appears in association with Buddhist wonder-workers outside of the context
of healing. In the abovementioned Liang hagiography, for example, a monk
named Zhu Fotucheng (also transcribed as Zhu Fotudeng) is said to have
been able to remove his intestines through a hole in his abdomen in order to
wash them out in a stream on a regular basis.[41]

This widespread trope probably originated in India, but tracking down
its origin or charting the direction of influence from narrative to narrative is
not necessarily the best use of our time (if it is even possible). The important
point for our purposes is that stories about Buddhist deities washing out the
intestines of a devotee would not have been read in a vacuum. Intestinal
washing and all sorts of other abdominal, cardiac, and cranial surgeries and
procedures abound in narratives about Yu Fu, Bian Que, Hua Tuo, Jīvaka,
Guanyin, and other wondrous healers authored during the late classical and
medieval periods. Plotlines and individual details about idealized medical
procedures were appropriated, shared, and emulated among religious and med-

ical hagiographers of all sorts. These obviously were compelling narrative elements, as they were borrowed and reworked again and again over the centuries by authors in many different religious and secular contexts.

By the time the tale about Fayi's miraculous dream was being written down, numinous surgery and intestinal washing were already closely linked with the life stories of a good number of model healers both in and outside of the Buddhist sphere. By composing narratives about Guanyin that featured the procedure, Buddhist authors both adapted the deity to fit into the prevailing cultural expectations of what divine healing entailed and also positioned their protagonist in competition with universally recognized medical heroes. What would have been seen as different and especially appealing about the Buddhist narratives is not so much the procedure, but the fact that these stories brought such "perfect" and "transformative" procedures into accessible range for the devout.[42] While wonder-working physicians such as Bian Que and Hua Tuo were associated with remote times and places, anyone who accepted, practiced, and patronized Buddhism could call upon Guanyin or another Buddhist deity and hope to receive a miraculous dream response here and now.

Healing Hagiographies

A third and final font of medieval healing narratives I will discuss in this chapter is the voluminous body of literature about the wondrous healing powers of monks. There are several overlapping genres of literature that include such tales. In this section, I will focus on four important texts that serve as representative examples. A number of healing tales are found in a compilation of "anomaly accounts" (zhiguai) by Wang Yan (b. ca. 454) called Records of Signs from the Unseen Realm.[43] This text was already mentioned several times above. Again, it is no longer extant as a separate composition, but large parts of it were incorporated into the Tripitaka by virtue of numerous quotations by other authors. Many of those quotes appear in Daoshi's Forest of Pearls, also already introduced above. This text's section on medicine (introduced in the previous chapter) contains a selection of fourteen anomaly accounts culled from Records of Signs as well as from other contemporary collections.[44] Even more important than either of these two sources, given their widespread influence and popularity, are a series of hagiographies of "eminent monks" (gaoseng). The first, entitled simply Biographies of Eminent

Monks (*Gaoseng zhuan*, T. 2059), was compiled around 530 by Huijiao (497–554), a leading monastic of the Liang dynasty. A second installment, called *Continued Biographies of Eminent Monks* (*Xu gaoseng zhuan*, T. 2060), was completed in the mid-seventh century by Daoxuan.[45]

Between them, the texts by Wang Yan, Huijiao, Daoxuan, and Daoshi include scores of narratives that hinge on the practice of divination, prophesy, rainmaking, exorcism, and other kinds of thaumaturgy (*ganying, shenyi₂*, or *gantong*)—of which tales involving healing form a significant portion. In compiling their collections, these four authors made use of a variety of sources, including oral interviews, local histories, biographical sketches, secular collectanea, and other miscellaneous writings.[46] Since most of these are now lost, we often cannot know how this source material presented Buddhist healing. But we can be sure that these four rewriters molded and pruned their own presentations of the source material strategically.[47] Unlike in the cases of the texts introduced in previous sections of this chapter, we know exactly who these individuals were and what kinds of social contexts they operated within. Most important, we know that all four were public figures who were personally committed to promulgating a positive image of Buddhist institutions and whose authorial activity was sponsored by elite or imperial patronage.[48] Though they drew material from a range of contemporary sources both in and outside of the Buddhist sphere, the end result of their recombining, reediting, and refashioning was an intentionally and carefully articulated argument that Buddhism was indispensable in assisting with the management of everyday problems, including matters of health and well-being. An important part of this public relations campaign involved billing the sangha as an unparalleled source of occult healing powers.

A handful of monks in these narratives are represented as masters of classical Chinese medical techniques. In the Liang hagiography of eminent monks, for example, the Han-era translator An Shigao is said to have been skilled in acupuncture and to have been knowledgeable of the Five Phases.[49] In the same text, Yu Fakai employs both acupuncture and pulse diagnosis.[50] Details such as these underscore both the sangha's prodigious learning and their willingness to assist the laity with worldly matters. Such stories also emphasize that the cure of illness is easy for eminent monks, contrasting their nonchalant success with the efforts of their rivals, who are inevitably portrayed as bumbling quacks unable to provide a successful cure. (Fakai's biography, for example, stresses that although his patient had received many unsuccessful treatments from others, the monk took one look, declared the condition "easy to cure," and quickly did so.)[51]

Most healing hagiographies, however, do not involve classical Chinese medicine, but rather seek to position Buddhist clerics against Daoists, popular spirit healers, and other ritual specialists and thaumaturges. In order to place Buddhist healing and healers within the same field of competition as their rivals, the authors of these hagiographies always prioritize domesticating translations. For example, monks are frequently portrayed as experts at driving out disease-causing demons with spells, and these techniques are always discussed using the metaphorical equivalents *zhou* or *shenzhou* rather than with transliteration or calques.[52] Among many other monks that are celebrated in the hagiographic collections for their spell-casting abilities, Fotucheng is perhaps the most exemplary. One of the most ambitious Buddhist healing narratives, the biography of Fotucheng is used by Huijiao to challenge the whole gamut of Chinese religiomedical practitioners all at once, weaving together tropes, plotlines, and individual details from multiple strains of rival literature. For example, when the biography tells that Fotucheng used a spell to bring a prince back from the dead, the story line not only positions its protagonist against rival spell casters, but also against Bian Que, who is said to have revived a prince from death with acupuncture.[53] Fotucheng is also said to be able to wash his intestines whenever he feels like it through a permanent hole in his side, which as mentioned above connects him with a range of deities and heroes (such as Yu Fu, Hua Tuo, Guanyin, and others) who were associated with organ washing. Fotucheng is also said able to read books at night thanks to the radiance that emanates through the same hole, a detail that serves not only to underscore his internal purity (i.e., his enlightenment), but also to position him among the many spirits, gods, and other numinous beings who emit light in Chinese religious tales.[54]

In addition to spell casting, the authors present monks as consummate healers in that they can help their patients tap into powers associated with Buddhist practice that are unavailable to rivals. As discussed in Chapter 3, therapeutic benefits were held to be inherent in even the most basic sorts of Buddhist activity. This idea is narrativized in the many stories where the stimulus for the patient's cure hinges on them undertaking a simple act of repentance or declaration of faith. In Daoxuan's biography of the monk Shi Chade, for example, the protagonist warns people to start practicing Buddhism in order to avoid being harmed by an epidemic. Those that take his advice and perform rites, participate in vegetarian feasts, meditate, and chant are healed, while ignoring him results in death.[55] In the same source, several monks establish reliquaries that grant miraculous healing boons to the local residents who venerate them.[56] Combining this trope with that of dream healing discussed in the previous section, a tale in the *Forest of Pearls* tells of a man who became ill and died, but is transported to another world where he takes refuge in the Three Jewels in front of some monks. Because of this action, the protagonist is able to travel back to his own funeral, reenter his body, and return to life.[57]

Monks also are exceptional healers by virtue of the fact that they can preach the sutras, which as already discussed in Chapter 3 are sources of beneficial power. Hearing monks chanting sutras provides protection from disease-causing demons in more than one story. One from the *Forest of Pearls* tells of a man whose "bones were disintegrating" and whose "flesh was emaciated" due to a long illness.[58] Many "spirit healers and physicians" (*wuyi*) had been unable to cure the illness. One night, his son has a dream in which some members of the sangha come to see him. Upon awakening, he invites monks to chant scriptures for his father. The next night, as the patient sleeps, he has a vision of dozens of demon children wearing five-colored clothing and bearing all manners of weapons attempting to enter the room. Suddenly, however, they retreat, announcing that they can return no more because of the presence of the monks. After this occurrence, says the text, the illness gradually improved. Many other narratives echo this one in suggesting that the apotropaic power of the recitation of Buddhist sutras is well known to the spirit world. In an episode from the Liang hagiography, the mere arrival of a monk in order to preach the sutras is enough to scare away a "flock of ghosts" that had been plaguing a laywoman.[59] While these particular stories do not necessarily specify which particular scriptures gave the monks their exorcistic powers, others mention that the Perfection of Wisdom (Ch. *bore*; Skt. *prajñāpāramitā*) scriptures, the *Śūraṃgama Sutra*, the *Guanyin Sutra*, and, especially, the *Lotus Sutra* could all be used for healing purposes.[60]

In addition to facilitating access to Buddhist practices and texts, another way in which monks are portrayed as being superior to their competition is their ability to easily invoke the presence of all-powerful deities for their own benefit or on behalf of their patrons. There are many stories in which the great buddhas and bodhisattvas appear in person in order to administer therapies or to dispense miraculous medicines as a direct result of the monks' engagement in prayer, chanting, offerings, repentance, or other types of rituals. Examples where Guanyin performs dream surgery and intestinal washing from the Liang hagiography, *Records of Signs*, and the *Forest of Pearls* have already been mentioned above, and Guanyin was a favorite in Daoxuan's collection as well. In one episode from that text, the crippled monk Shi Hongman recollects the *Guanyin Sutra* for three years, and his perseverance is rewarded by the apparition of the deity and the healing of his legs.[61] In another, a monk brings about the cure of his mother by chanting the name of Guanyin. As a result of his devotion, transformation buddhas appear upon the leaves of the trees around the residence, and her severe exhaustion (*weidun*) is alleviated.[62] Other deities besides Guanyin also play a role in healing. In the Liang hagiography, for example, the Buddha of Infinite Life cures one monk's illness by means of a bright light, while an unnamed buddha heals another with the touch of his hand.[63]

In these narratives about wondrous monks, divine intervention is depicted in ways that explicitly facilitate the positioning of Buddhist healing, healers, and deities within the Chinese cultural context. Their appearance is spoken of in the vocabulary of stimulus and response (*ganying*) and retribution (*fu* and *bao*), and there is a minimum of foreignizing language in the tales. In several cases, gods primarily associated with rival traditions are co-opted into the list of beings that can be invoked by Buddhist monks. In Daoxuan's collection, for example, the monk Shi Daoxian falls sick and is brought a "wondrous medicine" (*miaoyao*) by a celestial youth reminiscent of Daoist deities.[64]

Moreover, the whole gamut of occult therapies are routinely spoken of in these stories in terms of *shen*. The word "numinous spell" (*shenzhou*) is used throughout the collections as a translation for *dhāraṇī*. In a narrative appearing in both the Liang hagiography and the *Forest of Pearls*, An Huize prays to the "heavenly deities" (*tianshen*, a domesticating translation of *devas*) for relief during a time of pestilence and is answered by the appearance of two urns full of "numinous water" (*shenshui*) that he uses to eradicate the illness.[65] In the Tang hagiography, a "numinous spring" (*shenquan*) spontaneously flows when a reliquary is installed.[66] In more than one tale, the Buddha himself is referred to as a *shen*.[67] Flagging important plot elements with this richly laden term, these narratives capitalize upon associations between ritual purification, magical transformation, healing, and the spirit world that had been part of the domestic religiomedical culture since time immemorial.

Finally, these narratives also work their desired dramatic and rhetorical effects by transforming influences traditionally held to be ominous or downright malefic into beneficial forces. This logic is behind the many anomalous stories in Buddhist collections that turn conventional Chinese tropes on their head. A narrative from the Liang hagiography, for example, says that the monk Zhu Fakuang had "dozens of ghosts and spirits protecting him, both before and behind,"[68] suggesting that nefarious entities could be tamed by members of the sangha and turned to good. Another tale from the same source that is repeated in the *Forest of Pearls* tells of the time that the monk Shi Tanying contracted a skin disease (*xianchuang*). His case was incurable, but he prayed to a statue of Guanyin all day for a remedy all the same. Eventually, a snake comes out from behind the statue and regurgitates a rat in front of Tanying. He scrapes the snake saliva off the rat with a piece of bamboo and spreads it onto his sores. The rat then revives, and within two days, the monk's illness is healed.[69] This episode capitalizes on the folkloric connotations of snakes and rats but represents a creative twist on conventional archetypes.[70] The animals, which in Chinese popular literature would ordinarily represent dangerous demonic entities, are agents of healing that save the monk's life. The narrative thus underscores how evil portents are turned into blessings by the power of the monk's *gongyang*.

All of the stories discussed here about the wondrous healing powers of monks—and many more like them—had a crucial role to play in promoting Buddhism in China. While the beneficial effects of Buddhist devotion may be explained in some medieval literature as deriving from the accumulation of karmic benefit as discussed in Chapter 3, the tales recounted here invariably direct the reader's attention instead to the powers of spontaneous transformation unlocked by Buddhist practice. Such narratives gave devotees compelling reasons to flock to temples and pilgrimage sites, to treat Buddhist objects with reverence, to bestow offerings upon Buddhist statues, and to recopy sutras or to pay to have them chanted. They also gave aspirants motivation to undergo repentance rituals, to convert to Buddhism, or even to ordain into the sangha in order to access its occult secrets.

Even more than spurs to devotion or practice, however, these narratives serve primarily to extol the desirability of supporting monastics and to promote their reputation as uniquely capable conduits of cosmic powers. The hagiographies stress the contrast between the helplessness of the patients (even when they are emperors) versus the ease with which Buddhist clerics vanquish disease on their behalf. Such is their power that even an object that had come in contact with a monk—a tooth-cleaning twig or an alms bowl, perhaps—could be imbued with disease-vanquishing and demon-dispelling powers.[71] The hagiographers' emphasis remains on how—through their practice of meditation, disciplinary precepts, repentance, and so forth—monks accumulated a numinous power that could be shared in the form of apotropaic and purifying influences.[72] Unlike scholarly masters of classical learned medicine or Daoist celestial bureaucrats who negotiate the spiritual hierarchies, idealized monks use their powers to circumvent the normal order of the cosmos and to spontaneously overcome the forces of darkness.

* * *

Of course, all of the texts discussed throughout this entire book engage in resituating Indian medical knowledge and practice in the Chinese cultural and social landscape in some way or another. However, more than any other type of literature discussed in this book, authors of healing narratives were the most willing to reframe Buddhist medicine to fit with indigenous ideas about magical transformation, cosmic retribution, and the spirit world. Tapping into the language, idioms, symbols, plot elements, and other resources of the popular culture was vital to establish the credibility of the sangha as healers. These stories thus cue us in to what authors thought the most persuasive approaches would be when attempting to appeal to the general public. Healing narratives do not center around the Four Elements, the *tridoṣa*, or other Indian anatomical and physiological doctrines favored in exegetical treatises. In fact, these ideas are rarely, if ever, mentioned. Although the authors of the narratives discussed in this chapter include exoticizing details that stress Buddhism's uniqueness and novelty (such as surgical procedures or references to the foreign origins of healing monks), taken as a whole, they share an obvious preference to frame their subject in the most accessible and domesticating terms.

Stories originally intended to showcase Buddhist healing might have been told or read in the context of religious proselytism or moral edification, to provide inspiration, or simply for entertainment, and could have been enjoyed in both sacred and secular environments. However, plotlines that were particularly well constructed, tropes that appealed broadly, or themes that touched a nerve transcended whatever ideological boundaries they were first composed within and rapidly gained currency in a whole range of new social settings. While medieval Buddhist authors readily repurposed narrative elements from a range of rival sources, their contemporaries had no more compunction about incorporating metaphors, tropes, plot elements, and literary conventions that debuted in Buddhist writings into their own competing literature. This trend of appropriation and counterappropriation became so pervasive, and the syncretism so thoroughgoing, that at our historical remove it is rarely possible to tell what is being borrowed from where. Wondrous boons, powerful spirits,

dream adventures, magical implements, divine surgery, instantaneous metamorphosis, sudden revival from death—all of these pervade medieval Chinese popular literature of all sectarian inclinations and are the exclusive
"intellectual property" of none. Through their use of domesticating translation, authors of Buddhist healing narratives played a critical role in pollinat-
ing these discourses with Indian therapeutic techniques, Buddhist occult
practices, novel plot twists, and new classes of divine and human healers.

Estimates for the total population of the Chinese empire during the medieval period are extremely tentative, but they range as high as 53 million in
the Tang.[73] Meanwhile, calculations of the total number of Chinese members of the sangha range from 150,000 in the sixth century to about 260,000
by the mid-ninth.[74] Even if these figures are only rough estimates, it is clear
that the sangha represented only a minuscule fraction of the total population
at any given time. The proportion who were able to read the specialized vocabulary of the Buddhist scriptures would have been far smaller. Even with
the increasing availability of resources for learning Sanskrit mentioned in the
previous chapter, the number of people that had even a cursory knowledge of
Indic scripts or languages always remained statistically insignificant. Given
these facts, it is obvious that far more people would have come in contact
with Buddhist medicine in the form of popular narratives than any other
type of source discussed in this book. Most of these narratives, of course,
would have circulated in oral form and are therefore beyond our capacity to
recover and analyze today. However, some proportion of these tales were written, collected, recanonized, and preserved to today. The narratives discussed
in this chapter can provide a valuable window onto the types of stories in
circulation and, by extension, onto how Buddhist medical discourses became
part of the larger religiomedical conversation in medieval China.

Conclusion

The first half of the Tang dynasty represents the peak of the Indo-Sinitic cross-cultural encounter. By that time, numerous Buddhist scriptures focusing on all aspects of medicine had been translated into Chinese. Disparate ideas from across the range of Buddhist literature available in China had been augmented, collated, and commented upon by generations of pseudo-translators, compilers, and exegetes. Sectarian authors were busily systematizing this body of knowledge, defending it against unorthodox intrusions, and encoding it in increasingly foreignizing language. Efforts to sell Indian medicine to the public had also proved highly successful: elite physicians, members of high society, and even rulers were turning to Buddhist healers and ritual specialists for assistance. Many foreign ideas had been integrated into the writings of medieval physicians, and Buddhist literary tropes, rhetorical conventions, and occult practices had significantly infiltrated the normative religiomedical vocabulary and popular literature. All of the above notwithstanding, a reconfiguration of Eurasian geopolitics in the mid-eighth century set in motion a chain of events that would significantly curtail China's engagement with Indian culture.[1]

In the seventh century and the first half of the eighth, Tang armies had incorporated significant portions of Central Asia into the empire. Though many of them personally favored Daoism and sometimes took measures to curb the power of the sangha, Chinese rulers had also utilized Buddhism in order to promote unity across ethnic and linguistic boundaries and to appeal to popular sensibilities in non-Han regions throughout their expanding territory. In 751, however, the Tang's westward expansion halted with defeat at the hands of Muslim armies at the Talas River in present-day Kazakhstan. Then, in 755, the military refocused on the Chinese heartland in response to the outbreak of a major rebellion led by the Sogdian-Turkish general An Lushan (703–57). The uprising was successfully put down, but the ruling house was severely weakened in the conflict. In the decades that followed, the government's attention increasingly turned to internal issues, and its influence in Central Asia began to wane. By the ninth century, many kingdoms in the region that were previously in the Chinese orbit were converting to Islam, and Buddhism was declining as a major cultural influence.[2] Meanwhile, the focus of Chinese international trade shifted from the unstable Silk Roads to the sea routes, but these were now also dominated by Muslim instead of Indian merchants. Consequently, although international traffic did not abate, commercial relationships began to replace Buddhism as the primary context for Indo-Sinitic exchange.

With both the overland and maritime lines of religious transmission compromised, the processes of localization long under way intensified significantly, and Chinese Buddhism became increasingly untethered from India. Both doctrinal systems and the terminology used to express them veered further away from South Asian precedents.[3] Buddhist holy sites were mapped onto the Chinese landscape, and fewer pilgrims traveled abroad.[4] By the tenth century, the three "cores" of the Buddhist world—eastern India, Sri Lanka, and China—were operating more or less independently.[5] Buddhism outside of India was increasingly local in flavor, no longer dependent on the motherland for guidance or inspiration.

Increasingly threatened both by neighboring peoples and non-Han insurgents, and no longer looking to India as a spiritual beacon, the latter half of the Tang not surprisingly saw a sharp increase in xenophobia and cultural chauvinism in China. Criticism of Buddhism had always been present in some quarters of society, but diatribes painting the religion as an unseemly barbarian tradition now gained increasing urgency and a more sympathetic ear. In the first half of the ninth century, leading intellectuals launched the "classical literature" (guwen) movement, which among other things advocated a return to Confucian values.[6] Proponents decried the religiosity and gullibility of the populace and attempted to debunk clerics' claims to possess magical powers. They also lambasted Buddhist monasteries, which as tax-exempt landholding institutions had increased their financial clout at the expense of the state. These attitudes gathered steam and culminated in the "Huichang Persecution" of Buddhism in 842–45 under Emperor Wuzong. The stated goal of this violent repression was the total destruction of Buddhism on Chinese soil, and similar measures were soon undertaken against Manichaeism and other foreign religions that had taken root in China. With increasing vehemence, the government destroyed texts and statues, and forcibly defrocked over a quarter million clerics.[7] During this time, the state also seized monastic land and formally appropriated the Buddhist medical charities.[8]

The decimation of the sangha, the destruction of monastic infrastructure, and the withdrawal of the financial underpinnings for Buddhist charitable institutions all were devastating to China's engagement with Indian medicine. Abortive attempts to control or eliminate Buddhist healing activities in different contexts had been undertaken before that point: a government edict had outlawed the practice of healing and divination by Buddhist and Daoist clerics as early as 653, and the monastic medical charities had been placed under secular supervision during the reign of Empress Wu.[9] But such efforts had always had little impact on China's enthusiasm for Buddhist medicine. The disruptions of the ninth century would be different, however, with a longer-lasting deleterious effect.

One major consequence of the Huichang Persecution was the discontinuation of the translation assemblies for the span of about 160 years. In the interim, the Tang dynasty collapsed and gave way to six decades of internecine warfare. Not until the Song dynasty reunified the realm in the second half of the tenth century did significant imperial patronage of Buddhism begin again.[10] Emperor Taizong (r. 976–97) resumed sponsoring the translation of sutras; however, the gap of so many years as well as the institutional disruption meant that the oral and tacit knowledge handed down among members of the translation bureaus had been lost. Members of the new assembly constantly complained about their lack of resources and expertise. Centrally managed by the state, the project was intended more to demonstrate the new dynasty's prestige to an international audience than as an earnest attempt to learn from Indian culture. The textual output of this revived translation effort was large, consisting of 1,028 texts in 564 scrolls, which were circulated both inside China and around East Asia. Nevertheless, the new translations were largely ignored by the Chinese Buddhist establishment, which by that time had already significantly diverged from Indian models.

At the same time that it was regulating Buddhist translation, the reconstituted central government of the Song also began regulating medicine. Historians of Chinese medicine have noted that the state's involvement in this period had the effect of "sharpening the lines between heterodox and orthodox healing."[11] Medical education became increasingly standardized across the realm, while enthusiastic officials engaged in local campaigns to suppress spirit healers and other popular practitioners. In 1076, the state also entered into the pharmaceutical industry with centrally administered dispensaries. Although Song rulers and elites did patronize Buddhist charitable activities, the institutionalized care for the poor and the sick had lost its exclusive association with Buddhism and had become a regular feature of government administration.

A significant aspect of the Song medical reform was the creation in 1057 of the Bureau for Editing Medical Treatises (*jiaozheng yishu ju*). In the second half of the eleventh century, this bureau reedited, printed, and promulgated Han-era medical classics such as the *Inner Canon* and the *Treatise on Cold Damage*. As discussed in Chapter 1, by this point in time, many foreign medicines had been absorbed into the Chinese pharmaceutical literature and many points of Indian doctrine had become inextricably integrated into Chinese medical thought. Famous works by medieval writers that engaged with Buddhist knowledge—such as Sun Simiao and Wang Tao—were even part of the corpus edited and published by the government. These facts notwithstanding, as classical works became increasingly valorized, official support waned for competing models explicitly associated with foreign sources. Names of deities, Sanskrit terminology, and other foreign elements appearing in medical texts were sometimes deliberately obscured or downplayed.[12] Some medical texts listed in the dynastic bibliographies of the post-Tang period continued to nominally attribute medical knowledge to foreign masters, but a closer look at the contents of their writings reveals little or no engagement with Indian doctrine.[13] The two-hundred-volume official encyclopedia of medical doctrine from 1122, the *Comprehensive Records of Sagely Benefaction from the Zhenghe Reign Period*, barely mentions Buddhism at all.

Meanwhile, Buddhist writings from this period continued to showcase Buddhism's relevance for health, longevity, and curing illness.[14] But while newly translated sutras continued to mention Indian medical doctrines such as the Four Elements, *tridoṣa*, and so forth, writings by Song-era exegetes show signs that these ideas exerted far less of an intellectual influence. Instead of attempting to translate or explain these doctrines for their readers, authors of Buddhist secondary sources often fell into the desultory citation of stock phrases from scripture or simply parroting Daoxuan and Daoshi.[15] As a whole, Buddhist writings on healing from the post-Tang period betray a palpable shift away from language or imagery that might call attention to the foreignness of Buddhist ideas and practices.[16]

Despite the competition from new government institutions, Buddhist ritual and merit-making activities by all accounts continued to play a major role in community health care and civic life in the Song.[17] In addition, many of the basic orientations associated with Buddhist medicine had—in domesticated translation—become part of the common stock of popular healing knowledge, known across all segments of society in the Song. The pantheon of healing deities, the range of curative rites, the use of magical incantations and talismans, and the recognition of monks as healers and as guardians of medical knowledge continued to play major roles in the religiomedical landscape.[18] But due to the shifts in the reception environment, these conversations were conducted in ever more domesticated terminology.

Recent studies have provided a series of snapshots of various historical contexts in which certain aspects of Buddhist healing remained socially and culturally relevant throughout the later imperial period. In the Ming, for example, monasteries have been shown to have been important in caring for women whose therapeutic needs were not adequately addressed by male physicians.[19] In another example, some Buddhist monks in the Qing were keepers of prized gynecological knowledge, and they organized merit-publishing groups to disseminate their therapies in print.[20] The success of the contemporary Taiwanese Buddhist charitable association Tzu Chi Foundation demonstrates the continuing importance of healing in Chinese Buddhist proselytizing even today.[21] However, in none of these cases were Buddhist institutions or clerics forwarding Indian medical doctrines. Even while many aspects of Buddhist healing proved enormously popular in China over the *longue durée*, serious study and engagement with the Elements, *tridoṣa*, and other Indian doctrines fell by the wayside in the ninth century, never to regain anywhere near the cultural cachet they enjoyed in the first half of the Tang.[22]

*   *   *

Why did some aspects of the Buddhist medical transmission become permanent parts of Chinese religiomedical culture, while the core doctrines of Indian anatomy, etiology, and therapy did not? The variability of the Chinese reception raises important questions for historians. It tells us that "Buddhist medicine," while perhaps useful as a term of convenience, is not a monolithic entity. The story of its global transmission is nuanced and historically contingent. In an attempt to explain the complexities of this example of cross-cultural exchange, some historians have wanted to bracket off the "religious" aspects of Buddhist healing, which, they argue, were more easily accepted by the Chinese, from the "scientific" ideas, which were not.[23] However, this book has argued that the reception of Buddhist medical ideas and their impact on Chinese society and culture can be better understood by examining contemporary practices of translation than by imposing anachronistic dichotomies such as "religion" versus "science."

Our investigation into the Chinese translation of Buddhist medicine and the role of translated knowledge in the medieval Chinese religiomedical landscape began with a wide-angle view of the transmission of Buddhist medical texts from India to China along the transregional networks that flourished in the first millennium C.E. Then, we zoomed in on some of the individual authors involved in the reinterpretation and repackaging of this knowledge in China and examined their translation practices more closely. Admittedly, we still have only scratched the surface of a massive undertaking. There is more work to be done tracing the origins and development of Buddhist medical ideas, as well as refining and elaborating our understanding of the social dynamics of translation and religiomedical competition locally in China. Yet, even at these beginning stages of our exploration, we have discovered that we can learn much about the nexus of religion and medicine in medieval Chinese society from the examination of Buddhist translations.

For one, our study has demonstrated that medicine is inseparable from an operating definition of "religion" in this historical setting, and vice versa. Medieval China was characterized by intense competition between healers of many religious persuasions, and medical knowledge played a crucial role in legitimating and popularizing competing religious paradigms. The ability to explain health, disease, and the body was of vital ideological importance to sectarian writers of all varieties and was a key variable in their struggles for social and cultural capital. These facts both complicate modern scholarly categories and invite the interdisciplinary investigation of the overlaps between what are traditionally held to be separate fields of inquiry.

Second, we also have learned much about the human agency behind India's influence in China and Indo-Sinitic syncretism. We have seen that this cross-cultural exchange was a process replete with both tension and creativity, where the ingenuity of individual authors played a decisive role in the local reception of foreign ideas. We have seen that imported knowledge was translated strategically in dialogue with a variety of domestic standards, norms, and preferences, and was put to specific sociopolitical purposes in the target culture. Translators and authors frequently made choices to couch certain types of Buddhist medical knowledge in foreignizing, exoticizing terms in order to mark it as novel, unique, or specialized. Just as often, and within the same texts, they decided to deploy familiar Chinese concepts and vocabularies in order to explain foreign ideas to their readers in ways that would both appeal and seem accessible. Over the course of the medieval period, the linguistic and conceptual connections between Indian and Chinese medicine established by such translation decisions allowed Buddhist authors to absorb indigenous practices of self-cultivation, divination, demonology, and healing into their writings. Meanwhile, they also allowed Buddhism's textual and paratextual practices, foreign terminology, doctrines, practices, and frames of authority to be reciprocally appropriated by rival religiomedical groups.

Third, and finally, we have also gained insight into the connections between translation and the long-term successes or failures of particular aspects of Indian medical knowledge in China. What the most historically influential aspects of Buddhist medicine have in common is that they represent those parts of the Indian transmission that were most enthusiastically molded to fit with native Chinese idioms and cultural expectations. Authors who were interested in furthering the propagation and popularization of Buddhism in wider society developed blends of foreignizing and domesticating translation strategies that made Buddhist ideas seem accessible, relevant, and exciting for broader Chinese audiences. Meanwhile, discourses that appeared in specialized ascetic texts and secondary sources—compositions that were not intended to be widely circulated and that prioritized fidelity to the source context—remained less relevant in the long run. When stated so succinctly, this conclusion might seem overly simple. However, it is significant that we have refocused our attention on how individuals make meaning within the context of cross-culturally transmitted traditions, instead of simply studying the contents of the traditions themselves.

To conclude, I will note that, while this book has proposed answers to some of these questions about the medical exchange between India and China in the medieval period, I believe that the methodologies employed in this study could be just as fruitfully applied to other times and places. Whatever historical period we are studying, we cannot approach instances of cross-cultural exchange simply as the result of the collision or encounter of cultures writ large. Exploring cross-cultural exchange through the lens of translation allows us to appreciate both the impact of transmitted cultural-linguistic structures and also the creativity and agency of the individuals involved in their reception, adaptation, and continual reinterpretation. At the end of the day, integrating the two is critical for historians if we are going to bring our historical actors—and the worlds of meaning in which they lived, thought, and expressed themselves—back to life within our own translations of the past.

ABBREVIATIONS

Asian Medicine	*Asian Medicine: Tradition and Modernity.*
Bulletin of SOAS	*Bulletin of the School of Oriental and African Studies.*
CBETA	Chinese Buddhist Electronic Text Association. *Dianzi fodian jicheng.* http://www.cbeta.org/ and on CD-ROM (CBReader 2010 v. 1.0).
EASTM	*East Asian Science, Technology, & Medicine.*
EBTEA	Charles D. Orzech, Henrik H. Sørensen, and Richard K. Payne (eds.). 2011. *Esoteric Buddhism and the Tantras in East Asia.* Leiden: Brill.
DDB	Charles Muller (ed.). *Digital Dictionary of Buddhism.* http://buddhism-dict.net/ddb.
HJAS	*Harvard Journal of Asiatic Studies.*
HDW	Institute of History and Philology, Academia Sinica. *Scripta Sinica (Hanji dianzi wenxian).* http://hanchi.ihp.sinica.edu.tw.
Hōbōgirin	Paul Demiéville et al. 1929–2003. *Hōbōgirin: Diction-naire encyclopédique du Bouddhisme d'après les sources chinoises et japonaises.* Tokyo: Maison Franco-Japonaise.
JAOS	*Journal of the American Oriental Society.*
JIABS	*Journal of the International Association of Buddhist Studies.*
P.	Dunhuang manuscripts, Pelliot Chinese Collection, Bibliothèque Nationale de France.
Pacific World	*Pacific World: Journal of the Institute of Buddhist Studies.*
SCC	Joseph Needham et al. 1954–2004. *Science and Civilisation in China,* vols. 1–7. Cambridge: Cambridge University Press.

T.   *Taishō Tripitaka*. All citations and quotes from this
            source come from CBETA's corrected digitized
            edition. The left side of the citation (before the colon)
            consists of text number, optionally followed by a
            decimal and a chapter number. The right side consists
            of the page number, register, and line number.

X.   *Continued Tripitaka (Xu zangjing)*. Also accessed
            through CBETA.

NOTES

INTRODUCTION

1. T. 2145: 5b27, cited in Cheung 2006. All citations marked "T." refer to CBETA, and all translations are my own unless otherwise credited.

2. I use the term "Indo-Sinitic" to indicate the flow of tangible and intangible goods from India to China, as opposed to "Sino-Indian," which emphasizes the flow in the opposite direction. The former is copiously documented in historical sources, though much less is known about the latter. Recent monographs focusing on the broader cultural impact of Buddhism in China include Kieschnick 2003 and Sanping Chen 2012. While the transmission of Chinese ideas to India will not be discussed here, some ruminations on this subject can be found in Pelliot 1912; Chatterji 1959; Filliozat 1969; Bagchi 1981: 247–54; White 1996: 61–66; Samuel 2008: 278–82; Alter 2009; *SCC* 2: 427–30.

3. Studies of medical knowledge in early Indian Buddhist sources are available in Haldar 1977, 1992; Mitra 1985; Zysk 1998; Ṭhānissaro 2007: 54–68. An excellent introduction with annotated bibliography of primary and secondary sources is available in Mazars 2008. For studies of Chinese Buddhist medicine in Western languages, see the very useful overview in *Hōbōgirin* 3: 224–65 (English translation in Demiéville 1985), as well as Filliozat 1934; Birnbaum 1989a, 1989b; Deshpande 1999, 2000, 2003–4, 2008; Salguero 2009, 2010, 2010–11, 2012, 2013. For East Asian scholarship on the topic, see Obinata 1962, 1965; Fukunaga 1972, 1990; Ma, Gao, and Hong 1993: 113–83; Tso 1980, 1994; Tu 2001; Xue 2002: 500–727; Ma Zhonggeng 2005: 75–169; the numerous publications by Chen Ming listed in the references; and other works cited throughout this book. (Chen Ming 2013 and Deshpande and Fan 2012 were published while this manuscript was in final stages of preparation, and I have not had the opportunity to integrate them fully into the arguments and data presented here.)

4. The word "medieval" is derived from the European historical experience, and its application to Chinese history has been controversial (see, e.g., Barrett 1998; Luo 2005). Most of these debates concern comparisons between Chinese and European feudal or aristocratic social features, and hinge on related disagreements over what we mean by "modernity" in the Chinese context. I will not repeat these arguments here. I use the word "medieval" because it is in many quarters accepted as a convenient label for the period from the collapse of the Han dynasty in the early third century to the establishment

of the Song dynasty in the late tenth. Occasionally, I use the term "early medieval" to refer to the Period of Division, 220–589 C.E.

5. Although I refer to various "traditions" of religion and medicine throughout this book, I do not mean to imply that these are monolithic or unchanging bodies of knowledge handed down from time immemorial. Rather, I understand traditions as intergenerational social processes involving many individual acts of transmission, reception, reinterpretation, and retransmission. They are dynamic, continually "negotiated, reformulated, abandoned, reinvented, and concealed" over time (Engler and Grieve 2005: 2). On "tradition" in Chinese medicine, see especially Scheid 2006, 2007.

6. See, e.g., Edward L. Davis 2001; Strickmann 2002; Lo and Cullen 2005; Despeux 2010; Deshpande and Fan 2012.

7. See, e.g., Shi Wangcheng 1992; Zhu Jianping 1999; Shen 2001; essays in Rahman 2002; and numerous works by Chen Ming and Vijaya Deshpande cited in the references.

8. This position was most influentially articulated in Unschuld 1979a; repeated in Unschuld 2010: 132–53.

9. Examples of this approach include Wright 1959; Ch'en 1964, 1973; Wales 1967. See discussion and critiques of this mode of scholarship in Gimello 1978; Canepa 2010; Stephen Teiser's introduction in Zürcher 2007.

10. The cultural systems theory was most influentially expressed in Geertz 2000 [1973]. For scholarship relevant to Buddhist healing, see especially the works cited in the references by Michel Strickmann, whose French dissertation title included the word "syncrétismes," and whose many publications rely on this model.

11. See discussion in Mollier 2008: 1–22.

12. Examples of the discourse-centered approach in the study of medieval Chinese Buddhism include Sharf 2002; Campany 2003, 2012a; Cole 2009. Specifically on the term "repertoires," see discussion in Campany 2009: 28–30, 2012b: 37–43.

13. Sharf 2002: 16.

14. See discussion of these two modes in the social sciences and humanities more generally in Sewell 1999.

15. See Mair 2006 for a strong defense of this approach.

16. See, e.g., Teiser 2006; and essays by Matthew Canepa and others in *Ars Orientalis* 38 (2010). Sophisticated approaches to cross-cultural exchange in historical contexts other than medieval China include Aravamudan 2006; Heinrich 2008; Zhan 2009; Puente-Ballesteros 2011; Chan 2012; Hill 2013.

17. I have been greatly influenced by works on Chinese Buddhist translation by Erik Zürcher, Jan Nattier, and Daniel Boucher listed in the references and cited throughout this book. Two essays written by Charles Orzech (Orzech 2002, 2002–3) came to my attention after I had already worked out my basic theoretical framework and begun writing, and inspired me to push even further into translation studies. A broad and readable introduction to the field of translation studies is available in Bellos 2011.

18. Note that I do not intend to invoke the connotations of the term "cultural translation" currently in vogue in the fields of anthropology, postcolonial studies, or cultural studies (see Asad 1986; Bachmann-Medick 2006; discussion in Trivedi 2007).

19. On the terms "interlingual" and "intralingual" translation, see Jakobson 2004. (Jakobson also proposes the category of "intersemiotic" translation, or the translation between verbal and non-verbal signs, which is not relevant to this book.)

20. Throughout this book, I use male-gendered language in discussions of authors and translators due to the fact that the authorship of Buddhist texts was almost exclusively a male undertaking (the exceptions that prove this rule are discussed in Campany 1991b: 44–46, 1993a). The same, of course, cannot be assumed in the case of the oral storytelling discussed in Chapter 5.

21. This perspective is discussed in much more detail in Snell-Hornby 1995.

22. Friedrich 1992.

23. Nida 1964: 159–60. More recent studies of translation equivalence have built upon this basic binary. Scholars have now introduced a range of additional types of equivalence, each with their own logic and rationale (see, e.g., Koller 1989; Baker 1992).

24. Studies in this mold that explicitly focus on translation equivalence include Link 1957, 1969–70; Wright 1953a; Zürcher 1980.

25. The current state of the field of the neuroscience of translation is briefly reviewed in Tymoczko 2012.

26. The relevant translation studies literature is immense, but I am particularly influenced by Toury 1995. Studies focusing specifically on China include Lydia Liu 1995; Hill 2013; Pritzker, forthcoming. Other works have been cited throughout the remainder of this section and elsewhere in the book.

27. These two terms were most influentially developed in Venuti 1992, 2008.

28. On translation norms, see Toury 1995: 53–69, 2004.

29. See general discussion of the formation of the Chinese Buddhist canon in Mizuno 1995; Lancaster 2012; Hureau 2010.

30. Cf. Mollier 2008: 12; Zürcher 1982a: 168; and see also many sections of Cole 2009.

31. Such issues are discussed in Hayashiya 1945; Makita 1976; Okabe 1980; Zürcher 1982a; Buswell 1990; Nattier 2008 (especially pp. 9–11). I have primarily relied upon the collaborative and constantly updated *DDB* for the attributions in this book, using Lancaster and Park 1979 for texts not listed there.

32. Chen Shu-fen 2004a.

33. The earliest layer of the Pāli Canon was written down in the first century B.C.E. in Sri Lanka, but it is traditionally attributed to a third century B.C.E. oral transmission from northern India. On the history of the Pāli texts, see Collins 1990; Bechert 1991; Norman 2006. Translation of this canon is available at http://www.accesstoinsight.org. Discussion of the medical content in these sources is found in Haldar 1977, 1992; Mitra 1985; Zysk 1998; Ṭhānissaro 2007: 54–68; Mazars 2008.

34. The most influential Āyurvedic classics include the *Compendium of Caraka* (*Caraka-saṃhitā*) compiled between approximately 100 B.C.E. and 200 C.E., the *Compendium of Suśruta* (*Suśruta-saṃhitā*) compiled by the fifth century C.E., and the *Heart of Medicine* (*Aṣṭāṅgahṛdaya-saṃhitā*) composed by Vāgbhaṭa around 600 C.E. For dating and bibliographic information of these texts, see relevant sections of Meulenbeld 1999; Wujastyk 2003. Discussion of the contents of the Āyurvedic texts can be found in Filliozat 1964; Kutumbiah 1974; Jolly 1977; Mitra 1974. Translations are available in Sharma 2004–5, 2007–8; Wujastyk 2003; Murthy 2012.

35. Toury 1995: 23–39.

36. On pseudotranslation, see Toury 1995: 40–52. For studies of Chinese Buddhist "apocrypha," see Buswell 1990; Strickmann 2002; Mollier 2008; Hureau 2010.

37. See Lefevere 1992.

38. Alter 2009: 228. A more detailed discussion of the integration of religion and medicine in cultures other than medieval China is beyond the scope of this book. However, see theoretical discussions problematizing and historicizing the categories of "religion" and "science" in more general terms in Tambiah 1990; Harrison 2006.

39. On the modern formation of TCM and its global spread, see Sivin 1987; Taylor 2005; Zhan 2009; sections of Hinrichs and Barnes 2013; Pritzker, forthcoming.

40. For a recent survey of the history of Chinese medicine that does an admirable job of including a range of healers and multiple medical models, see Hinrichs and Barnes 2013. Note, however, that this book still uses the words "healing" and "medicine" to indicate separate categories of practitioners.

41. See discussion of this term in Sivin 1987: 22.

42. The vast majority of the instances of the term appearing in premodern sources consist of references to a Buddhist text called the *Foyi jing* (T. 793). Although the title of this text is today widely translated as the *Sutra on Buddhist Medicine*, medieval catalogs often give it the alternative name *Fo yiwang jing*, which means something closer to the "Sutra on the Buddha, King of Physicians." (As I will discuss below, *yiwang* [Skt. *vaidyarāja*] is an honorific title given to many Buddhist healing figures.) Since in all likelihood *yi* should be translated as "physician" in the shortened version of the title as well, I render that title as "Sutra on the Buddha as Physician."

43. See Asad 1986.

44. On the issues raised in this paragraph, see Lancaster 2012.

45. See discussion of the names of Jīvaka in Salguero 2009: 191–92.

CHAPTER I

1. Kuriyama 1993. For surveys of the history of Chinese medicine, see Ma Boying 1994; Unschuld 2010; Hinrichs and Barnes 2013. For reviews of the scholarly literature, see Hinrichs 1998; Lee Jen-der 2004; Lo 2009.

2. See von Glahn 2004: 98–129. On early Chinese ghost and demon lore more generally, see also Campany 1991a; Poo 2000, 2004, 2010. *Shen* is a word with wide semantic range that in this context might be translated as "deity," "divine being," or "spirit." I will discuss it in Chapter 3 as an adjective meaning something more like "numinous" or "paranormal." The Chinese term *gui* translates as "demon" or "ghost." It can refer both to deceased people who haunt the living as well as to other types of malevolent spirits.

3. Unschuld 2010: 19.

4. Yang 1957; Seidel 1987; overview in Brokaw 1991: 28–32.

5. On Daoist healing practices, see, inter alia, Strickmann 1993, 1995, 2002; Boken-kamp 1997: 230–74; Despeux 2000; Gai 2001; Xue 2002: 312–499; Campany 2002: 47–75; Mollier 2003; Sakade 2007; Lin 2008; Chi-Tim Lai 2010; Shih-shan Susan Huang 2010; Sivin 2011; Bumbacher 2012: 57–80; Stanley-Baker 2013.

6. For studies of these practitioners, see Stein 1979; Tsukamoto 1985: 119–23; Ma Boying 1994: 138–77; Lin 1994, 2008, 2009, 2010; von Falkenhausen 1995; Chi-Tim Lai 1998; Mollier 2008: 55–99. On the use of *wu* as a pejorative term, see Sivin 1995b: 31.

7. See Harper 1985, 1996, 1997, 1998.

8. Bodde 1975: 75–138; Eliasberg 1984; von Glahn 2004: 104–9.

9. See description of medieval medical bureaus in Hinrichs and Barnes 2013: 89–90.

10. *Comprehensive Records of Sagely Benefaction from the Zhenghe Reign Period* (*Zhenghe shengji zonglu*), compiled 1122, fascicles 195–97. See other examples of the continuity of spirit-based healing practices in the Song in Katz 1995: 39–75; Edward L. Davis 2001.

11. See discussion in Harper 1997; Li Jianmin 2009.

12. Kuriyama 2000: 3. On the diversity of opinion in the period, see Nylan 1999.

13. Introductions to sympathetic resonance can be found in *SCC* 2: 216–345; Lloyd and Sivin 2002: 193–203, 253–71; Sharf 2002: 78–97; Puett 2002: 145–200; Lewis 2006: 36–61; Unschuld 2010: 51–100; and articles in *Museum of Far Eastern Antiquities* 72 (2000). Qi has variously been translated as "vapor," "energy," and "vital force." Yin represents the forces of shadow, receptivity, femininity, and interiority, while yang represents the forces of light, activity, masculinity, and externality. For discussion of basic Chinese medical concepts, see Sivin 1987. Note that the character *ren*, which I have translated here as "Mankind," is not gendered in Chinese.

14. Sharf 2002: 83. On musical resonance as a primary metaphor in early Chinese cosmology, see Brindley 2012 (specifically in medicine, see pp. 131–56). See also discussion of *ganying* in Kieschnick 1997: 97–101.

15. Early and medieval Chinese arts of self-cultivation are discussed in Maspero 1981: 443–554; Kohn and Sakade 1989; Wile 1992; Sakade 2005, 2007; Kohn 1993, 2000, 2006, 2008; Lo 2000a, 2000b, 2001, 2002a, 2002b; Campany 2002: 18–47, 2005a, 2005b, 2005d, 2009; Despeux 2006; Arthur 2009; Stanley-Baker 2013; articles in *Asian Medicine* 7, no. 1 (2012). Major studies of Chinese alchemy include Sivin 1968; Strickmann 1979; Pregadio 2000, 2006a, 2006b; Ho Peng Yoke 2007; *SCC* 5.2–5.5.

16. While the core of the *Inner Canon* was composed in the classical period, the three extant versions of the text (the *Suwen*, *Taisu*, and *Lingshu*) all date from the seventh century. On the formation of the text and its ideas, see Yamada 1979, 1998; Epler 1980; Kegan 1988; Sivin 1993, 1995c; Li Jianmin 2000; Unschuld 2003. See translation of the *Suwen* in Unschuld and Tessenow 2011.

17. *Inner Canon: Lingshu* 71 (translated in de Bary and Bloom 1999: 275–78).

18. The political implications of correlative cosmology are discussed in Sivin 1995a; Lloyd and Sivin 2002: 16–81, 214–26; Lewis 2006: 36–61.

19. *Inner Canon: Suwen* 8 (translated in Unschuld and Tessenow 2011: 155–62).

20. On the historical development of the therapies of acupuncture and moxibustion, see Yamada 1998; Lu and Needham 2002.

21. See *Inner Canon: Suwen* 2 (translated in Unschuld and Tessenow 2011: 45–57).

22. See discussion of interplay between these models in Li Jianmin 2009. For a translation of an imperial physician's writings on demon-induced illnesses, see excerpts of Chao Yuanfang's *Treatise on Origins and Symptoms of Disease* (*Zhubing yuan hou lun*) in Unschuld 2010: 300–302. On ghosts made from qi, see Strickmann 2002: 12, 72–73, 304n51; Sterckx 2002: 74.

23. On the range of adepts in early China, see Campany 2009 (especially pp. 158–63). An assortment of medieval healers are introduced in various popular tales translated in DeWoskin 1983; Mather 2002; Campany 2002, 2012b. For discussion of a similar range of practitioners in later periods, see Kleinman 1980; Thompson 1990; Cullen 1993; Berg 2002: 61–168. Hinrichs and Barnes 2013, a survey of Chinese medical history from the Shang to the present, particularly focuses on the diversity of models, practices, and practitioners throughout Chinese history.

24. Zürcher 1980: 146. Of course, I do not wish to forward an oversimplified bifurcation between "great" and "little" traditions (cf. Redfield 1956; and see Sered 2007–8 for other possible ways of modeling a spectrum of practitioners).

25. Research has demonstrated a great number of ancient connections between the eastern and western halves of Eurasia. (See, e.g., Mair 2006; Kuzmina 2008; and numerous issues of the *Sino-Platonic Papers*. Specifically on possible ancient connections between Chinese, Greek, and Indian corporeal knowledge, see Mair 1990: 140–48; Libbrecht 1990). However, such contact was infrequent and indirect when compared with the ease of transportation and communication after the consolidation of the Silk Road and maritime routes between the second century B.C.E. and third century C.E. For comparisons of the very different scientific and medical cultures of early China and Greece, see Lloyd and Sivin 2002; Kuriyama 2002.

26. These events are chronicled in *Records of the Grand Historian* 123 (translated in Watson 1993b: 2:231–46).

27. See discussion of the term "Silk Road(s)" in Whitfield 2007. Coined by the German scholar Ferdinand von Richthofen, the term refers not to any specific route, but to the network as a whole. While many scholars expand the meaning of the term to cover the maritime networks as well, in this book I use "Silk Road" to indicate only land-based

trade routes. For studies on trade between first-millennium South and East Asia, see Xinru Liu 1991, 1996; Ting 1996; Wang Gungwu 1998; Tansen Sen 2003; Juliano and Lerner 2002. The spread of Buddhism along the trade routes is examined in Scott 1985; Zürcher 1990; Hansen 1998, 2004, 2012; Heirman and Bumbacher 2007; Zieme and Kudara 2008; Elverskog 2010; Deeg 2010; and the special issues of *Diogenes* 43, no. 171 (1995); *Pacific World* 4 (2002); and *Sino-Platonic Papers* 222 (2012). Specifically on cross-cultural medical exchange, see also Wang Xiaoxian 1994; Chen Ming 2003a, 2003d, 2005a, 2005b, 2007, 2009, 2013.

28. While I use modern disease categories here, the Chinese understanding of these diseases, of course, was expressed in indigenous medical language and concepts. For a discussion of epidemic diseases in Chinese history, see Hanson 2011.

29. McNeill 1998: 145–49; timeline of epidemics in China on pp. 297–306.

30. Ågren 1986; Hanson 2011: 5–6. See translation of *Treatise on Cold Damage* in Mitchell, Ye, and Wiseman 1999.

31. On Chinese characterizations of foreigners as demons, see Mollier 2006: 93–95. For historical studies of the medieval period more generally, see Twitchett 1979a; Holcombe 1994; Bielenstein 1996; Pearce, Spiro, and Ebrey 2001; Graff 2002; Dien 2007; Lewis 2009a, 2009b.

32. On perceptions of the South, see Schafer 1967: 130–34; Xiao 1993; von Glahn 2004: 78–97.

33. Population figures are discussed in Bielenstein 1947; de Crespigny 1968; Twitchett 1979b. Climactic factors also may have played a role in the disruptions of the early medieval period (Barrett 2007; Connie Chin 2008).

34. Holcombe 1994: 13, 127–29; Berkowitz 2000, 2010.

35. Rudolf G. Wagner 2003; essays in Chan and Lo 2010.

36. On Chinese Buddhists suffering from a "borderland complex" in light of their distance from the holy land, see Forte 1985; Tansen Sen 2003: 6–12. A general history of the Gupta is available in Thapar 2004: 280–325.

37. Thapar 1975: 46–47. The "seven treasures" were gold, silver, lapis lazuli, crystal or quartz, pearl, and two other substances that have alternately been understood as red coral, ammonite, agate, ruby, carnelian, amber, diamond, or emerald (Xinru Liu 1991: 93–94).

38. For the history of the introduction of Buddhism to China and its development during the medieval era, see Wright 1959; Tang Yongtong 1962; Ch'en 1964, 1973; Tsukamoto 1985; Zürcher 2007.

39. Wu Hung 1986; Rhie 1999: 27–95. The debate between advocates of the idea that Buddhism first arrived in China via land and via sea is outlined in Rong 2004. It is clear that both were important avenues for religious exchange with neighboring peoples. The current scholarly consensus is that Buddhism's initial spread to China occurred not as a result of gradual expansion from Central Asia, but via long-distance transmission directly from India (Neelis 2011).

40. Lancaster 2012: 226–31.

41. Zürcher 1989: 119, 2012: 7. While Zürcher characterizes the diversity of the Buddhist transmission as confusing to contemporaries, other scholars have suggested that doctrinal diversity contributes to Buddhism's cross-cultural appeal by providing more flexibility in its interpretation (Freiberger 2004: 274).

42. Zürcher 1991: 277. Early Chinese translations are discussed in more detail in Tsukamoto 1985: 78–112; Nattier 2008; Park 2012: 5–36; and the numerous publications by Erik Zürcher and Daniel Boucher cited in the references.

43. Zürcher 2012: 17.

44. Cited in Wilkinson 2012: 62. Estimates are under one hundred in Bose 1923: 146–48; and Zürcher 2012: 13. See also Bagchi 1981: 36–74, 255–77.

45. Cited in Wilkinson 2012: 68.

46. Tang Yijie 1991: 265.

47. Erik Zürcher (2012: 2) suggests that the textual output of "obscure monks or *upāsakas* [laypeople] producing primitive texts with limited circulation" may in fact have been extensive. He also notes that 90 percent of the anonymous Buddhist translations listed in the earliest catalog were subsequently lost (p. 9).

48. A sample of the existing historical studies of scientific or technical fields other than medicine include Birnbaum 1980; Bagchi 1981: 181–216; Chin Keh-mu 1982; Deshpande 1987, 1991–92; Tansen Sen 1995; Mazumdar 1998; Rahman 2002; Ma Zhonggeng 2005; and relevant sections of *SCC*.

49. These searches were conducted using the digitized edition of the *Taishō Tripitaka* made available by the Chinese Buddhist Electronics Texts Association via their jCBReader 2010 v. 1.0 (accessed 17 April 2012, searching vols. 1–55, 85).

50. T. 2043: 145a–b (translated in Li Rongxi 1993: 67–68). See discussion of a similar story in Indian sources in Mitra 1974: 57–60. On dissection in early Indian sources more generally, see Zysk 1986.

51. While the term is often translated in English as "worm," the semantic range of both the Chinese character *chong* and the original Sanskrit term are broader, connoting a range of creatures or bugs of varying size and appearance (for example, T. 620: 335c22–29 describes *chong* with twelve heads, twelve mouths, and ninety-eight eyes). I have chosen "parasites" as a more inclusive translation term, but I do not intend to invoke any modern medical connotations.

52. Many of these healing deities are discussed in Birnbaum 1989a, 1989b; Kuo 1994: 149–67. On the names of Amitābha/Amitāyus in Chinese sources, see Nattier 2006. On Guanyin, see especially Yü 2001. Readers unfamiliar with the sexual transformation of Guanyin should realize that he is a male deity in the period discussed in this book (see Yü 2001: 293–351).

53. See translations in Watson 1993a; Birnbaum 1989b, respectively.

54. These two bodhisattvas are mentioned at T. 665: 403b15–16.

55. Edward L. Davis 2001: 126–41; Strickmann 2002: 156–61.

56. For discussion of the relationship between the sangha and the spirit world in early Indian Buddhism, see DeCaroli 2004.

57. Strickmann 2002: 62–79.

58. Edward L. Davis 2001: 130–31, 140–41, 149–50. Much scholarly ink has been spilled deciphering the historicity of Nāgārjuna in the Indian context (see, e.g., White 1996: 66–70; Mabbett 1998; Meulenbeld 1999: 363–65). On representations of Nāgārjuna in China, see Deshpande 2003–4; Deshpande and Fan 2012; Young forthcoming. The biography is found at T. 2047A–B (English translation in Corless 1995; Li Rongxi 2002).

59. For general discussions of the Chinese understanding of karma and associated merit-making practices in China, see Teiser 1988, 1994; Gernet 1995; Cole 1998; Strickmann 2002: 39–50; *EBTEA*: 245–50.

60. On medieval Buddhist charity, including caring for the sick, see Michibata 1957: 388–406; 1967: 178–86; Ch'en 1973: 158–71, 294–303; Demiéville 1985: 57–60; Whalen W. Lai 1992; Gernet 1995: 217–27; Fan Kawai 2005b; *SCC* 6.6: 54–55. For general studies of Buddhist monastic institutions in medieval China, see also Kieschnick 2010; some essays in Benn, Meeks, and Robson 2010.

61. Ch'en 1973: 281–94; Tsukamoto 1985: 844–60; Whalen W. Lai 1987; Gernet 1995: 259–76; Liu Shufen 1995.

62. On the Longmen formulas, see Liu Shufen 2008: 152–57; Zhang 1999. On the Longmen grottoes more generally, see McNair 2007. On bathhouses in China, see Schafer 1956; *SCC* 6.6: 84; Heirman and Torck 2012: 46–51.

63. State-sangha relations are discussed in Ch'en 1973: 65–124; Weinstein 1973, 1987; Liu Shufen 2008, 2010; Li Gang 2010.

64. Ch'en 1973: 276–81; Janousch 1999; Chen Jinhua 2006; Ku 2010; Strange 2011.

65. Caswell 1988; Liu Shufen 1995; Tsiang 1996, 2002; Wong 2004; McNair 2007.

66. See discussions of anti-Buddhist polemics in Kohn 1995; Zürcher 2007: 254–85; Abramson 2008: 52–82; Assandri 2009. On suppressions of Buddhism in the Period of Division, see Ch'en 1952, 1954, 1964: 190–94; Liu Shufen 2002.

67. Wright 1957; Xiong 2006: 151–71. On the Aśokan legend itself, see Strong 1983: 134–61; Norman 2006: 147–69.

68. On Empress Wu's support for and use of Buddhism, see Forte 1976: 125–70, 1988; Guisso 1978; Weinstein 1987: 37–47; Tansen Sen 1995, 2003: 94–101; Barrett 2001; Chen Jinhua 2002a, 2002b; Twitchett 1979a: 290–332.

69. Evidence for the devotion to the Master of Medicines Buddha across various strata of medieval Chinese society is discussed in Ning 2004: 20–37, 130–33; Shi Zhiru 2013; Yao 2013: 496–99; *EBTEA*: 218–19.

70. *Record of the Sui Dynasty* (*Suishu*) 34.29 (see Wei 1973: 1047–48).

71. Such references occur in these authors' most influential works, including Tao Hongjing's so-called *Supplement to the Formulas to Keep Up One's Sleeve* (*Buji zhou hou fang*), Chao Yuanfang's *Treatise on the Origins and Symptoms of Disease,* Sun Simiao's *Essential Formulas Worth a Thousand in Gold for Every Emergency* (*Beiji qianjin yaofang*), and Wang Tao's *Secret Essentials from the Imperial Library* (*Waitai miyao*). See discussion in Lee T'ao 1953: 304–5; Demiéville 1985: 94–97; Shi Wangcheng 1992; Sakade 1998; Zhu Jianping 1999; Shen 2001; Strickmann 2002: 28–34; Deshpande 2008: 146–48; Unschuld

2010: 148–53. Sun's adoption of Buddhist ethics is discussed in Unschuld 1979b: 44–53. On the "Jīvaka formula" (*Qipo fang*), see Chen Ming 2001, 2003b, 2005a. On Chinese adoption of Indian ophthalmology, see Kovacs and Unschuld 1998: 37–42; Deshpande 1999, 2000, 2003–4; Fan Kawai 2005a; Deshpande and Fan 2012. On the Indian influence on Chinese embryology and other aspects of Chinese medicine, see, e.g., Shi Wangcheng 1992; Geng and Geng 1993; Shen 2001; Chen Ming 2005c, 2013; Li Qin-pu 2006.

72. Fan Xingzhun 1936; Schafer 1963: 184–94; Chen Ming 2007, 2013: 114–277. On tribute given to China by Buddhist kingdoms across Asia, see Bielenstein 2005.

73. For dating, discussion of contents, and account of the development of the genre, see Unschuld 1986: 44–52; Schmidt 2006.

74. Unschuld 2006: 25; Chen Ming 2007. See also discussion of developments in medieval pharmacology in Unschuld 1986; select essays in Lo and Cullen 2005.

75. On the medical content of these manuscripts, see Cong 1994; Kalinowski 2003; Chen Ming 2003a, 2003c, 2005a, 2005b; Lo and Cullen 2005; Li and Shi 2006; Despeux 2010. For overview of their cultural and historical context, see Mair 1989; Fraser 2004; Whitfield 2005.

76. Ostensibly Buddhist manuscripts pertaining to curing and preventing disease are discussed in Strickmann 2002; Wang 2005a, 2005b; Mollier 2008; Teiser 2009; Despeux 2010, vol. 2. A number of these texts have been incorporated into vol. 85 of the *Taishō Tripitaka* (see especially T. 2780, T. 2865, T. 2866, T. 2878, T. 2881, T. 2904, T. 2906, T. 2916).

77. Sakade 2005. On the symbolic and social meanings of special diets in Chinese culture, see Campany 2005a, 2005d, 2009: 62–88; Arthur 2009.

78. See discussion of these texts in Strickmann 2002; Mollier 2008.

79. Campany 2003: 319.

80. Sivin 1978: 319.

CHAPTER 2

1. Portions of this chapter were published previously in Salguero 2010–11.

2. The translocal character of East Asian Buddhism is discussed in Holcombe 2001: 94–108; Alter 2009.

3. I borrow this turn of phrase from Tryjarski 1995.

4. On the "invisibility" of the translator, see Venuti 2008.

5. Hitch 2009: 1; see also Sinor 1995.

6. Buddhist bibliographers modeled aspects of the Tripitaka on the indigenous canon of statecraft treatises and mimicked the imperial practices of housing, copying, and distributing texts (Lancaster 2012: 232).

7. For overviews of the foreign Buddhist missionaries in China, see Bagchi 1981: 36–74; Zürcher 2012.

8. A biography of one of the first significant pilgrims, Faxian (320?–420?), is found in Deeg 2005. Others are discussed below.

9. I have relied upon biographical sketches of many of these figures that are available in Bagchi 1981: 255–77; Buswell 2004; *DDB*. Additional sources are noted below for each individual.

10. Details of An Shigao's life, historical context, and translation career as well as discussion of his identity can be found in Forte 1995. See also Ch'en 1964: 43–44; Zürcher 2007: 30–43; Nattier 2008: 35–72.

11. Zürcher 1991; Nattier 2008.

12. On the attribution of this text to An Shigao, see Zürcher 1991: 298.

13. Dharmarakṣa's life and translation practice are discussed in Tsukamoto 1985: 193–229; Boucher 1996, 1998, 2006; Zürcher 2007: 65–70. On the multiethnic character of Dunhuang, see Mair 1989.

14. On the authorship of T. 701, see Demiéville 1985: 74; Boucher 1996: 278. On the authorship of the *Jīvaka Sutra*, see Salguero 2009: 186–94.

15. Biographical details in Ch'en 1964: 81–83; Robinson 1976: 71–73.

16. Biographical details in Li Rongxi 2000: 1–4.

17. Virtually all English translations of this sutra follow the modern meaning of the character zhi_1, translating it as "piles" or "hemorrhoids." From the text, however, which mentions zhi_1 occurring inside the nose, on the teeth, tongue, eyes, ears, hands, feet, and indeed all over the body, it is clear that it cannot be referring to these disorders. I am using the translation "sore" here in an attempt to capture the wide range of ulcers, abscesses, and festering lesions mentioned in the text. See brief discussion of this term and translation of the text in Veith and Minami 1966.

18. Forte 2002b.

19. For details of Amoghavajra's life, career, and patronage, see Chou 1945: 284–307; *EBTEA*: 351–59; Goble 2012.

20. The division of labor in various translation assemblies is discussed in Chen Jinhua 2004a, 2004b, 2005: 651–57; Cheung 2006: 8; Zürcher 2007: 31; Boucher 2008: 87–110; Park 2012: 5–36.

21. Many of these statements are collected in Cheung 2006.

22. Boucher 1996: 95–102, 2006: 31, 2008: 96.

23. Boucher 1996: 17n24; Zürcher 2007: 35, 332n91.

24. On Dharmarakṣa's increasing proficiency, see Boucher 2008: 94–96.

25. See biographical details in Waley 1952; Lusthaus 1995; Li Rongxi 1995; Wriggins 1996.

26. Weinstein 1987: 44.

27. Richards 1953: 250.

28. Early Buddhist languages and scripts are discussed in Brough 1961; Nattier 1990; Boucher 1998, 2000, 2008: 101–7; Norman 2006: 99–145.

29. On the high status of Sanskrit in first-millennium Asia, see Pollock 2006. On the "downward" translation from Sanskrit into Chinese, see Hsieh 2010: 253–93.

30. On the term *chu*₁, see Chen Jinhua 2005; Cheung 2006: 114–15n169; Boucher 2008: 93–94.

31. Mair 2013: 207–81.

32. On vernacularisms in early Buddhist translations, see Zürcher 1977, 1991, 1996; Pulleyblank 1983; Mair 2013: 207–81; Karashima 1996, 2013. Studies on the influence of Buddhist translation on the Chinese lexicon, language, and literary forms also include Tang Jian 1992; Zhu Qingzhi 1992, 1995; Liang 2000; and the many writings of Victor Mair cited in the references. An overview is given in Wilkinson 2012: 67–69.

33. The parameters of these debates are outlined in Cheung 2006: 10–13.

34. On Dao'an's life, thought, and ideas about translation, see Ui 1956; Link 1957, 1958, 1969–70; Tsukamoto 1985: 655–756; Cheung 2006: 69–86.

35. While the practice of *geyi* has received a large amount of scholarly attention (see especially Tang Yongtong 1968; Sharf 2002: 97–100; Itô 1996), Victor Mair (2013: 449–97) argues that its importance has been grossly overstated. According to Mair, it was an experimental exegetical method developed by a small number of early medieval authors that had only a limited utility and was swiftly abandoned.

36. T. 2145: 52b23–c21 (translated in Cheung 2006: 79–83); see also Zürcher 2007: 203.

37. Robinson 1976: 77–81; Cheung 2006: 81–83.

38. T. 2131: 1057c7–12 (translated in Cheung 2006: 157–59). For a detailed analysis of Xuanzang's practice of transliteration, see Chen Shu-fen 2004a. On Chinese Buddhist transliteration more generally, see Pulleyblank 1983; Mair 2013: 185–205; Karashima 1996: 36–38; Chen Shu-fen 2004b; Chaudhuri 2011.

39. Cheung 2006: 11.

40. Boucher 1996: 232.

41. Boucher 2008: 91. Boucher also notes that Dharmarakṣa may have translated proper names into Chinese as part of a strategy to market these texts to "a growing clientele of avant-garde sympathizers."

42. Nattier 2008: 17–18, 166–68.

43. Boucher 2008: 91.

44. Zürcher 2007: 34.

45. Nattier 2008: 24–25, 166–68. Karashima (2013) discusses evolution in the translation of certain sutras over the early medieval period as a result of the consolidation of norms; and Robinson (1976: 77–88) discusses Kumārajīva's engagement with the translation norms of his time.

46. See, e.g., chart of translation equivalents for the *tridoṣa* in Salguero 2010–11: 64–65. Translation equivalents for other Indian doctrines will be discussed in more detail in future publications. In addition to the literature cited elsewhere in this chapter, translation tactics used by specific translators for nonmedical vocabulary are discussed in more detail in Chen Shu-fen 2004b; and in articles in the special issue of *JIABS* 31, nos. 1–2 (2008).

47. See also Boucher 1996: 215–17, 197–214.

48. Demiéville 1985: 67; Unschuld 2010: 132–53; see discussion in Salguero 2010–11.

49. See detailed discussions of Dharmarakṣa's translation errors in Boucher 1998, 2008: 101–7.

50. See, e.g., Jakobson 2004 [1959]; Quine 1960.

51. These transliterations come from T. 310.13: 323a. As mentioned in the introduction, in the medieval period, the pronunciation of these characters would have matched the Sanskrit more closely.

52. T. 310.13: 324b26.

53. Boucher 1996: 214.

54. By the Tang, such reference materials indeed were commonly available, as we will see in Chapter 4.

55. The character is repeatedly used both independently and in conjunction with others (see first mention at T. 310.13: 322b9).

56. T. 310.13: 323c8–18.

57. T. 310.13: 323b24–25.

58. Stewart 2001; Orzech 2002, 2002–3; Salguero 2010–11. Metaphorical equivalence is not to be confused with the more formalized system of "categorizing concepts" (*geyi*) mentioned in note 35 above. While *geyi* is indeed an example of metaphorical equivalence, not all metaphorical equivalence should be considered *geyi*.

59. Glossing the ancient Chinese practice of *daoyin* (literally meaning "guiding and pulling") as "yoga-like exercises" strikes me as an apropos example (Hinrichs and Barnes 2013: 28). This translation of an unfamiliar Chinese practice makes perfect sense to most people in twenty-first-century America, since the Sanskrit term "yoga" has now become a fully domesticated part of our mainstream vocabulary. (For a long list of other Sanskrit terms that have entered common English usage, see Jackson 1982. See also Aravamudan 2006.)

60. On the *tridoṣa* in Indian texts, see Scharfe 1999. Chinese translations of the doctrine are discussed in detail in Salguero 2010–11.

61. See, e.g., Demiéville 1985: 67; Unschuld 2010: 142.

62. While Buddhist philosophers may discern shades of difference between *bhūta* and *dhātu*, these distinctions are not relevant to Chinese Buddhist texts on medicine, which seem to use the terms interchangeably.

63. The "medical marketplace" is an analytical tool that has enjoyed a great deal of currency among historians of European medicine when modeling the messy and competitive healing trades in early modern European societies (see especially Cook 1986; Loudon 1986; Pelling 1987; Porter 1989).

64. See Bourdieu 1977: 159–97, which describes struggle in a field in terms of "orthodox" and "heretical" positions—that is, the established dominant position and the new entrants who attempt to subvert the status quo.

65. Brokaw 1991: 28–32; Ching 1997: 35–66.

66. Bielenstein 1950; Twitchett 1979b: 40. Auspicious events also had political import (see Lippiello 2001).

67. On millenarian literature in medieval China, see Zürcher 1981, 1982b; Seidel 1984; Ownby 1999; Hubbard 2001; Strickmann 2002: 50–62. See broader discussion of Buddhist millenarianism in Nattier 1991.

68. Zürcher 2007: 150.

69. Three extant versions of this sutra are included in the *Taishō Tripitaka*. The earliest (T. 663) is a translation made between 414 and 421 by Dharmakṣema (see discussion of dating in Chen Jinhua 2004a). The second (T. 664) is a composite text composed in 597 made up of parts of Dharmakṣema's text and three other translations made in the sixth century. The third version (T. 665) is a completely new retranslation done in 703 by Yijing. See history of the text and its translations in Gummer 2000: 22–39; Zhou 2003: 33; Emmerick 2004: xi–xiii. See German translation of the Sanskrit text in Nobel 1958; English in Emmerick 2004. The medical content in this text is discussed below in Chapter 4, and see translation in Salguero 2013.

70. This text is held by tradition to be a translation by Kumārajīva, but actually represents a pseudotranslation of 470–80. The sutra became a mainstay of medieval state ritual under the southern Chen dynasty (557–89). In the Tang, Emperor Taizong had the sutra chanted on the twenty-seventh of each month for the benefit and protection of the state. An updated version called the *Sutra on the Perfection of Wisdom for Benevolent Kings to Protect the Country* (*Renwang huguo boreboluomiduo jing*, T. 246) was produced by Amoghavajra for the Emperor Daizong (r. 762–79). This text was given a central role in the reconstitution of the Tang dynasty after the An Lushan Rebellion and became a major part of the court ritual calendar in the late Tang. For a detailed study of the textual history and political context, see Orzech 1998. See also Chandra 1983; and consult Orzech 1998: 69–70n4 for further references.

71. These are T. 665 and T. 246 respectively.

72. For debates between Buddhists and Daoists in the medieval period, see Kohn 1995; Zürcher 2007: 254–85; Abramson 2008: 52–82; Assandri 2009. (For continuing friction in the Song, see also Strickmann 1978; Skonicki 2011.)

73. T. 2103: 147b (translated in Kohn 1995: 89–90).

74. On the *huahu* controversy, see Kohn 1993: 71–80, 1995: 6–17; Zürcher 2007: 288–320.

75. Ch'en 1964: 51.

76. Zürcher 2007: 262 (parenthesis in original).

77. Robson 2008: 139–40 (citing Mather 2002: 388).

78. T. 2122: 901a ff. (translated in Campany 2012b: 183).

79. T. 2122: 756b–c (translated in Campany 2012b: 114–16).

80. T. 2110: 539c (translated in Campany 2012b: 259).

81. Bourdieu stresses what he calls the "doxa," the underlying structure of the field that constrains and incentivizes the actions of all participants. He compares the role of doxa in structuring competition to a card game in which a given set of rules structure the competition among the participants (Bourdieu and Wacquant 1992: 98–100). These rules play a large part in determining the forms of competition that are acceptable, the lan-

guage and symbols employed in the competition, and the stakes associated with winning and losing.

82. This stereotype is discussed in Campany 2005c.

83. See many examples related to healing and protection in Strickmann 2002; Mollier 2008. Other types of Daoist borrowings are discussed in detail in Zürcher 1980; Bokenkamp 1983, 1990, 2001, 2004, 2006, 2007: 99–101, 400–401; Verellen 1992; Hsieh 2010: 63–124; Funayama 2011; Bumbacher 2012: 155–76.

84. See discussion in Chapter 5.

85. On the deification of Sun Simiao, see Unschuld 1994. On Sun's life and thought, see Sivin 1967.

86. Mutual borrowing, in fact, is likely to have intensified the rancor. As Bourdieu writes, "social identity lies in difference, and difference is asserted against what is closest, which represents the greatest threat" (Bourdieu 1984: 479; cf. Campany 2012a: 139).

87. Fuchs 2009: 33.

CHAPTER 3

1. The relevant literature is too extensive to adequately cite here, but see especially the seminal Lakoff and Johnson 2003 [1980].

2. Lakoff and Johnson 2003: 3–6.

3. The cross-cultural transmission of these metaphors will be discussed in further detail in future publications.

4. For definitions of "Tantra" and "Esoteric Buddhism" (*mijiao*), see White 2000: 7–18; Sharf 2002: 263–78; Strickmann 2002: 198–203; Payne 2006: 2–14; Orzech 2012; *EBTEA*: 3–24. Scholars are currently debating the parameters of exactly what these terms mean, and when these shifts occurred in China. While these debates are important to the history of East Asian Buddhism, they are not immediately relevant to my discussion here.

5. The South and Southeast Asian presentations of these ascetic discourses on bodies are discussed in Collins 1997; Mrozik 2007; Powers 2009: 112–40. On Indian bodies more generally, see Wujastyk 2009.

6. T. 375: 741c10–11 (cited in Demiéville 1985: 18–19).

7. Perspectives discussed in this paragraph are described in, e.g., T. 26.98: 583b–c; T. 310.13: 325a–b; T. 310.14: 331b–c; T. 1558.1–3; T. 1579.1.1–2; T. 1648.8. On the medical content in T. 1579, see Lusthaus 2013. For translation of T. 1648, see Ehara, Soma, and Kheminda 1961.

8. See extensive discussion of this type of meditation in Theravada Buddhism in Giustarini 2011.

9. Zysk 1986.

10. T. 310.16: 414b2–417b3. See other formulations of this doctrine at, e.g., T. 26.30: 464b–467a; T. 26.98: 583b.

11. T. 310.16: 416b16–18.

12. Chinese medical discourses on composite bodies are discussed in Lewis 2006: 36–61. See also Yamada 1991.

13. Mrozik 2007: 3; see also pp. 63–70.

14. T. 310.13. In addition to the translation by Bodhiruci discussed here, other translations of different versions of this text were done by Dharmarakṣa (T. 317) and Yijing (T. 310.14, T. 1451: 251a–262a). See also T. 606.5; T. 607.5; T. 1648.8 (translated in Ehara, Soma, and Kheminda 1961: 173). A German translation of Dharmarakṣa's sutra can be found in Huebotter 1932; and a translation of a Tibetan recension is in Langenberg 2008.

15. Kapani 1989; Das 2003; Kritzer 2009.

16. T. 310.13: 322b15–17. This convention is found in Pāli, Chinese, and Tibetan Buddhist sources alike (Boisvert 2000: 303; Kritzer 2009: 78).

17. T. 310.13: 324b6–23. See Kritzer 2006–7.

18. T. 310.13: 324c24–325a3.

19. T. 310.13: 322b10–14.

20. T. 310.13: 324c20–23.

21. T. 310.13: 325a4–11.

22. T. 310.13: 325a15–b28.

23. For discussions of these ideological positions in Buddhist embryologies from outside China, see Boisvert 2000; Garrett 2008, 2009; Langenberg 2008; Sasson 2009. Āyurvedic embryologies are discussed in Das 2003; Selby 2005.

24. T. 310.13: 323a6–8. The Five Aggregates represent the physical form, plus four aspects of mental function. The Form Aggregate is further divisible into the Four Elements.

25. The transliterations used by Bodhiruci for the stages of fetal development were already mentioned in Chapter 2. On names for the Winds, see discussion in Kritzer 2006–7.

26. The indigenous tradition of embryology begins with the writings of the Han physician Zhang Ji (see Furth 1999: 101–16). See a summary of fetal development in Chinese medical embryological narratives in Wilms 2005. Daoist embryology is discussed in Bokenkamp 2005: 157–62. Buddhist influence on Chinese embryology is discussed in Chen Ming 2005c.

27. See Leung 2009: 69–73.

28. Demiéville 1985: 74; Boucher 1996: 278; Heirman and Torck 2012: 56–57n39. This text survives today both as an independent sutra in the *Taishō Tripitaka* and embedded in commentaries from the Sui (T. 1793) and Tang (T. 2780). The latter was discovered at Dunhuang.

29. Buddhist bathhouses in general—and this text in particular—are discussed in Heirman and Torck 2012: 27–66. On bathhouses in ancient and medieval China, see Schafer 1956. Indian monastic bathing practices are described in Devi 1979; Rao 1982. Those appearing in Yijing's travelogue are discussed in Chapter 4.

30. T. 701: 803a1–2.

31. T. 701: 803a3–6.

32. These diseases appear in texts such as the *Inner Canon, Treatise on Cold Damage,* and *Treatise on the Origins and Symptoms of Disease.*

33. T. 701: 803a7–15.

34. The linking of good health, physical attractiveness, and other desirable attributes— themselves products of good karma—with the ability to perform further meritorious deeds in an upward spiral of beneficial karmic conditions is a common trope in Buddhist literature (Mrozik 2007: 70–73).

35. He will become a minister, a king, a celestial deva, a cakravartin, a bodhisattva, and eventually a Buddha (T. 701: 803a16–21).

36. See, e.g., T. 264.5; T. 374: 378a–379a (cited in Demiéville 1985: 17).

37. See, e.g., the short text *Sutra on the Medical Simile* (*Foshuo yiyu jing,* T. 219), which compares the Four Noble Truths that are the cornerstone of Buddhist philosophy to a good physician's understanding of particular illnesses, their causes, their treatments, and their eradication. See additional citations in Demiéville 1985: 9–14.

38. T. 262: 54c25–26 (translated in Watson 1993a: 288). See discussion of the numinous powers of sacred Buddhist scripture in Campany 1991b; Bumbacher 2012: 134–54.

39. T. 1161: 666b15, b6. Discussion and translation in Birnbaum 1989b: 115–48; see notes on authorship in Fujita 1990.

40. T. 475.5 (see translation in Watson 1997: 64–74). Other Chinese translations of the text are found in T. 474, T. 476.

41. T. 475: 544c–545a.

42. T. 475: 550a7–20. On the development of the doctrine of the docetic bodies of the enlightened, see Radich 2007.

43. See discussion in Demiéville 1985: 26–30.

44. See, for example, T. 747A: 562b–c, which promises "a long life without illness and a strong, robust body" as a reward for following the precepts, and freedom from illness for practicing compassion. Significantly, the text refers to the karmic results of one's actions with the metaphorical equivalents *fu* and *bao.* The therapeutic benefits of Buddhist practice are a significant focus of miracle tales and other Buddhist narratives (see Chapter 5). On Buddhist repentance rituals, see Kuo 1994, 1998; Yamabe 2005; Chappell 2005. For the Daoist context, see also Pei-yi Wu 1979; Masaaki 2002.

45. Demiéville 1985: 83–84.

46. See, e.g., T. 793, discussed below.

47. The *Lotus Sutra,* for example, warns in no uncertain terms that disparaging the faithful who venerate the text will lead to severe karmic consequences, including leprosy, physical deformities, malignant sores, and other afflictions (T. 262: 62a16–23; translated in Watson 1993a: 324). See similar threats mentioned in the Dunhuang manuscript *Sutra on Good and Bad Karmic Results* (*Shan'e yingguo jing,* T. 2881), as well as in the influential pseudotranslation from the mid-fifth century entitled the *Sutra of Trapuṣa and Bhallika* (*Tiwei boli jing*), translated in Tokuno 1994 (see especially pp. 305–6, but elsewhere as well).

48. See, e.g., T. 317: 890a18–20; T. 663: 351c26, 352a9–11; T. 665: 447c25–26; additional references and fuller discussion in Salguero 2010–11.

49. Some highlights in the extensive literature on winds in Chinese tradition include Kuriyama 1994; Unschuld 2003: 183–94; Chen Hsiu-fen 2005; Hsu 2007; Kleeman 2009. For India, see Zysk 2007.

50. This sutra is translated in Satiranjan Sen 1945 (cf. Unschuld 2010: 309–14). See discussion of its title in Introduction, note 42.

51. The medical sections of the Vinayas are found at T. 1421.3.7; T. 1425: 455a–457b; T. 1428.3.4; T. 1435.4.9.6; T. 1448. See discussion in Jaworski 1927; Tso 1980; Chen Ming 2008b.

52. T. 793: 737a25–27.

53. The terms "qi," "Heat," and "Cold" in this passage are likely to be translating the *tridoṣa*, but one cannot be certain in this case.

54. T. 793: 737b2–5.

55. T. 793: 737b6–14.

56. I borrow the term "transcreations" from Lal 1964.

57. Demiéville 1985: 14–18, 90.

58. Significantly, some of these Buddhist epithets were influential enough to be used outside of Buddhist circles. The title "King of Medicine," for example, is commonly used to refer to Sun Simiao and other famous physicians, as well as the legendary discoverer of the Chinese materia medica, the Divine Husbandman Shennong. The honorific "King of Physicians" was given to a number of heroes of classical Chinese medicine and was even adopted by emperors who fancied themselves models of compassion and charity—such as Emperor Fei (r. 566–68) of the Chen dynasty (Lee T'ao 1953: 314). On the history of the term "Medicine King" in China, see Chen Ming 2013: 43–56.

59. Healing rites are described in T. 449–451, T. 665.15, and most of the texts in the T. 867–1420 range cited in the references.

60. On the apparition of deities, see Campany 1993b; Bumbacher 2012: 142–43. Discussion of Buddhist visualization can be found in Yamabe 2005; *EBTEA*: 141–45.

61. T. 953: 297b9–10 (cited in Strickmann 1988: 40).

62. Many of these texts are collected in volume 20 of the *Taishō Tripiṭaka*. See discussion of Guanyin healing rituals in Strickmann 1996: 136–59; Yü 2001: 37–72; *EBTEA*: 94–99. See translations of Guanyin healing rites from T. 1059 in Satiranjan Sen 1945 (cf. Unschuld 2010: 314–21).

63. See, inter alia, T. 867, T. 895, T. 1097, T. 1200, T. 1202, T. 1248, T. 1277. Chinese Buddhist rituals of spirit possession and their textual sources are discussed in Strickmann 1990–91: 116–19, 1996: 213–14, 2002: 194–227; Edward L. Davis 2001: 115–52; Orzech 2011; *EBTEA*: 213–14, 251–54. Sections of T. 895 are translated in Strickmann 2002: 211–14. A comprehensive overview of Indian traditions of spirit possession can be found in Smith 2006.

64. Strickmann 1990–91: 117, 2002: 211; Edward L. Davis 2001: 123–24.

65. On this term, see Orzech 1998: 58; Sharf 2002: 118–19.

66. The best known of the Buddha-body doctrines is that of the "threefold body" (Ch. *sanshen*; Skt. *trikāya*). In this model a Buddha possesses a Dharma body (Ch. *fashen*; Skt. *dharmakāya*) synonymous with enlightenment itself, a reward body (Ch. *baoshen*; Skt. *saṃbhogakāya*) that resides in paradise, and a transformation or response body (Ch. *huashen*; Skt. *nirmāṇakāya*) by which he temporarily manifests in our world. See discussion of these terms and Buddha bodies more generally in Sharf 2002: 100–111, 119–24; Radich 2007; Boucher 2008: 3–19.

67. On the authorship of this text, see Yamabe 1999: 108–11; Greene 2012. See also Strickmann 2002: 119–22.

68. The *nāga* and *garuḍa* appear ubiquitously in Buddhist literature across Asia. The *nāga* (which the text translates as "dragon" [*long*]) is a mythic serpent that is often metaphorically equated with indigenous dragon lore. The *garuḍa* (translated in this source as "golden-winged bird" [*jinchi niao*] or "bird king" [*niaowang*]) is a gigantic bird-like spirit. Rawlinson 1986 argues that, in Indian Buddhism, *nāgas* are mainly representative of the Fire Element, and secondarily of Water. Lalou 1938 examines the extensive connections between *nāgas* and healing rites. On Indian healing traditions associated with *garuḍas*, see Slouber 2012.

69. T. 620: 334b–335a (translated in Greene 2012: 556–60).

70. T. 620: 334c21–22 (Greene 2012: 558).

71. See similar sequences in Robinet 1993: 55–96; Jane Huang 1987: 236–39; discussion in Shih-shan Susan Huang 2010. *Secret Essential Methods* is different from these Daoist depictions in that does not follow the logic of the Viscera, the Five Phases, or any other discernible indigenous system.

72. There has been considerable scholarly debate over the term "magic" in the Buddhist context. While theorists from inside and outside the Chinese sphere have stressed the term's pejorative connotations (e.g., Tambiah 1990; Burchett 2008; Bumbacher 2012: 179–86), many scholars of Chinese Buddhism have continued to characterize the techniques I mention in this section as magical (see, e.g., *EBTEA* 197–207). I have decided to use the terms "numinous" and "occult" instead, intending these not as rigorously defined analytical categories, but rather as everyday language that may elicit the preternatural and arcane aura surrounding these practices in medieval China.

73. See, e.g., the *dhāraṇī* taught by the Mother of Devil Children in the *Lotus Sutra*, which is explicitly approved by the Buddha in T. 262: 59b19–20 (translated in Watson 1993a: 310–11).

74. See, e.g., T. 1238, T. 1248, T. 1264B, T. 1265, T. 1277.

75. Harrison and Coblin 2012: 68. See discussions of the *dhāraṇī* literature in Strickmann 2002; McBride 2005; Mollier 2008; *EBTEA*: 176–80, 208–14; and works by Paul Copp cited in the references. As scholars have noted (Strickmann 2002: 103; Copp 2008b: 499), medieval Chinese sources do not obey the supposed distinction between spells and *dhāraṇīs*, nor do they make consistent distinctions between *dhāraṇīs* (i.e., the

ritually potent syllables particular to Buddhism) and mantras (i.e., the sacred pronouncements common to all Indian religions since the Vedic times).

76. *EBTEA*: 161. *Dhāraṇīs* do not play a major role in the first Chinese translation of the text in the third-century by Dharmarakṣa (T. 263), but do in the early fifth-century translation by Kumārajīva (T. 262: 58b–59b; translated in Watson 1993a: 307–11).

77. See titles listed in the 515 catalog by Sengyou (T. 2145: 31c12–21). Many of these spells are likely to be the same as those currently preserved in T. 1326–1329.

78. See T. 1028A–B, T. 1323–1325, T. 1691. Spells associated with the Master of Medicines Buddha appear in T. 449–451, T. 922–924. Additional spells texts for healing include T. 1043, T. 1059, T. 1136.

79. *EBTEA* 209.

80. See examples of therapeutic Buddhist talismans in, among other texts, T. 1229, T. 1238, T. 1265, T. 1307, T. 1420, T. 2904, T. 2906.See further discussion in Strickmann 1993, 1995, 2002: 132–78; Mollier 2008: 84–89, 123–32; Robson 2008; Copp 2008a; *EBTEA*: 225–29.

81. This formula appears as part of T. 1326, T. 1327, and T. 1329. The first part of the phrase featured in an exchange between Daoist polemicists and Buddhist apologists that was discussed in Chapter 2. It also is explained in an idiosyncratic domesticating translation in the *Sutra of Trapuṣa and Bhallika* (Tokuno 1994: 280).

82. See Overbey 2008; Copp 2012 on the hidden meanings of Chinese *dhāraṇīs*.

83. See van Gulik 1980: 52–53. This system, described in T. 880, has remained in use to contemporary times.

84. On the history of *siddhaṃ* in China, see van Gulik 1980; Chaudhuri 2011. Meanwhile, other authors developed arcane scripts for writing healing talismans based on Chinese characters (Robson 2008).

85. On these contradictory impulses in esoteric discourses, see Campany 2006, 2009: 88–129. On the sociology of secrecy, see also Alter 2009.

86. The pseudotranslation T. 905 (translated in White 2000: 370–80) does incorporate some indigenous Chinese medical knowledge into the esoteric ritual context, but this is now thought to be a Japanese rather than a Chinese composition (see Chen Jinhua 1998).

87. Copp 2008b.

88. Amoghavajra, predictably, does not use the metaphorical equivalent in his translation of T. 1323 and T. 1324. However, even he speaks of spells as *miyan* or *zhenyan*, which are domesticating translations that use ordinary Chinese terms meaning "esoteric words" and "true words" respectively.

89. Therapeutic *mudrās* are introduced in, e.g., T. 924A; T. 1097; T. 1265; T. 1277. See discussion and additional citations in Strickmann 2002; *EBTEA* 76–88.

90. Mollier 2008: 89–91; Robson 2008: 138. Alternative, less domesticating, explanations for the efficacy of *dhāraṇīs* are discussed in the writings of exegetes (Overbey 2008; Copp 2012), but to my knowledge such theorizing is not found in the healing *dhāraṇī* texts under discussion here.

91. See many examples in Mollier 2008.

92. Cf. Bagchi 1981: 217–46; Sujata Reddy 2002. This general perspective, and Bagchi's book in particular, is critiqued in Alter 2009.

CHAPTER 4

1. See discussion of such systems in Weinstein 1973: 283–91; Gregory 1991: 93–114; Ming-Wood Liu 1993; Mun 2006.

2. Biographical information is available in Ch'en 1964: 134–35; Paul 1984; Funayama 2008.

3. Zhiyi's life, ideas, and political connections are discussed in Hurvitz 1962; Weinstein 1973: 274–91; Chen Jinhua 1999.

4. Introductions to Jizang's life and his contributions to philosophy can be found in Chen Jinhua 1999; Ming-Wood Liu 1993.

5. See bibliographic details in Chen Jinhua 2004a.

6. T. 663.15. See discussion in Nobel 1951; English translation in Salguero 2013; translation of comparable chapter from the Sanskrit in Emmerick 2004: 75–80.

7. These are T. 1785 and T. 1787 respectively. As quotations are not always marked clearly in the compositions, I have had difficulties determining the original author of any given passage. Note also that, although I use the word "author" here for Zhiyi, several of his most well-known compositions, including this one, were in fact lectures that were transcribed by his disciple Guanding (561–632). While these frequently contain passages appropriated from other systematizing exegetes (such as, in this case, Paramārtha), scholars feel that they are still likely to reflect Zhiyi's ideas (Swanson 1997).

8. T. 1785: 80c–81a; T. 1787: 172a–b.

9. T. 1785: 81b15–18; T. 1787: 171c19–21.

10. The *Sutra on the Buddha as Physician* lists "eating what should not be eaten," "immoderate eating," and "eating contrary to custom" among the nine causes of untimely death (T. 793: 737b18–22). The latter is defined as eating excessive quantities of unfamiliar foods or eating familiar foods at unusual hours.

11. T. 1785: 81b17–20; T. 1787: 171c21–25. For specific food taboos leading to leprosy in medieval Chinese medical treatises, as well as the disease's regional associations, see Leung 2009: 57–59. Note that my translation of *lai* as "leprosy" is not meant to assert a connection between this condition and the modern category of Hansen's disease, but rather to bring out the moral and religious connotations of this severe skin condition. On medieval Chinese foodways more generally, see Engelhardt 2001; *SCC* 6.5: 116–48. North-South stereotypes in early Chinese medicine are discussed in Hanson 2011: 25–37.

12. T. 1785: 81c1–3; see similar passage at T. 1787: 172c9–11. Compare with *Inner Canon: Suwen* 3 (translated in Unschuld and Tessenow 2011: 71–73).

13. T. 1785: 81c10–11, 14–15; T. 1787: 172c14–15, 19.

14. T. 1785: 81a28–b3. Compare with *Inner Canon: Suwen* 2 and 42 (translated in Unschuld and Tessenow 2011: 45–57, 629).

15. T. 1785: 81b22–23; T. 1787: 172c7–9.

16. A detailed discussion of Zhiyi's medical thought is available in Yamano 1985; Huang Boyuan 2000; see also some brief comments in parts of Demiéville 1985; Birnbaum 1989a. The chapter of the treatise under consideration in this section is closely related to a similar chapter of Zhiyi's *A Step-by-Step Teaching for Understanding Dhyāna-Pāramitā* (*Shi chan boluomi cidi famen*, T. 1916). His most well-known work, *The Great [Treatise on] Śamatha and Vipaśyanā Meditation* (*Mohe zhiguan*, T. 1911), includes a section on medicine that is somewhat similar in structure and content to the text discussed here (T. 1911:106a–111c, translation by Paul Swanson forthcoming from Nanzan Institute for Religion and Culture).

17. This text is found in the *Taishō Tripitaka* under the title *Essentials of Practicing Śamatha and Vipaśyanā Meditation* (*Xiuxi zhiguan zuochan fayao*, T. 1915; medical content at 471b–472b). Sekiguchi (1954: 356–60) provides a critical edition based on the extensive comparison of early manuscripts (cited in Swanson 2007; translated in Salguero 2012). Either edition could be used to make the arguments I present in this section.

18. T. 1915: 471b12–20.

19. T. 1915: 471b20–29.

20. T. 1915: 471c13–15.

21. T. 1915: 471c15–17.

22. T. 1915: 471c20.

23. T. 1915: 471c23–24, loosely quoting T. 475: 545a17–20.

24. T. 1915: 471c26–472a1. Appearing as early as the second-century B.C.E. manuscripts from Mawangdui, healing syllables are a common feature of Chinese religiomedical literature. The Six Breaths are described in the writings of Chao Yuanfang and Sun Simiao, appear in multiple texts in the Daoist canon, and are found in Dunhuang manuscripts as well (Maspero 1981: 495–99; Despeux 1995, 2006; Strickmann 2002: 123–32; Sakade 2005: 281). The brief description of the Six Breaths in the *Taishō Tripitaka* version of Zhiyi's manual is followed by two interpolated lines of seven-character verses (T. 1915: 472a2–3) that are thought to possibly date from the Song (Despeux 2006: 50). The corresponding section of Sekiguchi 1954 is more detailed.

25. T. 1915: 472a04–7. While I have thus far been unable to find Indian terms matching all twelve of Zhiyi's techniques, many items in this list are recognizable translations of common Indian breathing practices, including *ujjāyī prāṇāyāma* ("upwards and retained breath exercise"), *nirvāṇa prāṇāyāma* ("dissipating breath exercise"), *śītalī* or *śītakārī prāṇāyāma* ("cooling breath exercise"), *bhastrikā prāṇāyāma* ("forced" or "bellows breath exercise"), *mūrchā prāṇāyāma* ("retained breath exercise"), and *anuloma prāṇāyāma* ("harmonizing breath exercise"). On the development of *prāṇāyāma* in Indian history, see Zysk 2007.

26. T. 1915: 472a8–13.

27. T. 1915: 472a13–16.

28. A note in the text says, "This is like what is explained in detail in the 'Seventy-two Secret Methods of Treating Illness' from the *Saṃyuktāgama*" (T. 1915: 472a15–16).

No such section of the *Saṃyuktāgama* (*Za ahan jing*, T. 99) exists, and I have been unable to find a detailed description of seventy-two methods of healing in any Āgama text. I conclude that Zhiyi's source for this healing technique is probably the *Secret Essential Methods for Treating the Maladies of Meditation*, which discusses meditations on the Four Elements extensively and also refers to the *Saṃyuktāgama* in its byline (T. 620: 333a10–11). See discussion in Greene 2012: 136–38.

    29. T. 1915: 472a16–17.

    30. T. 1915: 472a23–24.

    31. T. 1915: 472a29–472b13.

    32. T. 1915: 472a20–23. This passage does not appear in Sekiguchi's reconstruction. On grain avoidance practices, see Campany 2005a, 2005d, 2009: 62–88. For an example of the sort of syncretism this commentator is arguing against, see P. 2637 (discussed in Sakade 2005).

    33. Chen Ming 2005b: 107–25.

    34. Chen Jinhua 2002b.

    35. Tansen Sen 2001, 2003: 44–53.

    36. Forte 2002a.

    37. Adamek 2007; Yifa 2002.

    38. Biographical information and intellectual background in Satō 1986: 67–207; Chen Huaiyu 2007.

    39. Chen Huaiyu 2007: 159–62. See, e.g., T. 1804.18.

    40. This chapter has been examined in detail in Shinohara 2007. On the commentary more generally, see Satō 1986: 229–98.

    41. The first complete Chinese Vinaya, the *Vinaya in Ten Sections* of the Sarvāstivāda school (*Shisong lü*, T. 1435), was translated by Kumārajīva and Puṇyatāra in the first decade of the fifth century and proved to be the most important monastic code in the South during the Period of Division. The Dharmaguptaka Vinaya, or the *Four-Part Vinaya* (*Sifen lü,* T. 1428), translated a few years later by a team headed by the Kashmiri monk Buddhayaśas and the Chinese Zhu Fonian, became authoritative in the North and after reunification became the official code empire-wide. The Mahāsāṃghika Vinaya (*Mohesengqi lü*, T. 1425) translated by Faxian and Buddhabhadra in 416, the Mahīśāsaka Vinaya (*Mishasaibu hexi wufen lü*, T. 1421) translated by Buddhajīva and Daosheng in 423–24, and the Mūlasarvāstivāda Vinaya (*Genben shuoyiqieyoubu pinaiye*, T. 1442–1457) translated by Yijing in 703, all had more limited influence in China. A sixth Vinaya, that of the Kāśyapīya School, was only partially translated in 543 (T. 1460; cited in Funayama 2004: 97n2). Some scholars have additionally suggested that a translation of the Pāli Vinaya may have taken place in the fifth or sixth century (Zürcher 2012: 7n6; Heirman 2007: 190–92), although this has been debated. On the Chinese Vinaya, see Frauwallner 1956; Tso 1982; Yifa 2002: 5–7; Heirman 2007.

    42. T. 1804: 143a27–b6. The full narrative is located at T. 1428: 861b21–c10 (translated in Shinohara 2007: 107–8). See alternate version of the tale at T. 1425: 455a–457b. For a parallel story from the Mūlasarvāstivāda Vinaya, see Schopen 2004: 8. For the Pāli,

see discussion in Zysk 1998: 41; translation in Ṭhānissaro 2007: 54–57. See also a modified version of the tale that was incorporated into a Chinese translation of the *Dharmapāda* at T. 211: 591b9–c16. In some of these versions of the narrative, the Buddha orders an assistant to care for the monk instead of doing so himself.

43. T. 1804: 143b2, quoting T. 1428: 861c9–10.

44. T. 1804: 143b4–6.

45. T. 1804: 143b19–c3.

46. T. 1804: 143c8–12.

47. T. 1804: 143c19–20.

48. T. 1804: 143c20–144a9.

49. As Daoxuan's perspectives on these topics have been examined in detail in Shinohara 2007: 116–22, I will only briefly cover them here.

50. T. 1804: 144a13–27 (translated in Shinohara 2007: 108–9). Jetavana is one of the most important locations associated with the life of Śākyamuni Buddha. Just before his death, Daoxuan composed the *Illustrated Sutra of the Jetavana Monastery in Śrāvastī, Central India* (*Zhong tianzhu sheweiguo qihuansi tujing*, T. 1899), a fantastical description of the Indian monastery in large part based upon his own visionary experiences (translated in Tan 2002: 337ff.; discussed in Forte 1988: 39–52; Ho Puay-peng 1995; McRae 2005). An accompanying map of Jetavana is found in T. 1892 (redrawn in Ho Puay-peng 1995: 2–3).

51. T. 1804: 144a–145c.

52. Shinohara 1990, 1991: 203–24.

53. The two encyclopedias are discussed and outlined in Kawaguchi 1975; Teiser 1985.

54. Daoshi's other encyclopedia, *Collection of Essentials from the Scriptures* (*Zhujing yaoji*, T. 2123), presents similar medical perspectives. The chapter "Section on Sending Off the Dead" (*songzhong bu*) takes up all of the nineteenth fascicle (*juan*) of that text, but see especially the first five sections (T. 2123.29.1–5), which parallel the organization of *Forest of Pearls*. Scholars disagree on which encyclopedia was completed first. In this chapter I discuss the latter because of its greater length and influence.

55. T. 2122: 984a–c; cf. T. 2103: 309c–310a. (I thank Alexander O. Hsu, who is preparing a dissertation on *Forest of Pearls* that examines the range of Daoshi's sources in this chapter, for sharing this observation with me as well as the connection with Sun Simiao in note 57 and other details in this section.)

56. T. 2122: 987c–989c.

57. The only comment that mentions Chinese doctrines in any detail appears at T. 2122: 986a24–b2, in Daoshi's introductory remarks to the section on therapeutics. This passage appears to be quoting the biography of Sun Simiao, who is said to have been an acquaintance of Daoxuan's.

58. Some of the passages in the encyclopedia appear in the same order as they do in the Vinaya commentary, some of the language used in the encyclopedia's section titles are similar, and the decision to combine hospice and death practices along with healing and nursing is also derivative of the earlier commentary.

59. See discussion in Barrett 1998.

60. T. 2125: 224c (translation by Li Rongxi 2000: 125; see also Takakusu 1966).

61. T. 2125: 224c (Li Rongxi 2000: 126).

62. T. 2125: 224a–225a (Li Rongxi 2000: 121–27). See also Subba Reddy 1938.

63. T. 2125: 220c–221a (Li Rongxi 2000: 104). See also Devi 1979; Rao 1982; Heirman and Torck 2012: 27–66.

64. T. 2125: 209a (Li Rongxi 2000: 32–34). See discussion in Heirman and Torck 2012: 109–35. Similar practices in the Theravada Vinaya are discussed in Ṭhānissaro 2007: 7–8. The use of such plants for cleaning the teeth is still widespread in modern India (e.g., Farooqi and Srivastava 1968; Punjani 1998).

65. T. 2125: 207b (Li Rongxi 2000: 26). Cow dung, a sacred substance used in many purification rituals, was considered cleansing.

66. T. 2125: 208c–209a (Li Rongxi 2000: 34).

67. T. 2125: 218a–b (Li Rongxi 2000: 88–89). See discussion in Heirman and Torck 2012: 67–107.

68. T. 2125: 207a–208b, 221b–c (Li Rongxi 2000: 24–32, 107–8).

69. T. 2125: 225a (Li Rongxi 2000: 128). Yijing was surely aware of domestic critiques of the practice in China as well (see Ch'en 1964: 51).

70. On the use of "fermented urine medication" (*pūtimukta-bhaiṣajya*), see *Hōbōgirin* 4: 329a–335b; Ṭhānissaro 2007: 57–58. In the Pāli Vinaya, fermented urine is counted among the monk's four essential necessities along with food, robes, and shelter. Gombrich (2003: 100) posits that the rules requiring its use were never strictly enforced.

71. The equation between eyewitnessing and claims of authenticity is a well-worn trope dating back to the earliest layers of Buddhist literature. The classical opening phrase for the sutras, "thus have I heard" (Ch. *rushi wo wen*, or a similar combination of characters), frames the entire contents of the text as a report from a reliable source, who is claiming to have heard the Buddha's teaching on such-and-such an occasion (on this phrase, see Silk 1989; Lopez 1995; Zürcher 1996: 2). The eyewitness in the case of the sutra text is usually either Ānanda, the attendant of the Buddha celebrated as an having infallible memory, or a deity. While not possessing quite as lofty credentials, by characterizing himself as an eyewitness reporter of Indian Buddhist practice, Yijing was indeed claiming a unique status among his contemporaries as an arbiter of authenticity.

72. The description of medical facilities is located at T. 1899: 893c–894a; see references in note 50.

73. T. 1899: 882c–883b.

74. T. 2066: 6a15.

75. The literature is too vast to begin to cite adequately here, but I would be remiss not to mention Douglas 2005. Specifically on the Buddhist version of this "physiomoral discourse," see Mrozik 2007; Heirman and Torck 2012.

76. T. 665.24 (translated in Salguero 2013).

77. On Wu Zetian's mobilization of Buddhist ideology, see references in Chapter 1, note 68.

78. Didactic writings on Indic languages were not entirely new, some examples having been produced by well-known Chinese scholars and translators long before Huizhao's time. While little of the pre-Tang material has survived to the present day, the basic outline of this literature has been reconstructed from titles appearing in medieval Buddhist catalogs and excerpts quoted in Japanese Buddhist literature (van Gulik 1980: 12–36; Chaudhuri 2011: 16–53). The earliest text we know about is a treatise thought to be an exercise book on the *siddhaṃ* script listed in a fourth-century Buddhist catalog. Moving forward in time, the sources become more plentiful and the authors more well known: a text called the *Siddhaṃ Primer* (*Xitan zhang*) is attributed to Kumārajīva in the early fifth century; the famous poet Xie Lingyun (385–433) offered his reflections on Sanskrit and *siddhaṃ*; Paramārtha translated a Sanskrit dictionary in the late sixth century; even Emperor Wu of the Liang dynasty composed a commentary on Indian language. Such references hint that there was a certain amount of prestige associated with the study of the Indian script and language even in early medieval China.

79. van Gulik 1980: 22–24, 33–35; Chaudhuri 2011: 54–61. See also T. 2133, compiled by Yijing.

80. T. 1788: 325c2–5.

81. T. 1788: 325b22–24.

82. T. 1788: 325b27–c1, 325c26–29, 326a4–5.

83. T. 1788: 325b27–29.

84. T. 1788: 326a6–9.

CHAPTER 5

1. On narratives in South and Southeast Asian Buddhist traditions more generally, see Schober 1997 and essays in *JIABS* 33, nos. 1–2 (2010).

2. Benn 1998, 2007a, 2007b. For Indian precedents of these types of stories, see Ohnuma 2007.

3. Campany 1993b, 1996a; Shinohara 1998; Yü 2001: 151–94.

4. See Li and Dalia 2002; Young forthcoming; and citations in the section on hagiographies below.

5. Tsai 1994; Georgieva 1996; De Rauw 2005.

6. For accounts of the medical activities of early missionaries, see Fu and Ni 1996: 3–14.

7. Storch 1993; Nattier 2003: 58–59n11.

8. On medieval popular narratives in general, see the many publications cited in the references by Robert Ford Campany, upon whose methodological insights I have drawn extensively throughout this chapter. See also Gjertson 1978, 1981, 1989; Mair 1983; DeWoskin 1983; Shinohara 1994, 1998; Poo 1995, 2000; DeWoskin and Crump 1996; Lippiello 2001: 165–77; Bumbacher 2000; and literature cited elsewhere throughout this chapter.

9. Campany 1996b: 175–77, 2012b: 17–30.

10. Campany (2002: 93) states that healing is the chief means by which Daoist adepts assist the laity in Ge Hong's *Traditions of Divine Transcendents* (*Shenxian zhuan*). Tales focusing on the activities of popular spirit healers are introduced and translated in Lin 1994: 25–60. Healers also feature in other medieval collections translated in Mather 2002; DeWoskin 1983; Campany 2012b.

11. See Chapter 4, note 41.

12. See Rotman 2008: 27–30.

13. On the basis of the existing quotations, *Record of Signs* has been reconstructed and translated in Campany 2012b. See this particular narrative at T. 2059: 347a–b; T. 2122: 988a (translation and additional citations in Campany 2012b: 97–98).

14. Zysk 1998: 52–53, 151n9.

15. T. 1428: 850c–855a.

16. T. 553; T. 554; cf. T. 2121: 166c–170a.

17. The authorship of this text is discussed in Salguero 2009.

18. See discussion of Chinese representations of Jīvaka in Liu Mingshu 1996; Chen Ming 2005a: 77–97; Salguero 2009: 194–201.

19. On Jīvaka's trephination, see also Zysk 1993: 67–68, 1998: 120–21. On the appeal of the exotic in Chinese tales more generally, see Campany 2005c.

20. T. 553: 897c25; T. 554: 903a22–23.

21. Compare T. 553: 898a24–25 and T. 554: 903b3 with *Records of the Grand Historian* 105 (translated in Berkowitz 2005: 175).

22. T. 1428: 852a08–b08; further discussion in Salguero 2009: 198–99.

23. T. 1428: 853b26–854c10.

24. T. 2059: 388a–c (partially translated in Salguero 2010: 104–5); T. 2122: 491b–c (translated in Campany 2012b: 88–91).

25. Translated in Mair 1994: 688–96. See discussion of the Indian influence on the biography of Hua Tuo in Chen Yinke 1930; Demiéville 1985: 97–99; Lang 1986; Mair 1994: 688n1, 689n4, 696n22; Liu Mingshu 1996.

26. Chen Ming 2005a: 213ff., Salguero 2009: 209–10. See also Chen Ming 2001, 2003b.

27. Some scholars have objected to the use of the term "miracle" in the Buddhist context, although many others find it to be unobjectionable (see discussion in Robert L. Brown 1998; Gómez 2010). By electing to use this term, I do not mean to invoke Christian doctrine or connotations.

28. Maspero 1910; Ch'en 1964: 29–31; Tsukamoto 1985: 41–51; Nattier 2008: 35–37. See translations of versions of this story in Lippiello 2001: 187; Campany 2012b: 68. For various perspectives on dreams in Chinese culture, see essays in Carolyn T. Brown 1988; on medieval Chinese Buddhism in particular, see Strickmann 1988.

29. T. 2122: 988b18–27 (translated in Campany 2012b: 251–52). Other stories from the same source are preserved in T. 2122: 569a15ff.; T. 2110: 539c (translated in Campany 2012b: 219–20, 259, respectively).

30. From T. 2060: 680a21–27 (translated in Benn 2006: 456). On auto-cremation and self-immolation more generally, see Benn 1998, 2007a, 2007b. The Medicine King story is found at T. 262.23 (translated in Watson 1993a: 280–89); T. 263.21; 264.22.

31. *History of the Northern Dynasties* 84; T. 2122: 761b1–11 (discussed in Ning 2004: 35).

32. See discussion and an image of this implement in Demiéville 1985: 90.

33. See Wright 1954: 388–89; Verellen 1992; Chen Yuzhen 1993; Campany 1993b, 1996b: 322–23; discussion of historical belief in miracles in Campany 2009: 259–65.

34. Yü 2001: 75–7, 113–4. The chapter on Guanyin appears at T. 262.25 (translated in Watson 1993a: 298–306); T. 263.23; T. 264.24.

35. See examples in Yü 2001; Campany 1993b, 1996a, 2013: 49–51; Kieschnick 1997: 103–5.

36. See Strickmann 1996: 136–59; *EBTEA*: 94–99; texts collected in vol. 20 of the *Taishō Tripitaka*.

37. T. 2059: 350c16–a5; T. 2122: 998b7–17 (translated in Campany 2012b: 132–33). See discussions and translations of various versions of this story in Gjertson 1989: 18–19; Campany 1991b: 61n32, 1996a: 90; Yü 2001: 172–73; Salguero 2010: 101.

38. T. 2122: 988b9–12.

39. See, e.g., *Caraka* 8; *Suśruta* 4 (translated in Sharma 2007–8, 2004–5, respectively).

40. *Records of the Grand Historian* 105 (see Berkowitz 2005).

41. T. 2059: 386c28–387a1 (translated in Wright 1948: 366; discussed in Salguero 2009: 202–5).

42. See similar argument for hagiography in Campany 2012b: 2–3.

43. For episodes concerning healing, see Campany 2012b: entries 8, 12, 23, 24, 33, 67, 71, 87, 95, 100, 122, 126, 127, 129—most of which involve members of the sangha.

44. T. 2122: 987c–989c. Daoshi may have collaborated with Daoxuan in the compilation of these tales (see Shinohara 1990, 1991: 203–24).

45. See discussion of this series as a whole in Kieschnick 1997. For more detailed discussion of the medical episodes in the Liang hagiography, see Salguero 2010. My citations to the medical content in Daoxuan's collection in this section are largely drawn from Robin Beth Wagner 1995: 166–87; and Kieschnick 1997: 67–111. A Japanese translation of the Liang hagiography is available in Yoshikawa and Funayama 2009–10. For partial translations in Western languages, see Wright 1948; Shih 1968; Hirai 1992, 1993, 1994. Other medieval Buddhist hagiographic collections—such as the *Accounts of Biographies of Famous Monks* (*Mingseng zhuan chao*, X. 1523) and the *Biographies of Nuns* (*Biqiuni zhuan*, T. 2063) attributed to Baochang (d. 516), or the *Collected Records of Buddhist Miracles in China* (*Ji shenzhou sanbao gantong lu*, T. 2106) completed by Daoxuan in 664—also contain episodes that showcase the healing activities of the sangha. Subsequent additions to the *Biographies of Eminent Monks* series were authored in the Song and Ming dynasties, but, as these were written in the post-medieval period, they do not concern us here.

46. See discussion in Wright 1954: 408–29; Kieschnick 1997: 10–11; Campany 2012b: 19. Daoshi's sources are cited in his text immediately following each episode.

47. See Lefevere 1992 on compiling as strategic "rewriting."

48. See biographical sketch of Wang Yan and discussion of his motivations for compiling these narratives in Campany 2012b: 7–17. Both Huijiao and Daoxuan freely acknowledged the importance of thaumaturgy for proselytizing (Kieschnick 1997: 68). For a discussion of the persuasive strategies of medieval Chinese hagiography more generally, see Campany 2009: 216–58.

49. T. 2059: 323a26 (cf. T. 2145: 43b19–21; translated in Forte 1995: 68).

50. T. 2059: 350a15–22 (translated in Salguero 2010: 98–99).

51. T. 2059: 350a16–17 (translated in Salguero 2010: 98).

52. See examples of therapeutic spell casting at T. 2059: 336b11–13, 389a6–7, 392a8–10, 407b14–17; T. 2060: 652a29–b1; T. 2122: 491b–c (translated in Campany 2012b: 88–91); discussion in Kieschnick 1997: 84–87.

53. Salguero 2010: 96–97, 105–6. See T. 2059: 384b21–24 (translated in Wright 1948: 345–46).

54. Birnbaum 2004.

55. T. 2060: 655a7–10.

56. T. 2060: 668b3, 670b21–23, 673a8–10, 674a13–15. On the role of relics in medieval China, see Chen Jinhua 2002a, 2002b; Chen Huaiyu 2007: 57–92; Tansen Sen 2003: 57–76.

57. T. 2122: 988c8–989a8 (translated in Campany 2012b: 128–29). Stories of conversion as a result of, or precursor to, healing include T. 2059: 326a3–10 (discussed in Salguero 2010: 107; translated in Hirai 1993); T. 2059: 384b24–26 (translated in Wright 1948: 346); T. 2122: 453b (translated in Campany 2012b: 225); T. 2110: 539c (translated in Campany 2012b: 259). See additional stories about the healing effects of basic Buddhist practice cited in Chapter 2, notes 78–80, and throughout this chapter. For a discussion of the trope of travel to the underworld and subsequent revival from death, see Campany 1995.

58. T. 2122: 987c14–23.

59. T. 2059: 339b29–c3 (translated in Salguero 2010: 108).

60. Further discussion of the numinous powers of sutra chanting is found in Campany 1991b; Bumbacher 2012: 134–76.

61. T. 2060: 663a6–13.

62. T. 2060: 643a12–14.

63. T. 2059: 395b28–c1, 356c12–15 (translated in Salguero 2010: 101, 106–7).

64. T. 2060: 651b13–15.

65. T. 2059: 389b10–13 (translated in Salguero 2010: 102–3).

66. T. 2060: 669b29–c1. See also 669c27–28.

67. T. 2122: 987c17; T. 2059: 326a7–8.

68. T. 2059: 357a2–3.

69. T. 2122: 989a9–19.

70. On snake saliva as a poison in Chinese thought, see de Groot 1982: 5: 365; on snakes as healing agents, see 6: 106, 120. Specifically on the uses of snake for treatment of skin disease, see Leung 2009: 54. It is also probable that this episode is capitalizing on the positive associations of the *nāga*, the serpent-like Buddhist deities associated with Chinese dragon lore and healing powers (see Lalou 1938). We might also detect an oblique reference to ambergris, a medicinal substance known in China as "dragon spittle aromatic" (*longxian xiang*).

71. Examples of healing with such implements are given in Salguero 2010.

72. See Zürcher 1982a: 170–73. Teiser (1988: 4) calls this the sangha's "ascetic energy."

73. Bielenstein 1947; Durand 1960; Twitchett 1979b.

74. Zürcher 1982a: 164–65.

CONCLUSION

1. These historical events are discussed in Tansen Sen 2003; Beckwith 2009: 140–62.

2. On the Islamicization of the Silk Road, see Elverskog 2010.

3. See, e.g., Gregory 1991; Anderl 2011.

4. On the development of Chinese holy sites, see, e.g., Tansen Sen 2003: 76–86, 132–41; Robson 2009; Yü 2001: 353–406; Birnbaum 1986, 1989–90, 2004.

5. Tansen Sen 2003: 239.

6. Abramson 2008: 52–82. See, e.g., Han Yu's (768–824) famous "Memorial on the Buddha's Relic" (translated in Xiong 2005), written in 819. Han Yu was censured for this memorial, but it captured the changing sentiments of the post–An Lushan period. See another memorial critical of Buddhism dated 806 in Ch'en 1973: 191–92. See overview of the *guwen* movement in Bol 1992.

7. Weinstein 1987: 114–36. The statistic comes from p. 134.

8. Weinstein 1987: 131.

9. Ch'en 1973: 101.

10. The scope and impact of these translation projects are discussed in Jan 1966; Tansen Sen 2002, 2003: 102–41; Orzech 2006, 2012; Chaudhuri 2011: 48–51.

11. Hinrichs and Barnes 2013: 114. On the Song-era reforms discussed here, see also Scogin 1978; Goldschmidt 2001, 2005, 2006, 2007, 2009; Hinrichs 2011.

12. See examples in Fan Kawai 2005a; Harper 2010: 73–81.

13. See discussion of texts attributed to Jīvaka listed in the Song dynastic library catalog in Chen Ming 2001, 2003b, 2005a.

14. See, e.g., T. 219, T. 1330, T. 1691.

15. An example of this trend is the *Essentials for Buddhists* (*Shishi yaolan*; T. 2127: 306a–307b), a glossary written by the monk Daocheng in 1019. The section on caring for the sick in this composition recycles most of its citations from the Tang exegetes, while misquoting several passages.

16. Post-Tang texts on Buddhist medicine are collected in Shi and Li 2011. Other scholars (e.g., Strickmann 1978: 346–48; Yü 2001: 223–62; Anderl 2011; Skonicki 2011; Orzech 2012: 315) have shown that this trend is generalizable to arenas of Buddhist cultural production beyond healing.

17. Liu Shufen 2008; Huang Minzhi 2005.

18. Edward L. Davis 2001; Teiser 2009.

19. Chen Yünu 2008.

20. Yi-Li Wu 2000, 2010: 54–83.

21. C. Julia Huang 2009.

22. Foreign medical knowledge from other parts of Asia would become influential in later Chinese history (particularly under the foreign Yuan and Qing dynasties), but sustained efforts to import and translate Indian medicine would never be revived. For cross-cultural medical and pharmacological exchange after the Tang, see, e.g., Ma, Gao, and Hong 1993; Song 2001; Chen Ming 2007; Haidar 2008; Nappi 2009; Buell and Anderson 2010; articles in *Asian Medicine* 3, no. 2 (2007).

23. See, e.g., Unschuld 2010: 148–53; a similar position is implied in *SCC* 2: 425.

CHINESE
AND JAPANESE CHARACTERS

ajiatuo　阿迦陀

Amituo Fo　阿彌陀佛

amoluojia　阿摩洛迦

an　安

An Huize　安慧則

An Shigao　安世高

anfutuo　安浮陀

anmoluo　菴摩羅

aweishe　阿尾捨

awuluojia　阿無羅迦

Azhapoju　阿吒婆拘

bailian she　白蓮社

bao　報

Baochang　寶唱

baoshen　報身

bashu　八術

ben　本

Bian Que　扁鵲

bianhua　變化

bianhuashen　變化身

bibo　畢鉢

bing　病

bingku　病苦

bingku pian　病苦篇

bishou$_1$　筆受

bishou$_2$　閉手

boluoshequ　般羅奢佉

bore　般若

bujing guan　不淨觀

Bujing Jin'gang　不淨金剛

bukkyō igaku　仏教医学

butiao　不調

buxi　補息

Cao Zhi　曹植

chang　腸

Changjuli　常瞿利

Chao Yuanfang　巢元方

chimu　齒木

chixi　持息

chong 虫，蟲

chongxi　衝息

chu$_1$　出

chu$_2$　除

chuanyu　傳語

cuse　麁澀

da fashi　大法師

dantian　丹田

danuo　大儺

dao　道

Dao'an　道安

Daocheng　道誠

daoren　道人

Daoshi　道世

Daoxuan　道宣

daoyin　導引

dayi　大醫

di　地

diandao　顛倒

douxie　豆屑

duan　斷

duyu　度語

e'ren　惡人

fa　法

fahui　法會

famie　法滅

fangshi　方士

fangzhong shu　房中術

fannao　煩惱

fashen　法身

Faxian　法顯

Fazang　法藏

feibing　肺病

feizhen feiyou　非眞非有

feng　風

fengbing　風病

fengjie　風界

fo　佛

fo bingfang　佛病坊

Fo yiwang jing　佛醫王經

fojiao yixue　佛教醫學

foshuo　佛說

foyi　佛醫

Foyi jing　佛醫經

fu　福

fuyin　符印

fuzhou　符咒

gantong　感通

ganying　感應

ganying yuan　感應緣

gaoseng　高僧

Ge Hong　葛洪

geluoluo　歌羅邏

geyi　格義

gongyang　供養

Guanding　灌頂

Guangming Bianzhao Baozang　光明遍照寶藏

Guanshiyin　觀世音

gui　鬼

guizhu　鬼注

guobao　果報

guwen　古文

han　寒

hanbing　寒冰

he　和

He Danzhi　何澹之

helilejia　訶梨勒迦

hexi   和息
hua   化
Hua Tuo   華陀
huafo   化佛
huahu   化胡
huang   黃
Huangdi   黃帝
huashen   化身
Huiguo   惠果
Huijiao   慧皎
Huiyuan   慧遠
Huizhao   慧沼
huojie   火界
jiabei   加備
jiachi   加持
jiahu   加護
jia'na   伽那
jiang   漿
jianian   加念
jiaoxi   燋息
jiaozheng yishu ju   校正醫書局
jie   結
jiejie   結界
jinchi niao   金翅鳥
jing₁   經
jing₂   淨
jingshi   靜室
jinyao fangfa   進藥方法
Jiumoluoshi   鳩摩羅什
Jizang   吉藏
juan   卷
Juqu Jingsheng   沮渠京聲
Kang Falang   康法朗
Kang Senghui   康僧鎧, 康僧會
kong   空
ku   苦
lai   癩
leishu   類書
leng   冷

lengxi 冷息

li₁ 離

li₂ 痢

liangyao 良藥

lianlei 聯類

liao 療

Liao Zhu Fannao Bing 療諸煩惱病

ling 令

liuce 流廁

liufu 六腑

liushi 六時

liuwei 六味

liuzhong qi 六重氣

long 龍

Longmen 龍門

Longshu 龍樹

Longshu changnian zhi shu 龍樹長年之術

longtang 龍湯

longxian 龍涎

lunhui 輪廻

luocha 羅剎

mai, mo 脈

manxi 滿息

maokong 毛孔

Mawangdui 馬王堆

menggan 夢感

miaoyao 妙藥

miehuaixi 滅壞息

mijiao 密教

mingwang 明王

miyan 密言

moshi 末世

Moxishouluotian 魔醯首羅天

namo biqiuseng 南無比丘僧

namo fa 南無法

namo fo 南無佛

nanhai 南海

Nanshan lü zong 南山律宗

neizai 內災

ni 膩

niaowang 鳥王

nuanxi 煖息

nüe 瘧

panjiao 判教

pi 箆, 錍

pipidejia 仳仳得迦

Pishamen Tianwang 毘沙門天王

pusa 菩薩

Putiliuzhi 菩提流志

Puxian 普賢

qi 氣

qibao 七寶

qijie 七界

qilun 臍輪

qinggui 清規

Qipo 耆婆

Qipo fang 耆婆方

qishu 氣術

Qiyu 耆域

Rangwuli 穰麌梨

re 熱

ren 人

reqi 熱氣

ruo you yu gongyang wo zhe, ying gongyang bingren 若有欲供養我者應供養病人

rushi wo wen 如是我聞

ruyi zhu 如意珠

san dabing 三大病

san neizai 三內災

sandu 三毒

sanguo 三果

sanjiao 三焦

sanlun 三輪

sanshen 三身

sanxin 三辛

sanzang 三藏

seng 僧

sengjia 僧伽

Sengyai 僧崖

Sengyou　僧祐

Shangqing　上清

shangxi　上息

shanyou　善祐

shen　神

sheng₁　聖

sheng₂　盛

shengren bingfang yuan　聖人病坊院

shengzang　生藏

Shennong　神農

shenquan　神泉

shenshui　神水

shenyi₁　神醫

shenyi₂　神異

shenzhou　神呪, 神咒

Shi Chade　釋叉德

Shi Daoxian　釋道仙

Shi Hongman　釋洪滿

Shi Tanying　釋曇穎

shiben　失本

shibi　濕痺

shi'er xi　十二息

shijie　識界

shiqi　時氣

Shiyao, shiyao　施藥

shui　水

shuiguofei　水過肺

Shuihudi　睡虎地

shuijie　水界

shuzang　熟藏

sibing　四病

sida　四大

sidi　四諦

sijie　四界

Sima Qian　司馬遷

sizhong　四种

songzhong bu　送終部

sun　損

Sun Simiao　孫思邈

Taishō shinshū daizōkyō　大正新脩大藏經

taiyi shu　太醫署

tan　痰

Tanmochen　曇摩讖

tanyin　痰廦

Tao Hongjing　陶弘景

tian　天

tianming　天命

tianshen　天神

tianshi dao　天師道

tianshu　天書

tiantai zong　天台宗

tiantongzi　天童子

tianzhu　天竺

tiao　調

tujie　土界

tuo　脫

tuoluoni　陀羅尼

wang　妄

Wang Tao　王燾

wangxiang　妄想

wanwu　萬物

wei　胃

weidun　委頓

wen　文

wu　巫

wuchang yuan　無常院

Wuchushamo　烏芻沙摩

wujinzang　無盡藏

Wuliangshou Fo　無量壽佛

wuming　五明

Wushusemo　烏樞瑟摩

wuxing　五行

wuyi　巫醫

wuzang　五臟, 五藏

xi_1　覡

xi_2　息

xian　仙

xianchuang　癬瘡

xiantuo　涎唾

Xiao zhiguan　小止觀

xiaxi　下息

xie　邪

Xie Lingyun　謝靈運

Xiongnu　匈奴

xitan　悉曇

Xitan zhang　悉談章

xiuliang　休糧

xiyu　西域

Xuanzang　玄奘

xue　穴

xukongjie　虛空界

yan　驗

yangsheng　養生

yao　藥

yaoshang　藥上

yaoshi　藥師

Yaoshi Fo　藥師佛

yaowang　藥王

ye　業

yecha　夜叉

yefeng　業風

yi　醫

yichang　譯場

yifang　醫方

yihui　義會

Yijing　義淨

yin　淫

ying　應

yingshen　應身

yin-yang　陰陽

yiqie bing　一切病

yiwang　醫王

Yixing　一行

yiyao　醫藥

yiyi　義邑

yongzhong　癰腫

youpose　優婆塞

youpoyi 優婆夷

youtuona 優陀那

yu 愈

Yu Fakai 于法開

Yu Fu 俞跗

Yue Tianzi 月天子

Yuezhi 月氏 or 月支

yufang 浴坊

zeng 增

zengchangxi 增長息

zhanbing 瞻病

Zhang Ji 張機

Zhang Qian 張騫

Zhang Ying 張應

zhen 眞

Zhendi 眞諦

zheng 正

zhengfa 正法

zhenyan 眞言

zhi$_1$ 痔

zhi$_2$ 質

zhi$_3$ 治

zhibing 治病

zhiguai 志怪

Zhiguang 智廣

Zhisheng 智昇

Zhiyi 智顗

Zhiyue 支越

Zhongguo benchuan 中國本傳

Zhongshan 中山

zhou 呪, 咒

zhoujin boshi 咒禁博士

Zhu Fahu 竺法護

Zhu Fakuang 竺法曠

Zhu Falan 竺法蘭

Zhu Fayi 竺法義

Zhu Fonian 竺佛念

Zhu Fotucheng (also transcribed as Zhu Fotudeng) 竺佛圖澄

Zhu Lüyan 竺律炎

zhuanlun shengwan 轉輪聖王

$zhuyi_1$ 逐疫

$zhuyi_2$ 主譯

ziwei 滋味

zong 宗

zongchi 總持

zuo 左

REFERENCES

LIST OF TEXTS FROM THE *TAISHŌ TRIPITAKA*, BY REFERENCE NUMBER

In certain cases below, I have given the best-known title in English or Sanskrit rather than a full translation of the Chinese.

T. 26.30, *Xiangji yu jing* (*Sutra on the Simile of the Elephant Footprint*). Translated by Gautama Saṃghadeva, 397–98.

T. 26.98, *Nianchu jing* (*Sutra on the Bases of Mindfulness*). Translated by Gautama Saṃghadeva, 397–98.

T. 99, *Za ahan jing* (*Saṃyuktāgama*). Translated by Guṇabhadra, 435–43.

T. 150A, *Foshuo qichu sanguan jing* (*Sutra on the Seven Bases and Three Modes of Investigation*). Translated by An Shigao (fl. 148–70).

T. 211, *Faju piyu jing* (*Dharmapāda*). Translated by Dharmatrāta et al., ca. 290–306.

T. 219, *Foshuo yiyu jing* (*Sutra on the Medical Simile*). Translated by Dānapāla, late tenth century.

T. 245, *Foshuo renwang boreboluomi jing* (*Sutra on the Perfection of Wisdom for Benevolent Kings*). Unknown author, late fifth century. Translation misattributed to Kumārajīva (344–413).

T. 246, *Renwang huguo boreboluomiduo jing* (*Sutra on the Perfection of Wisdom for Benevolent Kings to Protect the Country*). Amoghavajra (705–74).

T. 262, *Miaofa lianhua jing* (*Lotus Sutra*). Translated by Kumārajīva, 406.

T. 263, *Zheng fahua jing* (*Lotus Sutra*). Translated by Dharmarakṣa, 286.

T. 264, *Tianpin miaofa lianhua jing* (*Lotus Sutra*). Translated by Jñānagupta and Dharmagupta, 601–2.

T. 278, *Da fangguang fo huayan jing* (*Flower Ornament Sutra*). Translated by Buddhabhadra et al., 418–20.

T. 279, *Da fangguang fo huayan jing* (*Flower Ornament Sutra*). Translated by Śikṣānanda, ca. 699.

T. 293, *Da fangguang fo huayan jing* (*Flower Ornament Sutra*). Translated by Prajñā, ca. 800.

T. 310.13, *Fo wei Anan shuo chutai hui* (*Sutra Spoken to Ānanda on Abiding in the Womb*). Translated by Bodhiruci, 703–13.

T. 310.14, *Foshuo ru taizang hui* (*Sutra on Entering the Womb*). Translated by Yijing, 710.

T. 310.16, *Pusa jianshi hui* (*Sutra on the Bodhisattva's Perception of Truth*). Translated by Narendrayaśas (517–89).

T. 317, *Foshuo baotai jing* (*Sutra on the Embryo*). Translated by Dharmarakṣa, 281 or 303.

T. 374, *Da banniepan jing* (*Mahāparinirvāṇa-sūtra*). Translated by Dharmakṣema, ca. 421.

T. 375, *Da banniepan jing* (*Mahāparinirvāṇa-sūtra*). Translated by Huiyan (363–443) et al.

T. 449, *Foshuo Yaoshi rulai benyuan jing* (*Sutra on the Master of Medicines Buddha*). Compiled by Dharmagupta, 615.

T. 450, *Yaoshi liuli guang rulai benyuan gongde jing* (*Sutra on the Master of Medicines Buddha*). Translated by Xuanzang, 650.

T. 451, *Yaoshi liuli guang qifo benyuan gongde jing* (*Sutra on the Master of Medicines Buddha*). Translated by Yijing, 707.

T. 474, *Foshuo Weimojie jing* (*Vimalakīrti Sutra*). Translated by Zhi Qian, 223–28.

T. 475, *Weimojie suoshuo jing* (*Vimalakīrti Sutra*). Translated by Kumārajīva (344–413).

T. 476, *Shuo Wugoucheng jing* (*Vimalakīrti Sutra*). Translated by Xuanzang in 650.

T. 553, *Foshuo Nainü Qiyu yinyuan jing* (*Āmrapālī and Jīvaka Avadāna Sutra*). Unknown author, fifth century. Translation misattributed to An Shigao (fl. 148–70).

T. 554, *Foshuo Nainü Qipo jing* (*Āmrapālī and Jīvaka Sutra*). Unknown author, fifth century. Translation misattributed to An Shigao (fl. 148–70).

T. 606, *Xiuxing daodi jing* (*Sutra on the Stages of the Path of Cultivation*). Translated by Dharmarakṣa, 284.

T. 607, *Daodi jing* (*Sutra on the Stages of the Path [of Cultivation]*). Translated by An Shigao (fl. 148–70).

T. 620, *Zhi chanbing miyao fa* (*Secret Essential Methods for Treating the Maladies of Meditation*). Juqu Jingsheng, 455.

T. 663, *Jin guangming jing* (*Sutra of Golden Light*). Translated by Dharmakṣema, 414–21.

T. 664, *Hebu jin guangming jing* (*Sutra of Golden Light*). Compiled by Baogui, 597.

T. 665, *Jin guangming zuisheng wang jing* (*Sutra of Golden Light*). Translated by Yijing, 703.

T. 701, *Foshuo wenshi xiyu zhongseng jing* (*Sutra on Bathing the Sangha in the Bathhouse*). Translated by Dharmarakṣa (ca. 233–311), misattributed to An Shigao.

T. 747A, *Foshuo zuifu baoying jing* (*Sutra on the Retribution of Sins and Merits*). Translated by Guṇabhadra, 435–43.

T. 793, *Foshuo foyi jing* (*Sutra on the Buddha as Physician*). Translated by Zhu Lüyan and Zhiyue, after 230.

T. 867, *Jin'gangfeng louge yiqie yujia yuqi jing* (*Sutra on All the Yogas and Yogins of the Pavilion of Vajra Peak*). Translation attributed to Vajrabodhi (671–741).

T. 880, *Yujia jin'gangding jing shi zimu pin* (*Explanation of the Script in the Yoga Vajraśekhara Sutra*). Amoghavajra (705–74).

T. 895, *Supohu tongzi qingwen jing* (*Sutra on the Questions of the Youth Subāhu*). Translated by Śubhakarasiṃha (637–735).

T. 901, *Tuoluoni ji jing* (*Dhāraṇī Compilation*). Compiled by Atigupta, 654.

T. 905, *Sanzhong xidi po diyu zhuan yezhang chu sanjie mimi tuoluoni fa* (*Ritual of the Secret Dhāraṇī of the Three Siddhis for the Destruction of Hell, the Transformation of Karmic Hindrances, and Liberation from the Three Conditioned Worlds*). Possibly authored by Annen (841–915?), translation misattributed to Śubhakarasiṃha (637–735).

T. 922, *Yaoshi liuliguang rulai xiaozai chu'nan niansong yigui* (*Ritual Procedure for Recitation to the Master of Healing, the Lapis Lazuli Radiance Tathāgata, for Eliminating Disaster and Escaping Hardships*). Yixing (684–727).

T. 923, *Yaoshi rulai guanxing yigui fa* (*Ritual Procedure for Contemplation of the Master of Healing Tathāgata*). Vajrabodhi (671–741).

T. 924A–B, *Yaoshi rulai niansong yigui* (*Ritual Procedure for Recitation to the Master of Healing Tathāgata*). Amoghavajra (705–74).

T. 953, *Yizi qite foding jing* (*Sutra on the Buddha's Wondrous Uṣṇīṣa in One Syllable*). Translated by Amoghavajra (705–74).

T. 1028A, *Foshuo hu zhu tongzi tuoluoni jing* (*Dhāraṇī for the Protection of All Children*). Translated by Bodhiruci (d. 727).

T. 1028B, *Tongzi jing niansong fa* (*Method of Recitation of the Sutra on the [Dhāraṇī for the Protection of All] Children*). Translated by Śubhakarasiṃha (637–735).

T. 1043, *Qing Guanshiyin pusa xiaofu duhai tuoluoni zhoujing* (*Sutra of the Dhāraṇī Spell to Ask Guanyin Bodhisattva to Absorb Poisons*). Translated by Zhu Nanti (fl. ca. 419).

T. 1059, *Qianshou qianyan Guanshiyin pusa zhibing heyao jing* (*Sutra on the Use of Medicinal Herbs for Healing Illness by the Thousand-eyes, Thousand-hands Avalokiteśvara*). Translated by Bhagavatdharma, Tang.

T. 1097, *Bukongjuansuo tuoluoni Zizai wang zhoujing* (*Sutra on the Dhāraṇī of the Unerring Net of Avalokiteśvara*). Translated by Maṇicintana (d. 721).

T. 1136, *Foshuo yiqie zhu rulai xin guangming jiachi Puxian pusa yanming jin'gang zuisheng tuoluoni jing* (*Sutra on Samantabhadra's Adamantine and Superlative Dhāraṇī for Prolonging the Life Span, a Radiant Blessing Bestowed from the Hearts of All the Buddhas*). Translated by Amoghavajra (705–74).

T. 1161, *Foshuo guan Yaowang Yaoshang er pusa jing* (*Sutra on the Contemplation of the Two Bodhisattvas King of Medicine and Supreme Medicine*). Translated by Kālayaśas (fl. 424–42).

T. 1200, *Dilisanmeiye budongzun weinu wang shizhe niansong fa* (*Recitation Method for the Trisamaya of the Envoys of the Wrathful King Āryācalanātha*). Amoghavajra (705–74).

T. 1202, *Budong shizhe tuoluoni mimi fa* (*Secret Methods of the Dhāraṇī of the Messengers of Āryācalanātha*). Vajrabodhi (671–741).

T. 1229, *Huiji jin'gang jin baibian fa jing* (*Sutra on Ucchuṣma's Rite for the Exorcism of One Hundred Transformations*). Translated by Ajitasena, 732.

T. 1238, *Azhaboju guishen dajiang shangfo tuoluoni jing* (*Sutra of the Supremely Enlightened Dhāraṇī of Āṭavika the Demon General*). Unknown authorship.

T. 1248, *Beifang Pishamen tianwang suijun hufa zhenyan* (*Mantra for Protection of the Northern King Vaiśravaṇa, Whom Armies Follow*). Translated by Amoghavajra (705–74).

T. 1264B, *Foshuo Rangwuli tongnü jing* (*Sutra on the Maiden Jāṅgulī*). Translated by Amoghavajra (705–74).

T. 1265, *Foshuo Changjuli dunü tuoluoni zhoujing* (*Sutra on the Dhāraṇī Spell for Jāṅgulī the Poison Woman*). Translated by Quduo, Tang dynasty.

T. 1277, *Suji liyan Moxishouluotian shuo aweishe fa* (*The Rapid and Efficacious Āveśa Method Explained by Maheśvāra*). Translated by Amoghavajra (705–74).

T. 1307, *Foshuo beidou qixing yanming jing* (*Sutra on the Extension of the Life Span by the Seven Stars of the Northern Dipper*). Attributed to "an Indian monk," Tang.

T. 1323, *Chu yiqie jibing tuoluoni jing* (*Sutra on the Dhāraṇī to Eliminate All Illnesses*). Translated by Amoghavajra (705–74).

T. 1324, *Nengjing yiqie yan jibing tuoluoni jing* (*Sutra on the Dhāraṇī That Can Clear Up All Eye Ailments*). Translated by Amoghavajra (705–74).

T. 1325, *Foshuo liao zhibing jing* (*Sutra on the Treatment of Sores*). Translated by Yijing (635–713).

T. 1326, *Foshuo zhou shiqi bing jing* (*Sutra on the Spell for the Illness of Seasonal Qi*). Uncertain authorship, possibly Zhu Tanwulan (fl. 381–395).

T. 1327, *Foshuo zhou chi jing* (*Sutra on the Spell for the Teeth*). Translated by Zhu Tanwulan (fl. 381–95).

T. 1328, *Foshuo zhou mu jing* (*Sutra on the Spell for the Eyes*). Uncertain authorship, possibly Zhu Tanwulan (fl. 381–395).

T. 1329, *Foshuo zhou xiaoer jing* (*Sutra on the Spell for Children*). Uncertain authorship, possibly Zhu Tanwulan (fl. 381–395).

T. 1330, *Luomona shuo jiuliao xiaoer jibing jing* (*Sutra on the Cure of Childhood Illnesses Spoken by Rāvaṇa*). Translated by Faxian (d. 1001).

T. 1331, *Foshuo guanding qiwanerqian shenwang hu biqiu zhou jing* (*Sutra on the Consecration of 72,000 Devas for Protection of the Sangha*). Attributed to Śrīmitra, 317–22, probably compiled ca. 457.

T. 1332, *Qifo bapusa suoshuo da tuoluoni shenzhou jing* (*Sutra of the Great Dhāraṇī Spirit Spells Spoken by the Seven Buddhas and Eight Bodhisattvas*). Unknown authorship, late fourth to early fifth centuries.

T. 1336, *Tuoluoni zaji* (*Collection of Miscellaneous Dhāraṇī*). Unknown authorship, first half of the sixth century.

T. 1420, *Longshu wuming lun* (*Nāgārjuna's Treatise on the Five Sciences*). Unknown authorship. Translation attributed to Nāgārjuna and Aśvaghoṣa.

T. 1421, *Mishasaibu hexi wufen lü* (*Mahīśāsaka Vinaya*). Translated by Buddhajīva and Daosheng, 423–24.

T. 1425, *Mohesengqi lü* (*Mahāsāṃghika Vinaya*). Translated by Buddhabhadra and Faxian, 416.

T. 1428, *Sifen lü* (*Dharmaguptaka Vinaya*). Translated by Buddhayaśas and Zhu Fonian, 408–13.

T. 1435, *Shisong lü* (*Sarvāstivāda Vinaya*). Translated by Puṇyatāra and Kumārajīva, 404–6.

T. 1448, *Genben shuoyiqieyoubu pinaiye yaoshi* (*Mūlasarvāstivāda Vinaya: Medical Matters*). Translated by Yijing, 703.

T. 1451, *Genben shuoyiqieyoubu pinaiye zashi* (*Mūlasarvāstivāda Vinaya: Miscellaneous Matters*). Translated by Yijing, 703.

T. 1460, *Jietuo jie jing* (*Sutra of the Liberating Precepts*). Translated by Gautama Prajñāruci, 543.

T. 1508, *Ahan koujie shier yinyuan jing* (*Sutra on the Oral Explanation of the Twelve Causal Links in the Agamas*). An Shigao (fl. 148–70). Misattributed to Anxuan and Yan Fotiao (both of the Later Han).

T. 1509, *Dazhi du lun* (*Mahāprajñāpāramitā-śāstra*). Translated by Kumārajīva (344–413).

T. 1558, *Apidamo jushe lun* (*Abhidharmakośa-bhāṣya*). Translated by Xuanzang, 651–54.

T. 1579, *Yujia shidi lun* (*Yogācārabhūmi-śāstra*). Translated by Xuanzang, 646–48.

T. 1648, *Jietuo dao lun* (*Vimuttimagga*). Translated by Saṃghabhara, 515.

T. 1691, *Jiaye xianren shuo yi nüren jing* (*Sutra on Women's Medicine Spoken by the Sage Kāśyapa*). Translated by Faxian (d. 1001).

T. 1785, *Jin guangming jing wenju* (*Commentary on the Sutra of Golden Light*). Spoken by Zhiyi (538–97), transcribed by Guanding (561–632).

T. 1787, *Jin guangming jing shu* (*Commentary on the Sutra of Golden Light*). Jizang (549–623).

T. 1788, *Jin guangming zuisheng wang jing shu* (*Commentary on the Sutra of Golden Light*). Huizhao, 703–14.

T. 1793, *Wenshi jing yiji* (*Commentary on the Sutra on Saunas [and Baths of the Sangha]*). Shi Huiyuan (523–92).

T. 1804, *Sifenlü shanfan buque xingshi chao* (*Emended Commentary on Monastic Practices from the Dharmaguptaka Vinaya*). Daoxuan, 626–30.

T. 1892, *Guanzhong chuangli jietan tujing* (*Illustrated Sutra on the Construction of Ordination Platforms*). Daoxuan (596–667).

T. 1899, *Zhong tianzhu sheweiguo qihuansi tujing* (*Illustrated Sutra of the Jetavana Monastery in Śrāvastī, Central India*). Daoxuan (596–667).

T. 1911, *Mohe zhiguan* (*Great [Treatise on] Śamatha and Vipaśyanā Meditation*). Spoken by Zhiyi (538–97), transcribed by Guanding (561–632).

T. 1915, *Xiuxi zhiguan zuochan fayao* (*Essentials of Practicing Śamatha and Vipaśyanā Meditation*). Zhiyi, 575–85.

T. 1916, *Shi chan boluomi cidi famen* (*A Step-by-Step Teaching for Understanding Dhyāna-Pāramitā*). Spoken by Zhiyi (538–97). Transcribed by Fashen, edited by Guanding (561–632).

T. 2043, *Ayuwang jing* (*King Aśoka Sutra*). Translated by Saṃghabhara, 512.

T. 2047A–B, *Longshu pusa zhuan* (*Biography of Nāgārjuna Bodhisattva*). Translated by Kumārajīva, 402–12.

T. 2059, *Gaoseng zhuan* (*Biographies of Eminent Monks*). Compiled by Huijiao, ca. 530.

T. 2060, *Xu gaoseng zhuan* (*Continued Biographies of Eminent Monks*). Compiled by Daoxuan, 645.

T. 2063, *Biqiuni zhuan* (*Biographies of the Nuns*). Compilation attributed to Baochang (d. 516).

T. 2066, *Datang xiyu qiufa gaoseng zhuan* (*Tang Dynasty Biographies of Eminent Monks Who Traveled to the West Seeking the Dharma*). Yijing, 691.

T. 2103, *Guang hongming ji* (*Expanded Hongming ji*). Compiled by Daoxuan (596–667).

T. 2106, *Ji shenzhou sanbao gantong lu* (*Collected Records of Buddhist Miracles in China*). Compiled by Daoxuan (596–667).

T. 2110, *Bianzheng lun* (*On the Discernment of the Correct*). Compiled by Falin (572–640).

T. 2121, *Jinglü yixiang* (*Diverse Attributes of the Sutras and Vinayas*). Compiled by Baochang (d. 516).

T. 2122, *Fayuan zhulin* (*Forest of Pearls in the Garden of the Dharma*). Compiled by Daoshi, 668.

T. 2123, *Zhujing yaoji* (*Collection of Essentials from the Scriptures*). Compiled by Daoshi, ca. 659.

T. 2125, *Nanhai jigui neifa zhuan* (*Records of Buddhist Practices Sent Home from the Southern Seas*). Yijing, 691.

T. 2127, *Shishi yaolan* (*Essentials for Buddhists*). Compiled by Daocheng, 1019.

T. 2131, *Fanyi mingyi ji* (*Compilation of Explanations of Translated Buddhist Terms*). Compiled by Fayun, 1143.

T. 2132, *Xitan zi ji* (*An Explanation of Siddhaṃ Letters*). Zhiguang, before 806.

T. 2133, *Fanyu qianzi wen* (*Sanskrit Reader of One Thousand Characters*). Yijing, early eighth century.

T. 2145, *Chu sanzang jiji* (*Compilation of Notices on the Production of the Tripitaka*). Sengyou, 515.

T. 2154, *Kaiyuan shijiao lu* (*Kaiyuan-Era Catalog of Buddhist Teachings*). Compiled by Zhisheng, 730.

T. 2780, *Wenshi jing shu* (*Commentary on the Sutra on Saunas [and Baths of the Sangha]*). Huijing, seventh century, Dunhuang manuscript.

T. 2865, *Hu shenming jing* (*Sutra on Protection of the Life Span*). Unknown authorship, Dunhuang manuscript.

T. 2866, *Hu shenming jing* (*Sutra on Protection of the Life Span*). Unknown authorship, Dunhuang manuscript.

T. 2878, *Foshuo jiuji jing* (*Sutra on Deliverance from Disease*). Unknown authorship, Dunhuang manuscript.

T. 2881, *Shan'e yingguo jing* (*Sutra on Good and Bad Karmic Results*). Unknown authorship, Dunhuang manuscript.

T. 2904, *Qiqian fo shenfu jing* (*Sutra on the Spirit Talismans of the Seven-Thousand Buddhas*). Unknown authorship, Dunhuang manuscript.

T. 2906, *Sanwanfo tonggen shenmi zhi yin bing fa longzhong shangzun wangfo fa* (*Mañjuśrī's Methods for the Numinous Secret Seals and Rites of the Combined Faculties of Thirty-Thousand Buddhas*). Unknown authorship, Dunhuang manuscript.

T. 2916, *Quanshan jing* (*Sutra Urging Goodness*). Unknown authorship, Dunhuang manuscript.

OTHER HISTORICAL TEXTS

Aṣṭāṅgahṛdaya-saṃhitā (*Heart of Medicine*). Vāgbhaṭa, ca. 600. Translated in Murthy 2012.

Beiji qianjin yaofang (*Essential Formulas Worth a Thousand in Gold for Every Emergency*). Sun Simiao, 650–59. Taipei: Zhongguo yiyao yanjiusuo, 1990 (in *HDW*). Partially translated in Wilms 2008.

Beishi (*History of the Northern Dynasties*). Li Yanshou, 659. Taipei: Dingwen shuju, 1980 (in *HDW*).

Bencao shiyi (*Supplement to the Materia Medica*). Chen Zangqi, 739. Hehui: Anhui kexue jishu chubanshe, 2003.

Buji zhou hou fang (*Supplement to the Formulas to Keep Up One's Sleeve*). Tao Hongjing (456–536). Hefei: Anhui kexue jishu chubanshe, 1983.

Caraka-saṃhitā (*Compendium of Caraka*). Compilation attributed to Caraka, by 200 C.E. Translated in Sharma 2007–8.

Fojia bigu fang (*Buddhist Formulas for Grain Avoidance*). Unknown authorship. Dunhuang manuscript, P. 2637.

Haiyao bencao (*Overseas Materia Medica*). Li Xun, ninth to tenth centuries. Beijing: Renmin weisheng chubanshe, 1997.

Houhan shu (*Records of the Later Han*). Fan Ye, 445. Taipei: Dingwen shuju, 1981 (in *HDW*).

Hu bencao (*Foreign Materia Medica*). Zheng Qian, ca. 875. No longer extant.

Huangdi neijing (*Inner Canon of the Yellow Emperor*). Authorship unknown, first century B.C.E. Translated in Unschuld and Tessenow 2011.

Mingxiang ji (*Records of Signs from the Unseen Realm*). Wang Yan, ca. 490. Reconstructed and translated in Campany 2012b.

Sanguo zhi (*Records of the Three Kingdoms*). Chen Shou, 297. Taipei: Dingwen shuju, 1980 (in *HDW*).

Shanghan lun (*Treatise on Cold Damage*). Zhang Ji, 196–220. Translated in Mitchell, Ye, and Wiseman 1999.

Shennong bencao jing (*Materia Medica of the Divine Husbandman*). Unknown authorship, first to second century. Taipei: Xueyuan chubanshe, 1995 (in *HDW*).

Shenxian zhuan (*Traditions of Divine Transcendents*). Ge Hong, ca. 317. Reconstructed and translated in Campany 2002.

Shiji (*Records of the Grand Historian*). Sima Qian, 104–87 B.C. Taipei: Dingwen shuju, 1981 (in *HDW*). Partially translated in Watson 1993b.

Shishuo xinyu (*A New Account of Tales of the World*). Compiled by Liu Yiqing (403–44). Translated in Mather 2002.

Suishu (*Record of the Sui Dynasty*). Wei Zheng, 636. Taipei: Dingwen shuju, 1980 (in *HDW*).

Suśruta-saṃhitā (*Compendium of Suśruta*). Compilation attributed to Suśruta, by fifth century C.E. Translated in Sharma 2004–5.

Waitai miyao (*Secret Essentials from the Imperial Library*). Wang Tao, 752. Beijing: Huaxia chubanshe, 1993.

Xinxiu bencao (*Newly Revised Materia Medica*). Su Jing, 650–59. Hehui: Anhui kexue jishu chubanshe, 2005.

Zhenghe shengji zonglu (*Comprehensive Records of Sagely Benefaction from the Zhenghe Reign Period*). Shen Fu et al., 1122. Taipei: Xinwen fang, 1978.

Zhubing yuan hou lun (*Treatise on the Origins and Symptoms of Disease*). Chao Yuanfang, 610. Beijing: Renmin weisheng chubanshe, 1996 (in *HDW*).

MODERN SOURCES

Abramson, Marc S. 2008. *Ethnic Identity in Tang China*. Philadelphia: University of Pennsylvania Press.

Adamek, Wendi Leigh. 2007. *The Mystique of Transmission: On an Early Chan History and Its Contexts*. New York: Columbia University Press.

Ågren, Hans. 1986. "Chinese Traditional Medicine: Temporal Order and Synchronous Events." In J. T. Fraser, N. Lawrence, and F. C. Haber (eds.), *Time, Science, and Society in China and the West*. Amherst: University of Massachusetts Press.

Alter, Joseph. 2009. "Yoga in Asia—Mimetic History: Problems in the Location of Secret Knowledge." *Comparative Studies of South Asia, Africa and the Middle East* 29 (2): 213–29.

Anderl, Christoph. 2011. "Coming to Terms with Terms: The Rhetorical Function of Technical Terms in Chán Buddhist Texts." In Christoph Anderl (ed.), *Zen Buddhist Rhetoric in China, Korea, and Japan*. Leiden: Brill.

Aravamudan, Srinivas. 2006. *Guru English: South Asian Religion in a Cosmopolitan Language*. Princeton, N.J.: Princeton University Press.

Arthur, Shawn. 2009. "Eating Your Way to Immortality: Early Daoist Self-Cultivation Diets." *Journal of Daoist Studies* 2: 32–63.

Asad, Talal. 1986. "The Concept of Cultural Translation in British Anthropology." In J. Clifford and G. E. Marcus (eds.), *Writing Culture: The Poetics and Politics of Ethnography*. Berkeley: University of California Press.

Assandri, Friederike. 2009. "Inter-religious Debate at the Court of the Early Tang: An Introduction to Daoxuan's *Ji gujin Fo Dao lunheng*." In Friederike Assandri and

Dora Martins (eds.), *From Early Tang Court Debates to China's Peaceful Rise*. Amsterdam: Amsterdam University Press.

Bachmann-Medick, Doris. 2006. "Meanings of Translation in Cultural Anthropology." In Theo Hermans (ed.), *Translating Others*. Manchester: St. Jerome.

Bagchi, Prabodh Chandra. 1981. *India and China: A Thousand Years of Cultural Relations.* Calcutta: Saraswat Library.

Baker, Mona. 1992. *In Other Words: A Coursebook on Translation*. London: Routledge.

Barrett, T. H. 1998. "China and the Redundancy of the Medieval." *Medieval History Journal* I (1): 73–89.

———. 2001. "Stūpa, Sūtra, and Śarīra in China, c. 656–706 CE." *Buddhist Studies Review* 18 (1): 1–63.

———. 2007. "Climate Change and Religious Response: The Case of Early Medieval China." *Journal of the Royal Asiatic Society* 17 (2): 139–56.

Bechert, Heinz. 1991. "Methodological Considerations Concerning the Language of the Earliest Buddhist Tradition." *Buddhist Studies Review* 8 (1–2): 3–20.

Beckwith, Christopher I. 2009. *Empires of the Silk Road: A History of Central Eurasia from the Bronze Age to the Present*. Princeton, N.J.: Princeton University Press.

Bellos, David. 2011. *Is That a Fish in Your Ear? Translation and the Meaning of Everything.* New York: Faber and Faber.

Benn, James A. 1998. "Where Text Meets Flesh: Burning the Body as an Apocryphal Practice in Chinese Buddhism." *History of Religions* 37 (4): 295–322.

———. 2006. "Written in Flames: Self-Immolation in Sixth-Century Sichuan." *T'oung Pao* 92: 410–65.

———. 2007a. *Burning for the Buddha: Self-Immolation in Chinese Buddhism*. Honolulu: University of Hawai'i Press.

———. 2007b. "Spontaneous Human Combustion: Some Remarks on a Phenomenon in Chinese Buddhism." In Phyllis Granoff and Koichi Shinohara (eds.), *Heroes and Saints: The Moment of Death in Cross-cultural Perspectives*. Newcastle: Cambridge Scholars Publishing.

Benn, James A., Lori Rachelle Meeks, and James Robson. 2010. *Buddhist Monasticism in East Asia: Places of Practice*. London: Routledge.

Berg, Daria. 2002. *Carnival in China: A Reading of the Xingshi Yinyuan Zhuan*. Leiden: Brill.

Berkowitz, Alan J. 2000. *Patterns of Disengagement: The Practice and Portrayal of Reclusion in Early Medieval China*. Stanford, Calif.: Stanford University Press.

———. 2005. "Sima Qian, 'Accounts of the Legendary Physician Bian Que.'" In Mair, Steinhardt, and Goldin 2005.

———. 2010. "Social and Cultural Dimensions of Reclusion." In Chan and Lo 2010.

Bielenstein, Hans. 1947. "The Census of China During the Period 2–742 A.D." *Bulletin of the Museum of Far Eastern Antiquities* 19: 125–63.

———. 1950. "An Interpretation of the Portents in the Ts'ien-han-shu." *Bulletin of the Museum of Far Eastern Antiquities* 22: 127–43.

———. 1996. "The Six Dynasties, Vol. I." *Bulletin of the Museum of Far Eastern Antiquities* 68.

———. 2005. *Diplomacy and Trade in the Chinese World, 589–1276*. Leiden: Brill.

Birnbaum, Raoul. 1980. "Introduction to the Study of T'ang Buddhist Astrology: Research Notes on Primary Sources and Basic Principles." *Society for the Study of Chinese Religions Bulletin* 8: 5–19.

———. 1986. "The Manifestation of a Monastery: Shen-ying's Experiences on Mount Wu-t'ai in T'ang Context." *Journal of the American Oriental Society* 106 (1): 119–37.

———. 1989a. "Chinese Buddhist Traditions of Healing and the Life Cycle." In Lawrence E. Sullivan (ed.), *Healing and Restoring: Health and Medicine in the World's Religious Traditions*. New York: Macmillan.

———. 1989b. *The Healing Buddha*. Boulder, Colo.: Shambhala.

———. 1989–90. "Secret Halls of the Mountain Lords: The Caves of Wu-t'ai Shan." *Cahiers d'Extrême-Asie* 5: 115–40.

———. 2004. "Light in the Wutai Mountains." In Matthew Kapstein (ed.), *The Presence of Light: Divine Radiance and Religious Experience*. Chicago: University of Chicago Press.

Bodde, Derk. 1975. *Festivals in Classical China: New Year and Other Annual Observances During the Han Dynasty, 206 B.C.–A.D. 220*. Princeton, N.J.: Princeton University Press and Chinese University of Hong Kong.

Boisvert, Mathieu. 2000. "Conception and Intrauterine Life in the Pāli Canon." *Studies in Religion/Sciences Religieuses* 29 (3): 301–11.

Bokenkamp, Stephen R. 1983. "Sources of the Ling-Pao Scriptures." In Michel Strickmann and R. A. Stein (eds.), *Tantric and Taoist Studies in Honor of R. A. Stein*. Brussels: Institut belge des hautes études chinoises.

———. 1990. "Stages of Transcendence: The Bhūmi Concept in Taoist Scripture." In Buswell 1990.

———. 1997. *Early Daoist Scriptures*. Berkeley: University of California Press.

———. 2001. "Lu Xiujing, Buddhism, and the First Daoist Canon." In Pearce, Spiro, and Ebrey 2001.

———. 2004. "The Silkworm and the Bodhi Tree: The Lingbao Attempt to Replace Buddhism in China and Our Attempt to Place Lingbao Daoism." In Lagerwey 2004.

———. 2005. "Simple Twists of Fate: The Daoist Body and Its *Ming*." In Lupke 2005.

———. 2006. "The *Viśvantara-jātaka* in Buddhist and Daoist Translation." In Penny 2006.

———. 2007. *Ancestors and Anxiety: Daoism and the Birth of Rebirth in China*. Berkeley: University of California Press.

Bol, Peter K. 1992. *"This Culture of Ours": Intellectual Transitions in T'ang and Sung China*. Stanford, Calif.: Stanford University Press.

Bose, Phanindra Nath. 1923. *The Indian Teachers in China*. Madras: S. Ganesan.

Boucher, Daniel. 1996. "Buddhist Translation Procedures in Third-Century China: A Study of Dharmaraksa and His Translation Idiom." Ph.D. diss., University of Pennsylvania.

———. 1998. "Gāndhārī and the Early Chinese Buddhist Translations Reconsidered: The Case of the Saddharmapuṇḍarīkasūtra." *JAOS* 118 (4): 471–506.

———. 2000. "On Hu and Fan Again." *JIABS* 21 (1): 7–28.

———. 2005. "Buddhism and Language in Early-Medieval China." In Mair, Steinhardt, and Goldin 2005.

———. 2006. "Dharmarakṣa and the Transmission of Buddhism to China." *Asia Major* 19:13–37.

———. 2008. *Bodhisattvas of the Forest and the Formation of the Mahāyāna: A Study and Translation of the Rāṣṭrapālaparipṛcchā-sutra.* Honolulu: University of Hawai'i Press.

Bourdieu, Pierre. 1984. *Distinction: A Social Critique of the Judgement of Taste.* Trans. Richard Nice. Cambridge, Mass.: Harvard University Press.

———. 1977. *Outline of a Theory of Practice.* Trans. Richard Nice. Cambridge: Cambridge University Press.

Bourdieu, Pierre, and Loïc J. D. Wacquant. 1992. *An Invitation to Reflexive Sociology.* Chicago: University of Chicago Press.

Brindley, Erica Fox. 2012. *Music, Cosmology, and the Politics of Harmony in Early China.* Albany: State University of New York Press.

Brokaw, Cynthia Joanne. 1991. *The Ledgers of Merit and Demerit: Social Change and Moral Order in Late Imperial China.* Princeton, N.J.: Princeton University Press.

Brough, John. 1961. "A Kharoṣṭhī Inscription from China." *Bulletin of SOAS* 24 (3): 517–30.

Brown, Carolyn T. (ed.). 1988. *Psycho-Sinology: The Universe of Dreams in Chinese Culture.* Washington, D.C.: Woodrow Wilson International Center for Scholars.

Brown, Robert L. 1998. "Expected Miracles: The Unsurprisingly Miraculous Nature of Buddhist Images and Relics." In Richard H. Davis 1998.

Buell, Paul D., and Eugene N. Anderson. 2010. *A Soup for the Qan.* 2nd ed. Leiden: Brill.

Bumbacher, Stephan Peter. 2000. *The Fragments of the Daoxue zhuan: Critical Edition, Translation and Analysis of a Medieval Collection of Daoist Biographies.* Frankfurt: Peter Lang.

———. 2012. *Empowered Writing: Exorcistic and Apotropaic Rituals in Medieval China.* St. Petersburg, Fla.: Three Pines.

Burchett, Patton E. 2008. "The 'Magical' Language of Mantra." *Journal of the American Academy of Religion* 76 (4): 807–43.

Buswell, Robert E. (ed.). 1990. *Chinese Buddhist Apocrypha.* Honolulu: University of Hawai'i Press.

——— (ed.). 2004. *Encyclopedia of Buddhism.* New York: Macmillan.

Campany, Robert Ford. 1991a. "Ghosts Matter: The Culture of Ghosts in Six Dynasties Zhiguai." *Chinese Literature: Essays, Articles, Reviews* 13: 15–34.

————. 1991b. "Notes on the Devotional Uses and Symbolic Functions of Sūtra Texts as Depicted in Early Chinese Buddhist Miracle Tales and Hagiographies." *JIABS* 14 (1): 28–72.

————. 1993a. "Buddhist Revelation and Taoist Translation in Early Medieval China." *Taoist Resources* 4 (1): 1–29.

————. 1993b. "The Real Presence." *History of Religions* 32 (3): 233–72.

————. 1995. "To Hell and Back: Death, Near-Death, and Other Worldly Journeys in Early Medieval China." In J. J. Collins and M. Fishbane (eds.), *Death, Ecstasy, and Other Worldly Journeys*. Albany: State University of New York Press.

————. 1996a. "The Earliest Tales of the Bodhisattva Guanshiyin." In Lopez 1996.

————. 1996b. *Strange Writing: Anomaly Accounts in Early Medieval China*. Albany: State University of New York Press.

————. 2002. *To Live as Long as Heaven and Earth: A Translation and Study of Ge Hong's "Traditions of Divine Transcendents."* Berkeley: University of California Press.

————. 2003. "On the Very Idea of Religions (in the Modern West and in Early Medieval China)." *History of Religions* 42 (4): 287–319.

————. 2005a. "Eating Better Than Gods and Ancestors." In Roel Sterckx (ed.), *Of Tripod and Palate: Food, Politics and Religion in Traditional China*. London: Palgrave.

————. 2005b. "Living Off the Books: Fifty Ways to Dodge Ming in Early Medieval China." In Lupke 2005.

————. 2005c. "Long-Distance Specialists in Early Medieval China." In Eric Ziolkowski (ed.), *Journeys West and East*. Wilmington: University of Delaware Press.

————. 2005d. "The Meanings of Cuisines of Transcendence in Late Classical and Early Medieval China." *T'oung Pao* 91: 1–57.

————. 2006. "Secrecy and Display in the Quest for Transcendence in China, ca. 220 B.C.E.–350 C.E." *History of Religions* 45 (4): 291–336.

————. 2009. *Making Transcendents: Ascetics and Social Memory in Early Medieval China*. Honolulu: University of Hawai'i Press.

————. 2010. "Narrative in the Self-Presentation of Transcendence-Seekers." In Alan K. L. Chan and Yuet-Keung Lo (eds.), *Interpretation and Literature in Early Medieval China*. Albany: State University of New York Press.

————. 2012a. "Religious Repertoires and Contestation: A Case Study Based on Buddhist Miracle Tales." *History of Religions* 52 (2): 99–141.

————. 2012b. *Signs from the Unseen Realm: Buddhist Miracle Tales from Early Medieval China*. Honolulu: University of Hawai'i Press.

Canepa, Matthew P. 2010. "Theorizing Cross-Cultural Interaction Among the Ancient and Early Medieval Mediterranean, Near East, and Asia." *Ars Orientalis* 38: 7–30.

Caswell, James O. 1988. *Written and Unwritten: Buddhist Caves at Yungang*. Vancouver: University of British Columbia Press.

Chan, Alan K. L., and Yuet-Keung Lo (eds.). 2010. *Philosophy and Religion in Early Medieval China*. Albany: State University of New York Press.

Chan, Man Sing. 2012. "Sinicizing Western Science: The Case of Quanti xinlun." *T'oung Pao* 98: 528–56.

Chandra, Lokesh. 1983. "The Role of Tantras in the Defence Strategy of T'ang China." In E. R. Sreekrishna Sarma et al. (eds.), *Surabhi*. Tirupati: E. R. Sreekrishna Sarma Felicitation Committee.

Chappell, David W. 2005. "The Precious Scroll of the Liang Emperor: Buddhist and Daoist Repentance to Save the Dead." In Weinstein and Bodiford 2005.

Chatterji, Suniti Kumar. 1959. "India and China: Ancient Contacts—What India Received from China." *Journal of the Asiatic Society* 1: 89–122.

Chaudhuri, Saroj Kumar. 2011. *Sanskrit in China and Japan.* New Delhi: International Academy of Indian Culture and Aditya Prakashan.

Ch'en, Kenneth. 1952. "Anti-Buddhist Propaganda During the Nan-ch'ao." *HJAS* 15 (1–2): 166–92.

———. 1954. "On Some Factors Responsible for the Anti-Buddhist Persecution Under the Pei-ch'ao." *HJAS* 17: 261–73.

———. 1964. *Buddhism in China: A Historical Survey.* Princeton, N.J.: Princeton University Press.

———. 1973. *The Chinese Transformation of Buddhism.* Princeton, N.J.: Princeton University Press.

Chen Hsiu-fen. 2005. "Wind Malady as Madness in Medieval China: Some Threads from the Dunhuang Medical Manuscript." In Lo and Cullen 2005.

Chen Huaiyu. 2007. *The Revival of Buddhist Monasticism in Medieval China.* New York: Peter Lang, 2007.

Chen Jinhua. 1998. "The Construction of Early Tendai Esoteric Buddhism: The Japanese Provenance of Saichō's Transmission Documents and Three Esoteric Buddhist Apocrypha Attributed to Śubhākarasiṃha." *JIABS* 21 (1): 21–76.

———. 1999. *Making and Remaking History: A Study of Tiantai Sectarian Historiography.* Tokyo: International Institute for Buddhist Studies.

———. 2002a. *Monks and Monarchs, Kinship and Kingship: Tanqian in Sui Buddhism and Politics.* Kyoto: Scuola Italiana di Studi sull'Asia Orientale.

———. 2002b. "Śarīra and Scepter: Empress Wu's Political Use of Buddhist Relics." *JIABS* 25 (1–2): 33–150.

———. 2004a. "The Indian Buddhist Missionary Dharmaksema (385–433): A New Dating of His Arrival in Guzang and of His Translations." *T'oung Pao* 90: 215–63.

———. 2004b. "The Location and Chief Members of Śikṣānanda's (652–710) Avataṃsaka Translation Office: Some Remarks on a Chinese Collection of Stories and Legends Related to the Avataṃsaka Sutra." *Journal of Asian History* 38 (2): 121–40.

———. 2005. "Some Aspects of the Buddhist Translation Procedure in Early Medieval China: With Special References to a Longstanding Misreading of a Keyword in the Earliest Extant Buddhist Catalogue in East Asia." *Journal Asiatique* 293 (2): 603–62.

———. 2006. "Pañcavārṣika Assemblies in Liang Wudi's Buddhist Palace Chapel." *HJAS* 66 (1): 43–103.

Chen Ming. 2001. "Yindu gudai yidian zhong de Qipo fang." *Zhonghua yixue zazhi* 31 (4): 202–6.

———. 2003a. "'Bashu' yu 'sanju': Dunhuang Tulufan wenshu zhong de Yindu 'shengming feituo' yixue lilun." *Ziran kexueshi yanjiu* 22 (1): 26–41.

———. 2003b. "'Qianjin fang' zhong de 'Qipo yiyao fang.'" *Beijing ligong daxue xuebao (Shehui kexue ban)* 5 (2): 91–96.

———. 2003c. "Qipo de xingxiang yanbian jiqi zai Dunhuang Tulufan diqu de yingxiang." *Wenjin xuezhi* 1: 138–64.

———. 2003d. "Tulufan hanwen yixue wenshu zhong de wailai yinsu." *Xin shixue* 14 (4): 1–63.

———. 2005a. *Dunhuang chutu huhua yidian "Qipo shu" yanjiu* (English title: *A Study on Sanskrit Text of Jīvaka-Pustaka from Dunhuang*). Hong Kong: Xinwen feng.

———. 2005b. *Shufang yiyao: Chutu wenshu yu xiyu yixue* (English title: *Foreign Medicine in Medieval China: Medical Manuscripts Discovered in Dunhuang and Western Regions*). Beijing: Peking University Press.

———. 2005c. "Zhuan nü wei nan: Turning Female to Male, an Indian Influence on Chinese Gynaecology?" *Asian Medicine* 1 (2): 315–34.

———. 2006. "Hanyi mijiao wenxian zhong de shengming feituo chengfen bianxi—yi tongzi fang he yanyao fang weili." *Gujin lunheng* 14: 27–46.

———. 2007. "The Transmission of Foreign Medicine via the Silk Roads in Medieval China: A Case Study of the *Haiyao bencao*." *Asian Medicine* 3 (2): 241–64.

———. 2008a. "Daguwenshu 3436 hao canpian zhong de zhihan xiaokao—zhonggu wailai yaowu zhaji zhi yi." *Dunhuang xue* 27: 159–66.

———. 2008b. "'Genben shuoyiqie youbu pinaiye yaoshi' cihui xuanshi." *Dunhuang Tulufan yanjiu* 11: 391–405.

———. 2009. "Sichou zhi lu yu zhonggu wailai jieduxue zhishi de zhuanbo." *Wenshi* 87 (2): 73–94.

———. 2013. *Zhonggu yiliao yu wailai wenhua*. Beijing: Peking University Press.

Chen, Sanping. 2012. *Multicultural China in the Early Middle Ages*. Philadelphia: University of Pennsylvania Press.

Chen Shu-fen. 2004a. "On Xuanzang's Transliterated Version of the Sanskrit Prajñāpāramitāhṛdayasūtra (Heart Sutra)." *Monumenta Serica* 52: 113–59.

———. 2004b. *Rendition Techniques in the Chinese Translation of Three Sanskrit Buddhist Scriptures*. Devon: Hardinge Simpole.

Chen Yinke. 1930. "Sanguo zhi Cao Chong Hua Tuo zhuan yu fojiao gushi." *Qinghua xuebao* 6 (1): 17–20.

Chen Yunü. 2008. "Buddhism and the Medical Treatment of Women in the Ming Dynasty: A Research Note." *Nan Nü* 10: 279–303.

Chen Yuzhen. 1993. "'Fayuan zhulin' suo yin waidian zhi yanjiu." *Zhonghua foxue xuebao* 6 (7): 303–28.

Cheung, Martha. 2006. *An Anthology of Chinese Discourse on Translation*. Vol. 1, *From Earliest Times to the Buddhist Project*. Manchester: St. Jerome.

Chin, Connie. 2008. "Climate Change and Migrations of People During the Jin Dynasty." *Early Medieval China* 2: 49–78.

Chin Keh-mu. 1982. "India and China: Scientific Exchange." In Debiprasad Chattopadhyaya (ed.), *Studies in the History of Science in India*. Vol. 2. New Delhi: Editorial Enterprises.

Ching, Julia. 1997. *Mysticism and Kingship in China: The Heart of Chinese Wisdom*. Cambridge: Cambridge University Press.

Chou Yi-Liang. 1945. "Tantrism in China." *HJAS* 8 (3–4): 241–332.

Cleary, Thomas, F. 1993 [1984]. *The Flower Ornament Scripture*. Boston: Shambhala.

Cole, Alan. 1998. *Mothers and Sons in Chinese Buddhism*. Stanford, Calif.: Stanford University Press.

———. 2009. *Fathering Your Father: The Zen of Fabrication in Tang Buddhism*. Berkeley: University of California Press.

Collins, Steven. 1990. "On the Very Idea of the Pāli Canon." *Journal of the Pali Text Society* 15: 89–126.

———. 1997. "The Body in Theravāda Buddhist Monasticism." In Sarah Coakley (ed.), *Religion and the Body*. Cambridge: Cambridge University Press.

Cong Chunyu. 1994. *Dunhuang zhongyiyao quanshu*. Beijing: Zhongguo guji chubanshe.

Cook, Harold J. 1986. *The Decline of the Old Medical Regime in Stuart London*. Ithaca, N.Y.: Cornell University Press.

Copp, Paul F. 2008a. "Altar, Amulet, Icon: Transformations in Dhāraṇī Amulet Culture, 740–980." *Cahiers d'Extrême-Asie* 17: 239–64.

———. 2008b. "Notes on the Term 'Dhāraṇī' in Medieval Chinese Buddhist Thought." *Bulletin of SOAS* 71 (3): 493–508.

———. 2011. "Manuscript Culture as Ritual Culture in Late Medieval Dunhuang: Buddhist Seals and Their Manuals." *Cahiers d'Extrême-Asie* 20: 193–226.

———. 2012. "Anointing Phrases and Narrative Power: A Tang Buddhist Poetics of Incantation." *History of Religions* 52 (2): 142–72.

———. Forthcoming. *The Body Incantatory: Spells and the Ritual Imagination in Medieval Chinese Buddhism*. New York: Columbia University Press.

Corless, Roger. 1995. "The Chinese Life of Nāgārjuna." In Donald S. Lopez (ed.), *Buddhism in Practice*. Princeton, N.J.: Princeton University Press.

Cuevas, Bryan J., and Jacqueline Stone. 2007. *The Buddhist Dead: Practices, Discourses, Representations*. Honolulu: University of Hawai'i Press.

Cullen, Christopher. 1993. "Patients and Healers in Late Imperial China: Evidence from the Jinpingmei." *History of Science* 31: 99–150.

Das, Rahul Peter. 2003. *The Origin of the Life of a Human Being: Conception and the Female According to Ancient Indian Medical and Sexological Literature*. Delhi: Motilal Banarsidass.

Davis, Edward L. 2001. *Society and the Supernatural in Song China*. Honolulu: University of Hawai'i Press.

Davis, Richard H. (ed.). 1998. *Images, Miracles, and Authority in Asian Religious Traditions*. Boulder, Colo.: Westview Press

de Bary, William Theodore, and Irene Bloom. 1999. *Sources of Chinese Tradition: From Earliest Times to 1600*. 2nd ed. New York: Columbia University Press.

de Crespigny, Rafe. 1968. "Prefectures and Population in South China in the First Three Centuries A.D." *Bulletin of the Institute of History and Philology* 40 (1): 139–54.

de Groot, J. J. M. 1982 [1892–1910]. *The Religious System of China: Its Ancient Forms, Evolution, History and Present Aspect; Manners, Customs, and Social Institutions Connected Therewith*. Vols. 1–6. Taipei: Southern Materials Center.

De Rauw, Tom. 2005. "Baochang: Sixth-Century Biographer of Buddhist Monks . . . and Nuns?" *JAOS* 125 (2): 203–18.

DeCaroli, Robert. 2004. *Haunting the Buddha: Indian Popular Religions and the Formation of Buddhism*. New York: Oxford University Press.

Deeg, Max. 2005. *Das Gaoseng-Faxian-zhuan als religionsgeschichtliche Quelle: Der älteste Bericht eines chinesischen buddhistischen Pilgermönchs über seine Reise nach Indien mit Übersetzung des Textes*. Wiesbaden: Harrassowitz Verlag.

———. 2010. "Maritime Routes in the Indian Ocean in Early Times According to Chinese Buddhist Texts." In Ralph Kauz (ed.), *Aspects of the Maritime Silk Road: From the Persian Gulf to the East China Sea*. Wiesbaden: Harrassowitz Verlag.

Demiéville, Paul. 1985 [1937]. *Buddhism and Healing: Demiéville's Article "Byō" from Hōbōgirin*. Trans. Mark Tatz. Lanham, Md.: University Press of America.

Deshpande, Vijaya. 1987. "Medieval Transmission of Alchemical and Chemical Ideas Between India and China." *Indian Journal of History of Science* 22 (1): 15–28.

———. 1991–92. "Chinese Sources for History of Indian Science." *Annals of the Bhandarkar Oriental Research Institute* 72–73: 229–42.

———. 1999. "Indian Influences on Early Chinese Ophthalmology: Glaucoma as a Case Study." *Bulletin of SOAS* 62 (2): 306–22.

———. 2000. "Ophthalmic Surgery: A Chapter in the History of Sino-Indian Medical Contacts." *Bulletin of SOAS* 63 (3): 370–88.

———. 2003–4. "Nāgārjuna and Chinese Medicine." *Stvdia Asiatica* 4–5: 241–57.

———. 2008. "Glimpses of Āyurveda in Medieval Chinese Medicine." *Indian Journal of History of Science* 43 (2): 137–61.

Deshpande, Vijaya, and Fan Ka-wai. 2012. *Restoring the Dragon's Vision: Nagarjuna and Medieval Chinese Ophthalmology*. Hong Kong: City University of Hong Kong.

Despeux, Catherine. 1995. "L'expiration des six souffles d'après les sources du canon taoïque: Un procédé classique du qigong." In Jean-Pierre Diény (ed.), *Hommage à Kwong Hing Foon: Études d'histoire culturelle de la Chine*. Paris: Collège de France, Institut des hautes études chinoises.

———. 2000. "Talismans and Sacred Diagrams." In Kohn 2000.

———. 2006. "The Six Healing Breaths." In Kohn 2006.

———— (ed.). 2010. *Médecine, religion et société dans la Chine médiévale: Étude de manuscrits chinois de Dunhuang et de Turfan.* 3 vols. Paris: Collège de France, Institut des hautes études chinoises.

Devi, Bibha. 1979. "I-tsing's Observation on Bathing and Its Medical Appraisal." In Shyam Kishore Lal and Arun M. Parkhe (eds.), *Chikitsa: Collection of Research Articles on Ayurveda,* vol. 1. Maharashtra: Dharmatma Tatyajimaharaj Memorial Medical Relief Trust.

DeWoskin, Kenneth J. 1983. *Doctors, Diviners and Magicians of Ancient China: Biographies of Fang-shih.* New York: Columbia University Press.

DeWoskin, Kenneth J., and J. I. Crump. 1996. *In Search of the Supernatural: The Written Record.* Stanford, Calif.: Stanford University Press.

Dien, Albert E. 2007. *Six Dynasties Civilization.* New Haven, Conn.: Yale University Press.

Douglas, Mary. 2005. *Purity and Danger: An Analysis of Concepts of Pollution and Taboo.* London: Routledge.

Durand, John D. 1960. "The Population Statistics of China, A.D. 2–1953." *Population Studies* 13 (3): 209–56.

Ehara, N. R. M., Soma Thera, and Kheminda Thera. 1961. *The Path of Freedom, by the Arahant Upatissa, Translated into Chinese (Gedatsu Dō Ron) by Tipiṭaka Sanghapāla of Funan.* Colombo: D. Roland D. Weerasuria.

Eliasberg, Danielle. 1984. "Quelques aspects du grand exorcisme No à Touen-Houang." In Michel Soymié (ed.), *Contributions aux études de Touen-Houang.* Vol. 3. Paris: Publications de l'École française d'Extrême-Orient.

Elverskog, Johan. 2010. *Buddhism and Islam on the Silk Road.* Philadelphia: University of Pennsylvania Press.

Emmerick, R. E. 2004 [1996]. *The Sūtra of Golden Light, Being a Translation of the Suvarṇabhāsottamasūtra.* 3rd ed. Oxford: Pali Text Society.

Engelhardt, Ute. 2001. "Dietetics in Tang China and the First Extant Works of Materia Dietetica." In Hsu 2001.

Engler, Steven, and Gregory P. Grieve (eds.). 2005. *Historicizing "Tradition" in the Study of Religion.* Berlin: Walter de Gruyter.

Epler, Dean C. 1980. "Bloodletting in Early Chinese Medicine and Its Relation to the Origin of Acupuncture." *Bulletin of the History of Medicine* 54 (3): 337–67.

Fairbank, John King (ed.). 1957. *Chinese Thought and Institutions.* Chicago: University of Chicago Press.

Fan Kawai. 2005a. "Couching for Cataract and Sino-Indian Medical Exchange from the Sixth to the Twelfth Century AD." *Clinical and Experimental Ophthalmology* 33: 188–90.

————. 2005b. "Han-Tang jian fojiao yu yiliao qiuji—yi laibing wei zhongxin." In Zhang and Liang 2005.

Fan Xingzhun. 1936. "Hufang kao." *Zhonghua yixue zazhi* 22 (12): 1235–66.

Farooqi, M. I. H., and J. G. Srivastava. 1968. "The Tooth-Brush Tree." *Quarterly Journal of Crude Drug Research* 8: 1297–99.

Filliozat, Jean. 1934. "La médicine indienne et l'expansion bouddhique en Extrême-Orient." *Journal Asiatique* 224: 301–7.

———. 1964. *The Classical Doctrine of Indian Medicine, Its Origins and Its Greek Parallels.* Delhi: Munshiram Manoharlal.

———. 1969. "Taoïsme et yoga." *Journal Asiatique* 257 (1–2): 41–87.

Forte, Antonino. 1976. *Political Propaganda and Ideology in China at the End of the Seventh Century: Inquiry into the Nature, Authors and Function of the Tunhuang Document S.6502, Followed by an Annotated Translation.* Naples: Istituto universitario orientale, Seminario di studi asiatici.

———. 1985. "Hui-Chih (fl. 676–703 A.D.), a Brahman Born in China." *Estratto da Annali dell'Istituto Universitario Orientale* 45: 106–34.

———. 1988. *Mingtang and Buddhist Utopias in the History of the Astronomical Clock: The Tower, Statue, and Armillary Sphere Constructed by Empress Wu.* Rome: Istituto Italiano per il Medio ed Estremo Oriente; and Paris: École française d'Extrême-Orient.

———. 1995. *The Hostage An Shigao and His Offspring: An Iranian Family in China.* Kyoto: Instituto Italiano di Cultura, Scuola di Studi sull'Asia Orientale.

———. 2002a. "Fazang and Śākyamitra, a Seventh-Century Singhalese Alchemist at the Chinese Court." In Xing Yitian (ed.), *Regional Culture, Religion, and Arts Before the Seventh Century: Papers from the Third International Conference on Sinology, History Section.* Taipei: Institute of History and Philology, Academia Sinica.

———. 2002b. "The South Indian Monk Bodhiruci (d. 727): Biographical Evidence." In Antonino Forte and Federico Masini (eds.), *A Life Journey to the East: Sinological Studies in Memory of Giuliano Bertuccioli (1923–2001).* Kyoto: Scuola Italiana di Studi sull' Asia Orientale.

Fraser, Sarah E. 2004. "An Introduction to the Material Culture of Dunhuang Buddhism: Putting the Object in Its Place." *Asia Major* 17 (1): 1–13.

Frauwallner, Erich. 1956. *The Earliest Vinaya and the Beginnings of Buddhist Literature.* Rome: Instituto italiano per il Medio ed Estremo Oriente.

Freiberger, Oliver. 2004. "The Buddhist Canon and the Canon of Buddhist Studies." *JIABS* 27 (2): 261–83.

Friedrich, Hugo. 1992 [1965]. "On the Art of Translation." In Rainer Schulte and John Biguenet (eds.), *Theories of Translation: An Anthology of Essays from Dryden to Derrida.* Chicago: University of Chicago Press.

Fu Fang and Ni Qing (eds.). 1996. *Zhongguo foyi renwu xiaozhuan.* Xiamen: Lujiang.

Fuchs, Martin. 2009. "Reaching Out; or, Nobody Exists in One Context Only: Society as Translation." *Translation Studies* 2 (1): 21–40.

Fujita Kōtatsu. 1990. "The Textual Origins of the Kuan Wu-liang-shou ching: A Canonical Scripture of Pure Land Buddhism." In Buswell 1990.

Fukunaga Katsumi. 1972. *Bukkyō igaku shōsetsu.* Tokyo: Yūzankaku.

———. 1990. *Bukkyō igaku jiten.* Tokyo: Yūzankaku.

Funayama Tōru. 2004. "The Acceptance of Buddhist Precepts by the Chinese in the Fifth Century." *Journal of Asian History* 38 (2): 97–120.

———. 2008. "The Work of Paramārtha: An Example of Sino-Indian Cross-cultural Exchange." *JIABS* 31 (1–2): 141–83.

———. 2011. "Buddhist Theories of Bodhisattva Practice as Adopted by Daoists." *Cahiers d'Extrême-Asie* 20: 15–34.

Furth, Charlotte. 1999. *A Flourishing Yin: Gender in China's Medical History, 960–1665.* Berkeley: University of California Press.

Gai Jianmin. 2001. *Daojiao yixue.* Beijing: Zongjiao wenhua.

Garrett, Frances. 2008. *Religion, Medicine and the Human Embryo in Tibet.* Abingdon: Routledge.

———. 2009. "Tibetan Buddhist Narratives of the Forces of Creation." In Sasson and Law 2009.

Geertz, Clifford. 2000. *The Interpretation of Cultures.* New York: Basic Books.

Geng Liutong and Geng Yinxun. 1993. *Foxue yu zhongyixue.* Fuzhou: Fujian kexue jishu.

Georgieva, Valentina. 1996. "Representation of Buddhist Nuns in Chinese Edifying Miracle Tales During the Six Dynasties and the Tang." *Journal of Chinese Religions* 24: 47–76.

Gernet, Jacques. 1995. *Buddhism in Chinese Society: An Economic History from the Fifth to the Tenth Centuries.* Trans. Franciscus Verellen. New York: Columbia University Press.

Gimello, Robert M. 1978. "Random Reflections on the 'Sinicization' of Buddhism." *Society for the Study of Chinese Religions Bulletin* 5: 52–89.

Giustarini, Giuliano. 2011. "The Truth of the Body: The Liberating Role of Physical (and Mental) Boundaries in Asubhabhāvanā." *Thai International Journal of Buddhist Studies* 2: 96–124.

Gjertson, Donald E. 1978. *Ghosts, Gods, and Retribution: Nine Buddhist Miracle Tales from Six Dynasties and Early T'ang China.* Amherst: University of Massachusetts Press.

———. 1981. "The Early Chinese Buddhist Miracle Tale: A Preliminary Survey." *JAOS* 101 (3): 287–301.

———. 1989. *Miraculous Retribution: A Study and Translation of T'ang Lin's Ming-pao chi.* Berkeley: Centers for South and Southeast Asian Studies, University of California.

Goble, Geoffrey C. 2012. "Chinese Esoteric Buddhism: Amoghavajra and the Ruling Elite." Ph.D. diss., Indiana University.

Goldschmidt, Asaf Moshe. 2001. "Changing Standards: Tracing Changes in Acumoxa Therapy During the Transition from the Tang to the Song Dynasties." *EASTM* 18: 75–111.

———. 2005. "The Song Discontinuity: Rapid Innovation in Northern Song Dynasty Medicine." *Asian Medicine* 1 (1): 53–90.

———. 2006. "Huizong's Impact on Medicine and on Public Health." In Patricia Buckley Ebrey and Maggie Bickford (eds.), *Emperor Huizong and Late Northern Song China: The Politics of Culture and the Culture of Politics.* Cambridge, Mass.: Harvard University Press.

———. 2007. "Epidemics and Medicine During the Northern Song Dynasty: The Revival of Cold Damage Disorders (Shanghan)." *T'oung Pao* 93: 53–109.

———. 2009. *The Evolution of Chinese Medicine: Song Dynasty, 960–1200.* London: Routledge.

Gombrich, Richard F. 2003. *Theravāda Buddhism: A Social History from Ancient Benares to Modern Colombo.* London: Routledge.

Gómez, Luis O. 2010. "On Buddhist Wonders and Wonder-Working." *JIABS* 33 (1–2): 513–54.

Graff, David A. 2002. *Medieval Chinese Warfare, 300–900.* London: Routledge.

Greene, Eric Matthew. 2012. "Meditation, Repentance, and Visionary Experience in Early Medieval Chinese Buddhism." Ph.D. diss., University of California, Berkeley.

Gregory, Peter N. 1991. *Tsung-mi and the Sinification of Buddhism.* Princeton, N.J.: Princeton University Press.

Guisso, R. W. L. 1978. *Wu Tse-t'ien and the Politics of Legitimation in T'ang China.* Bellingham: Western Washington University Press.

Gummer, Natalie. 2000. "Articulating Potency: A Study of the Suvarṇa(pra)-bhāsottamasūtra." Ph.D. diss., Harvard University.

Haidar, Mansura. 2008. "Medical Works of the Medieval Period from India and Central Asia." *Diogenes* 55 (218): 27–43.

Haldar, J. R. 1977. *Medical Science in Pali Literature.* Calcutta: Indian Museum.

———. 1992. *Development of Public Health in Buddhism.* Delhi: Indological Book House.

Hansen, Valerie. 1998. "The Path of Buddhism into China: The View from Turfan." *Asia Major* 11 (2): 37–66.

———. 2004. "Religious Life in a Silk Road Community: Niya During the Third and Fourth Centuries." In Lagerwey 2004.

———. 2012. *The Silk Road: A New History.* New York: Oxford University Press.

Hanson, Marta E. 2011. *Speaking of Epidemics in Chinese Medicine: Disease and the Geographic Imagination in Late Imperial China.* Abingdon: Routledge.

Harper, Donald. 1985. "A Chinese Demonography of the Third Century B.C." *HJAS* 45 (2): 459–98.

———. 1996. "Spellbinding." In Lopez 1996.

———. 1997. "Warring States, Qin, and Han Manuscripts Related to Natural Philosophy and the Occult." In Edward L. Shaughnessy (ed.), *New Sources of Early Chinese History: An Introduction to the Reading of Inscriptions and Manuscripts.* Berkeley:

Society for the Study of Early China and the Institute of East Asian Studies, University of California.

———. 1998. *Early Chinese Medical Literature: The Mawangdui Medical Manuscripts*. London: Kegan Paul.

———. 2010. "Précis de connaissance médicale le Shanghan Lun (Traité des atteintes par le froid) et le Wuzang Lun (Traité des cinq viscères)." In Despeux 2010.

Harrison, Paul, and W. South Coblin. 2012. "The Oldest Buddhist Incantation in Chinese? A Preliminary Study of the Chinese Transcriptions of the Mantra in the Druma-kinnara-rāja-paripr̥cchā-sūtra." *Sino-Platonic Papers* 222: 63–85.

Harrison, Peter. 2006. " 'Science' and 'Religion': Constructing the Boundaries." *Journal of Religion* 86 (1): 81–106.

Hayashiya Tomojirō. 1945. *Iyaku kyōrui no kenkyū*. Tokyo: Tōyō bunko.

Heinrich, Larissa N. 2008. *The Afterlife of Images: Translating the Pathological Body Between China and the West*. Durham, N.C.: Duke University Press.

Heirman, Ann. 2007. "Vinaya: From India to China." In Heirman and Bumbacher 2007.

Heirman, Ann, and Stephan Peter Bumbacher (eds.). 2007. *The Spread of Buddhism*. Leiden: Brill.

Heirman, Ann, and Mathieu Torck. 2012. *A Pure Mind in a Clean Body: Bodily Care in the Buddhist Monasteries of Ancient India and China*. Ghent: Academia Press.

Hill, Michael Gibbs. 2013. *Lin Shu, Inc.: Translation and the Making of Modern Chinese Culture*. New York: Oxford University Press.

Hinrichs, TJ. 1998. "New Geographies of Chinese Medicine." *Osiris* 13: 287–325.

———. 2011. "Governance Through Medical Texts and the Role of Print." In Lucille Chia and Hilde de Weerdt (eds.), *Knowledge and Text Production in an Age of Print: China, 900–1400*. Leiden: Brill.

———. Forthcoming. *Shamans, Witchcraft, and Quarantine: The Medicalizing of Transformative Governance and Southern Customs in Song China*. Cambridge, Mass.: Harvard University Press.

Hinrichs, TJ, and Linda L. Barnes (eds.). 2013. *Chinese Medicine and Healing: An Illustrated History*. Cambridge, Mass.: Belknap Press.

Hirai Shun'ei. 1992. "An Explanatory Study of the *Kaoseng chuan* (II)." *Komazawa University Journal of Buddhist Studies* 23: 1–14.

———. 1993. "An Explanatory Study of the *Kaoseng chuan* (III)." *Komazawa University Journal of Buddhist Studies* 24: 1–35.

———. 1994. "An Explanatory Study of the *Kaoseng chuan* (IV)." *Komazawa University Journal of Buddhist Studies* 25: 11–25.

Hitch, Doug. 2009. "The Special Status of Turfan." *Sino-Platonic Papers* 186.

Ho, Peng Yoke. 2007. *Explorations in Daoism: Medicine and Alchemy in Literature*. London: Routledge.

Ho Puay-peng. 1995. "The Ideal Monastery: Daoxuan's Description of the Central Indian Jetavana Vihāra." *East Asian History* 10: 1–18.

Holcombe, Charles. 1994. *In the Shadow of the Han: Literati Thought and Society at the Beginning of the Southern Dynasties.* Honolulu: University of Hawai'i Press.

———. 2001. *The Genesis of East Asia, 221 B.C.–A.D. 907.* Honolulu: Association for Asian Studies and University of Hawai'i Press.

Hsieh, Shu-wei. 2010. *Tianjie zhi wen: Wei Jin Nanbeichao lingbao jing yanjiu.* Taipei: Taiwan shangwu yinshuguan.

Hsu, Elisabeth (ed.). 2001. *Innovation in Chinese Medicine.* Cambridge: Cambridge University Press.

———. 2007. "The Experience of Wind in Early and Medieval Chinese Medicine." *Journal of the Royal Anthropological Institute* 13, Supp. 1: 117–34.

Huang Boyuan. 2000. "Zhiyi yixue sixiang zhi yanjiu—yi 'Mohe zhiguan' guanbing huanjing wei zhongxin." M.A. thesis, Huafan daxue.

Huang, C. Julia. 2009. *Charisma and Compassion: Cheng Yen and the Buddhist Tzu Chi Movement.* Cambridge, Mass.: Harvard University Press.

Huang, Jane. 1987. *The Primordial Breath.* Vol. 2, *An Ancient Chinese Way of Prolonging Life Through Breath Control.* Torrance, Calif.: Original Books.

Huang Minzhi. 2005. "Songdai de sengren yu yiliao." In Zhang and Liang 2005.

Huang, Shih-shan Susan. 2010. "Daoist Imagery of Body and Cosmos." *Journal of Daoist Studies* 3: 57–90.

Hubbard, Jamie. 2001. *Absolute Delusion, Perfect Buddhahood: The Rise and Fall of a Chinese Heresy.* Honolulu: University of Hawai'i Press.

Huebotter, Franz. 1932. *Die Sūtra Über Empfängnis und Embryologie.* Tokyo: Mitteilungen der Deutschen Gesellschaft für Natur- und Völkerkunde Ostasiens.

Hureau, Sylvie. 2010. "Translations, Apocrypha, and the Emergence of the Buddhist Canon." In Lagerwey and Lü 2010.

Hurvitz, Leon. 1962. "Chih-i (538–597)." *Mélange chinois et bouddhiques* 12.

Idema, W. L., and Erik Zürcher (eds.). 1990. *Thought and Law in Qin and Han China: Studies Dedicated to Anthony Hulsewé on the Occasion of His Eightieth Birthday.* Leiden: Brill.

Itô, Takatoshi. 1996. "The Formation of Chinese Buddhism and 'Matching the Meaning' (Geyi)." *Memoirs of the Research Department of the Toyo Bunko* 54: 65–91.

Jackson, Roger. 1982. "Terms of Sanskrit and Pāli Origin Acceptable as English Words." *JIABS* 5: 141–42.

Jakobson, Roman. 2004 [1959]. "On Linguistic Aspects of Translation." In Venuti 2004.

Jan Yün-Hua. 1966. "Buddhist Relations Between India and Sung China." *History of Religions* 6 (1): 24–42.

Janousch, Andreas. 1999. "The Emperor as Bodhisattva: The Bodhisattva Ordination and Ritual Assemblies of Emperor Wu of the Liang Dynasty." In Joseph Peter McDermott (ed.), *State and Court Ritual in China.* Cambridge: Cambridge University Press.

Jaworski, Jan. 1927. "La section des remèdes dans le Vinaya des Malūśāsaka et dans le Vinaya Pali." *Rocznik Orjentalistyczny* 5: 92–101.

Jolly, Julius. 1977. *Indian Medicine.* 2nd ed. Delhi: Munshiram Manoharlal.

Juliano, Annette L., and Judith A. Lerner. 2002. *Nomads, Traders and Holy Men Along China's Silk Road.* Turnhout, Belgium: Brepols.

Kalinowski, Marc (ed.). 2003. *Divination et société dans la Chine médiévale: Étude des manuscrits de Dunhuang de la Bibliothèque nationale de France et de la British Library.* Paris: Bibliothèque nationale de France.

Kapani, Lakshmi. 1989. "Upanishad of the Embryo / Note on the Garbha-Upaniṣad." In Michel Feher, Ramona Naddaff, and Nadia Tazi (eds.), *Fragments for a History of the Human Body*, Vol. 3. New York: Zone Books.

Karashima, Seishi. 1996. "On Vernacularisms and Transcriptions in Chinese Buddhist Scriptures." *Sino-Platonic Papers* 71: 32–42.

———. 2013. "A Study of the Language of Early Chinese Buddhist Translations: A Comparison Between the Translations by Lokakṣema and Zhi Qian." *Annual Report of the International Research Institute for Advanced Buddhology, Soka University* 16: 273–88.

Katz, Paul. 1995. *Demon Hordes and Burning Boats: The Cult of Marshall Wen in Late Imperial Chekiang.* Albany: State University of New York Press.

Kawaguchi Gishō. 1975. "Hōon jurin to Shokyō yōshū tono kankei." *Komazawa daigaku daigakuin bukkyōgaku kenkyūukai nenpo* 9: 139–46.

Kegan, David Joseph. 1988. "The 'Huang-ti Nei-ching': The Structure of the Compilation; the Significance of the Structure." Ph.D. diss., University of California, Berkeley.

Kieschnick, John. 1997. *The Eminent Monk: Buddhist Ideals in Medieval Chinese Hagiography.* Honolulu: University of Hawai'i Press.

———. 2003. *The Impact of Buddhism on Chinese Material Culture.* Princeton, N.J.: Princeton University Press.

———. 2010. "Buddhist Monasticism." In Lagerwey and Lü 2010.

Kleeman, Terry. 2009. "The Ritualized Treatment of Stroke in Early Medieval Daoism and the Secret Incantation of the Northern Thearch." In F. C. Reiter (ed.), *Foundations of Daoist Ritual: A Berlin Symposium.* Wiesbaden: Otto Harrassowitz.

Kleinman, Arthur. 1980. *Patients and Healers in the Context of Culture: An Exploration of the Borderland Between Anthropology, Medicine, and Psychiatry.* Berkeley: University of California Press.

Kohn, Livia. 1993. *The Taoist Experience: An Anthology.* Albany: State University of New York Press.

———. 1995. *Laughing at the Tao: Debates Among Buddhists and Taoists in Medieval China.* Princeton, N.J.: Princeton University Press.

——— (ed.). 2000. *Daoism Handbook.* Leiden: Brill.

————— (ed.). 2006. *Daoist Body Cultivation: Traditional Models and Contemporary Practices*. Magdalena, N.M.: Three Pines Press.

—————. 2008. *Chinese Healing Exercises: The Tradition of Daoyin*. Honolulu: University of Hawaiʻi Press.

Kohn, Livia, and Harold D. Roth (eds.). 2002. *Daoist Identity: History, Lineage, and Ritual*. Honolulu: University of Hawaiʻi Press.

Kohn, Livia, and Yoshinobu Sakade. 1989. *Taoist Meditation and Longevity Techniques*. Ann Arbor: Center for Chinese Studies, University of Michigan.

Koller, Werner. 1989 [1979]. "Equivalence in Translation Theory." In Andrew Chesterman (ed.), *Readings in Translation Theory*. Helsinki: Oy Finn Lectura Ab.

Kovacs, Jürgen, and Paul U. Unschuld. 1998. *Essential Subtleties on the Silver Sea: The "Yin-hai jing-wei"; A Chinese Classic on Ophthalmology*. Berkeley: University of California Press.

Kritzer, Robert. 2006–7. "The Names of Winds in the Various Versions of the *Garbhāvakrāntisūtra*." *Bulletin d'Etudes Indiennes* 24–25: 139–53.

—————. 2009. "Life in the Womb: Conception and Gestation in Buddhist Scripture and Classical Indian Medical Literature." In Sasson and Law 2009.

Ku, Kathy Cheng-Mei. 2010. "The Buddharāja Image of Emperor Wu of Liang." In Chan and Lo 2010.

Kuo Li-ying. 1994. *Confession et contrition dans le bouddhisme chinois du Vᵉ au Xᵉ siècle*. Paris: Publications de l'École française d'Extrême-Orient.

—————. 1998. "Maṇḍala et rituel de confession à Dunhuang." *Bulletin de l'École française d'Extrême-Orient* 85: 227–56.

Kuriyama, Shigehisa. 1993. "Concepts of Disease in East Asia." In Kenneth Kiple (ed.), *The Cambridge World History of Human Disease*. Cambridge: Cambridge University Press.

—————. 1994. "The Imagination of Winds and the Development of the Chinese Conception of the Body." In Angela Zito and Tani E. Barlow (eds.), *Body, Subject and Power in China*. Chicago: University of Chicago Press.

—————. 2000. "Epidemics, Weather, and Contagion in Traditional Chinese Medicine." In Lawrence I. Conrad and Dominik Wujastyk (eds.), *Contagion: Perspectives from Pre-Modern Societies*. Aldershot: Ashgate.

—————. 2002. *The Expressiveness of the Body and the Divergence of Greek and Chinese Medicine*. New York: Zone Books.

Kutumbiah, P. 1974. *Ancient Indian Medicine*. Bombay: Orient Longman.

Kuzmina, E. E. 2008. *The Prehistory of the Silk Road*. Philadelphia: University of Pennsylvania Press.

Lagerwey, John (ed.). 2004. *Religion and Chinese Society*. Vol. 1, *Ancient and Medieval China*. Hong Kong: Chinese University Press.

Lagerwey, John, and Lü Pengzhi (eds.). 2010. *Early Chinese Religion, Part Two: The Period of Division (220–589 AD)*. Leiden: Brill.

Lagerwey, John, and Marc Kalinowski (eds.). 2009. *Early Chinese Religion, Part One: Shang Through Han (1250 BC–220 AD)*. Leiden: Brill.

Lai, Chi-Tim. 1998. "The Opposition of Celestial-Master Taoism to Popular Cults During the Six Dynasties." *Asia Major* 11 (1): 1–20.

———. 2010. "The Ideas of Illness, Healing, and Morality in Early Heavenly Master Daoism." In Chan and Lo 2010.

Lai, Whalen W. 1987. "The Earliest Folk Buddhist Religion in China: *T'i-wei Po-li Ching* and Its Historical Significance." In David W. Chappell (ed.), *Buddhist and Taoist Practice in Medieval Chinese Society: Buddhist and Taoist Studies II*. Honolulu: University of Hawai'i Press.

———. 1992. "Chinese Buddhist and Christian Charities: A Comparative History." *Buddhist-Christian Studies* 12: 5–33.

Lakoff, George, and Mark Johnson. 2003 [1980]. *Metaphors We Live By*. Chicago: University of Chicago Press.

Lal, P. 1964. *Great Sanskrit Plays, in New English Transcreations*. New York: New Directions.

Lalou, Marcel. 1938. "Le culte des nāga et le thérapeutique." *Journal Asiatique* 230: 1–19.

Lancaster, Lewis R. 2012 [1999]. "The Movement of Buddhist Texts from India to China and the Construction of the Chinese Buddhist Canon." *Sino-Platonic Papers* 222: 226–38.

Lancaster, Lewis R., and Sung-bae Park. 1979. *The Korean Buddhist Canon: A Descriptive Catalogue*. Berkeley: University of California Press.

Lang Xucai. 1986. "Lao zheng mafeisan he zailun Hua Tuo de guoji." *Zhonghua yishi zazhi* 16 (2): 88–92.

Langenberg, Amy Paris. 2008. "The Buddhist Rhetoric of Childbirth in an Early Mahāyāna Sūtra." Ph.D. diss., Columbia University.

Lee, Jen-der. 2004. "The Past as a Foreign Country: Recent Research on Chinese Medical History in Taiwan." *Gujin lunheng* 11: 37–58.

Lee T'ao. 1953. "Achievements of Chinese Medicine in the Sui (589–617 A.D.) and T'ang (618–907 A.D.) Dynasties." *Chinese Medical Journal* 71: 301–20.

Lefevere, André. 1992. *Translation, Rewriting, and the Manipulation of Literary Frame*. London: Routledge.

Leung, Angela Ki Che. 2009. *Leprosy in China: A History*. New York: Columbia University Press.

Lewis, Mark Edward. 2006. *The Construction of Space in Early China*. Albany: State University of New York Press.

———. 2009a. *China Between Empires: The Northern and Southern Dynasties*. Cambridge, Mass.: Belknap Press.

———. 2009b. *China's Cosmopolitan Empire: The Tang Dynasty*. Cambridge, Mass.: Belknap Press.

Li Gang. 2010. "State Religious Policy." In Lagerwey and Lü 2010.

Li Jianmin. 2000. *Si-sheng zhi yu: Zhou Qin Han maixue zhi yuanliu.* Taipei: Institute of History and Philology, Academia Sinica.

————. 2009. "They Shall Expel Demons: Etiology, the Medical Canon and the Transformation of Medical Techniques Before the Tang." In Lagerwey and Kalinowski 2009.

Li Rongxi. 1993. *The Biographical Scripture of King Aśoka.* Berkeley, Calif.: Numata Center.

————. 1995. *A Biography of the Tripitaka Master of the Great Ci'en Monastery of the Great Tang Dynasty.* Berkeley, Calif.: Numata Center.

————. 2000. *Buddhist Monastic Traditions of Southern Asia: A Record of the Inner Law Sent Home from the South Seas.* Berkeley, Calif.: Numata Center.

————. 2002. "The Life of Nāgārjuna Bodhisattva." In Li and Dalia 2002.

Li Rongxi and Albert Dalia (eds.). 2002. *Lives of Great Monks and Nuns.* Berkeley, Calif.: Numata Center.

Li Qin-pu. 2006. "Yindu qiri zhutai lun ji qi zai hanyi de yige biaoxian." *Bulletin of the Institute of History and Philology* 77 (4): 729–89.

Li Yingcun and Shi Zhenggang. 2006. *Dunhuang fo ru dao xiangguan yishu shiyao.* Beijing: Minzhu chubanshe.

Liang Xiaohong. 2000. *Fojiao yu hanyu cihui.* Taipei: Foguang wenhua shi.

Libbrecht, U. 1990. "Prāṇa=Pneuma=Ch'i?" In Idema and Zürcher 1990.

Lin Fu-shih. 1994. "Chinese Shamans and Shamanism in the Chiang-Nan Area During the Six Dynasties Period (3rd–6th Century A.D.)." Ph.D. diss., Princeton University.

————. 2008. *Zhongguo zhonggu shiqi de zongjiao yu yiliao.* Taipei: Lianjing chubanshe.

————. 2009. "The Image and Status of Shamans in Ancient China." In Lagerwey and Kalinowski 2009.

————. 2010. "Shamans and Politics." In Lagerwey and Lü 2010.

Link, Arthur E. 1957. "Shyh Daw-An's Preface to Saṅgharakṣa's Yogācārabhūmi-Sūtra and the Problem of Buddho-Taoist Terminology in Early Chinese Buddhism." *JAOS* 77 (1): 1–14.

————. 1958. "The Biography of Shih Tao-An." *T'oung Pao* 46: 1–48.

————. 1969–70. "The Taoist Antecedents of Tao-An's Prajñā Ontology." *History of Religions* 9 (2–3): 181–215.

Lippiello, Tiziana. 2001. *Auspicious Omens and Miracles in Ancient China: Han, Three Kingdoms and Six Dynasties.* Sankt Augustin: Monumenta Serica Institute.

Liu, Lydia H. 1995. *Translingual Practice: Literature, National Culture, and Translated Modernity—China, 1900–1937.* Stanford, Calif.: Stanford University Press.

Liu, Ming-Wood. 1993. "The Chinese Madhyamaka Practice of P'an-chiao: The Case of Chi-Tsang." *Bulletin of SOAS* 56 (1): 96–118.

Liu Mingshu. 1996. "Bian Que yu Yindu gudai mingyi Qipo." *Zhengzhou daxue xuebao* 5: 100–101.

Liu Shufen. 1995. "Art, Ritual and Society: Buddhist Practice in Rural China During the Northern Dynasties." *Asia Major* 8 (1): 19–47.

———. 2002. "Ethnicity and the Suppression of Buddhism in Fifth-Century North China: The Background and Significance of the Gaiwu Rebellion." *Asia Major* 15 (1): 1–21.

———. 2008. "Tang-Song shiqi sengren, guojia he yiliao de guanxi: Cong yaofang dong dao huimin ju." In Li Jianmin (ed.), *Cong yiliao kan Zhongguo shi*. Taipei: Lianjing chuban gongsi.

———. 2010. "The Return of the State: On the Significance of Buddhist Epigraphy and Its Geographic Distribution." In Lagerwey and Lü 2010.

Liu, Xinru. 1991 [1988]. *Ancient India and Ancient China: Trade and Religious Exchanges, AD 1–600*. Delhi: Oxford University Press.

———. 1996. *Silk and Religion: An Exploration of Material Life and the Thought of People, AD 600–1200*. Delhi: Oxford University Press.

Lloyd, Geoffrey, and Nathan Sivin. 2002. *The Way and the Word: Science and Medicine in Early China and Greece*. New Haven, Conn.: Yale University Press.

Lo, Vivienne. 2000a. "Crossing the Neiguan 'Inner Pass': A Nei/Wai 'Inner/Outer' Distinction in Early Chinese Medicine." *EASTM* 17: 15–65.

———. 2000b. "Tracking the Pain: Jue and the Formulation of a Theory of Circulating Qi Through the Channels." *Sudhoffs Archiv* 83: 191–211.

———. 2001. "The Influence of Nurturing Life Culture on the Development of Western Han Acumoxa Therapy." In Hsu 2001.

———. 2002a. "Lithic Therapy in Early Chinese Body Practices." In Patricia Anne Baker and Gillian Carr (eds.), *Practitioners, Practices and Patients: New Approaches to Medical Archaeology and Anthropology*. Oxford: Oxbow Books.

———. 2002b. "Spirit of Stone: Technical Considerations in the Treatment of the Jade Body." *Bulletin of SOAS* 65 (1): 99–128.

———. 2009. "But Is It [History of] Medicine? Twenty Years in the History of the Healing Arts of China." *Social History of Medicine* 22 (2): 283–303.

Lo, Vivienne, and Christopher Cullen (eds.). 2005. *Medieval Chinese Medicine: The Dunhuang Medical Manuscripts*. London: RoutledgeCurzon.

Lopez, Donald S., Jr. 1995. "Authority and Orality in the Mahāyāna." *Numen* 42: 21–47.

——— (ed.). 1996. *Religions of China in Practice*. Princeton, N.J.: Princeton University Press.

Loudon, Irvine. 1986. *Medical Care and the General Practitioner, 1750–1850*. Oxford: Clarendon Press.

Lu, Gwei-Djen, and Joseph Needham. 2002 [1980]. *Celestial Lancets: A History and Rationale of Acupuncture and Moxa*. London: RoutledgeCurzon.

Luo Yinan. 2005. "A Study of the Changes in the Tang-Song Transition Model." *Journal of Song-Yuan Studies* 35: 99–127.

Lupke, Christopher (ed.). 2005. *The Magnitude of Ming: Command, Allotment, and Fate in Chinese Culture*. Honolulu: University of Hawai'i Press.

Lusthaus, Dan. 1995. "Xuanzang." In Ian McGreal (ed.), *Great Thinkers of the Eastern World*. New York: HarperCollins.

——. 2013. "A Note on Medicine and Psychosomatic Relations in the First Two *Bhūmis* of the *Yogācārabhūmi*." In Ulrich Timme Kragh (ed.), *The Foundation for Yoga Practitioners: The Buddhist Yogācārabhūmi Treatise and Its Adaptation in India, East Asia, and Tibet*. Cambridge, Mass.: Department of South Asian Studies, Harvard University.

Ma Boying. 1994. *Zhongguo yixue wenhua shi*. Shanghai: Shanghai renmin chubanshe.

Ma Boying, Gao Xi, and Hong Zhongli. 1993. *Zhong-wai yixue wenhua jiaoliu shi*. Shanghai: Wenhui.

Ma Zhonggeng. 2005. "Han-Tang fojiao yu kexue—jiyu fozang wenxian de yanjiu (English Title: Buddhism and Science from Han Dynasty to Tang Dynasty—A Study Based on the Chinese Tripitaka)." Ph.D. diss., Shandong University.

Mabbett, Ian. 1998. "The Problem of Historical Nagarjuna Revisited." *JAOS* 118 (3): 332–46.

Mair, Victor H. 1983. *Tun-Huang Popular Narratives*. Cambridge: Cambridge University Press.

——. 1989. "Dunhuang as a Funnel for Central Asian Nomads into China." In Gary Seaman (ed.), *Proceedings of the Soviet-American Academic Symposia in Conjunction with the Museum Exhibition "Nomads: Masters of the Eurasian Steppe."* Vol. 1, *Ecology and Empire: Nomads in the Cultural Evolution of the Old World*. Los Angeles: University of Southern California.

——. 1990. "[The] File [on the Cosmic] Track [and Individual] Dough[tiness]: Introduction and Notes for a Translation of the Ma-Wang-Tui Manuscripts of the *Lao Tzu* [Old Master]." *Sino-Platonic Papers* 20.

——. 1994. *The Columbia Anthology of Traditional Chinese Literature*. New York: Columbia University Press.

—— (ed.). 2006. *Contact and Exchange in the Ancient World*. Honolulu: University of Hawai'i Press.

——. 2013. *China and Beyond: A Collection of Essays*. Amherst, N.Y.: Cambria Press.

Mair, Victor H., Nancy S. Steinhardt, and Paul R. Goldin (eds.). 2005. *Hawai'i Reader in Traditional Chinese Culture*. Honolulu: University of Hawai'i Press.

Makita Tairyō. 1976. *Gikyō kenkyū*. Kyoto: Kyōto daigaku jinbun kagaku kenkyūjo.

Masaaki, Tsuchiya. 2002. "Confession of Sins and Awareness of Self in the Taiping Jing." In Kohn and Roth 2002.

Maspero, Henri. 1910. "Le songe et l'ambassade de l'empereur Ming: Étude critique des sources." *Bulletin de l'École française d'Extrême-Orient* 10: 95–130.

——. 1981. *Taoism and Chinese Religion*. Amherst: University of Massachusetts Press.

Mather, Richard B. 2002 [1976]. *Shih-shuo Hsin-yü: A New Account of Tales of the World*. 2nd ed. Ann Arbor: Center for Chinese Studies, University of Michigan.

Mazars, Sylvain. 2008. *Le bouddhisme et la médecine traditionnelle de l'Inde.* Paris: Springer.

Mazumdar, Sucheta. 1998. *Sugar and Society in China: Peasants, Technology, and the World Market.* Cambridge, Mass.: Harvard University Asia Center.

McBride, Richard D. 2005. "Dhāraṇī and Spells in Medieval Sinitic Buddhism." *JIABS* 28 (1): 85–114.

McNair, Amy. 2007. *Donors of Longmen: Faith, Politics and Patronage in Medieval Chinese Buddhist Sculpture.* Honolulu: University of Hawai'i Press.

McNeill, William. 1998 [1976]. *Plagues and People.* New York: Anchor Books.

McRae, John. 2005. "Daoxuan's Vision of Jetavana: The Ordination Platform Movement in Medieval Chinese Buddhism." In Weinstein and Bodiford 2005.

Meulenbeld, G. Jan. 1999. *A History of Indian Medical Literature.* Vol. 1A. Groningen: Egbert Forsten.

Michibata Ryōshū. 1957. *Tōdai bukkyō shi no kenkyū.* Kyoto: Hōzōkan.

———. 1967. *Chūgoku bukkyō to shakai fukushi jigyō.* Kyoto: Hōzōkan.

Mitchell, Craig, Feng Ye, and Nigel Wiseman. 1999. *Shang Han Lun: On Cold Damage.* Brookline, Mass.: Paradigm.

Mitra, Jyotir. 1974. *History of Indian Medicine from Pre-Mauryan to Kuṣāṇa Period.* Varanasi: Jyotiralok Prakashan.

———. 1985. *A Critical Appraisal of Ayurvedic Material in Buddhist Literature with Special Reference to Tripitaka.* Varanasi: Jyotiralok Prakashan.

Mizuno, Kogen. 1995. *Buddhist Sutras: Origin, Development, Transmission.* Tokyo: Kosei.

Mollier, Christine. 2003. "Talismans." In Kalinowski 2003.

———. 2006. "Visions of Evil: Demonology and Orthodoxy in Early Daoism." In Penny 2006.

———. 2008. *Buddhism and Taoism Face to Face: Scripture, Ritual, and Iconographic Exchange in Medieval China.* Honolulu: University of Hawai'i Press.

Mrozik, Susanne. 2007. *Virtuous Bodies: The Physical Dimension of Morality in Buddhist Ethics.* New York: Oxford University Press.

Mun, Chanju. 2006. *The History of Doctrinal Classification in Chinese Buddhism: A Study of the Panjiao Systems.* Lanham, Md.: University Press of America.

Murthy, K. R. Srikantha. 2012. *Vāgbhaṭa's Aṣṭāṅga Hṛdayam: Text, English Translation, Notes, Appendix, and Indices.* Varanasi: Chowkhamba Krishnadas Academic.

Nappi, Carla. 2009. "Bolatu's Pharmacy: Theriac in Early Modern China." *Early Science and Medicine* 14 (6): 737–64.

Nattier, Jan. 1990. "Church Language and Vernacular Language in Central Asian Buddhism." *Numen* 37 (2): 195–219.

———. 1991. *Once Upon a Future Time: Studies in a Buddhist Prophecy of Decline.* Berkeley, Calif.: Asian Humanities Press.

———. 2003. *A Few Good Men: The Bodhisattva Path According to the Inquiry of Ugra (Ugraparipṛcchā)*. Honolulu: University of Hawai'i Press.

———. 2006. "The Names of Amitābha/Amitāyus in Early Chinese Buddhist Translations (1)." *Annual Report of the International Research Institute for Advanced Buddhology, Soka University* 9: 183–99.

———. 2008. *A Guide to the Earliest Chinese Buddhist Translations: Texts from the Eastern Han and Three Kingdoms Periods*. Tokyo: International Research Institute for Advanced Buddhology, Soka University.

Neelis, Jason. 2011. *Early Buddhist Transmission and Trade Networks: Mobility and Exchange Within and Beyond the Northwestern Borderlands of South Asia*. Leiden: Brill.

Nida, Eugene Albert. 1964. *Towards a Science of Translation: With Special Reference to Principles and Procedures Involved in Bible Translating*. Leiden: Brill.

Nida, Eugene Albert, and Charles R. Taber. 2003 [1969]. *The Theory and Practice of Translation*. Leiden: Brill.

Nihonyanagi Kenji. 1994. *Bukkyō igaku gaiyō*. Kyoto: Hōzōkan.

Ning Qiang. 2004. *Art, Religion and Politics in Medieval China: The Dunhuang Cave of the Zhai Family*. Honolulu: University of Hawai'i Press.

Nobel, Johannes. 1951. "Ein alter Medizinischer Sanskrit-Text und seine Deutung." *JAOS*, Supp. 11.

———. 1958. *Survārṇaprabhāsottama-Sūtra: Das Goldglanz-Sūtra: Ein Sanskrittext des Mahāyāna-Buddhismus: I-Tsing's Chinesische Version und ihre Tibetische Übersetzung*. Leiden: Brill.

Norman, K. R. 2006. *A Philological Approach to Buddhism: The Bukkyō Dendō Kyōkai Lectures 1994*. 2nd ed. Lancaster: Pali Text Society.

Nylan, Michael. 1999. "A Problematic Model: The Han 'Orthodox Synthesis,' Then and Now." In Kai-wing Chow, On-cho Ng, and John B. Henderson (eds.), *Imagining Boundaries: Changing Confucian Doctrines, Texts, and Hermeneutics*. Albany: State University of New York Press.

Obinata Daijō. 1962. *Bukkyō eisei gaku*. Tokyo: Sanko.

———. 1965. *Bukkyō igaku no kenkyū*. Tokyo: Kazama shobō.

Ohnuma, Reiko. 2007. *Head, Eyes, Flesh, and Blood: Giving Away the Body in Indian Buddhist Literature*. New York: Columbia University Press.

Okabe, Kazuo. 1980. "The Chinese Catalogues of Buddhist Scriptures." *Journal of the Faculty of Buddhism of the Komazawa University* 38: 1–12.

Orzech, Charles D. 1998. *Politics and Transcendent Wisdom: The Scripture for Humane Kings in the Creation of Chinese Buddhism*. University Park: Pennsylvania State University Press.

———. 2002. "Fang Yankou and Pudu: Translation, Metaphor, and Religious Identity." In Kohn and Roth 2002.

———. 2002–3. "Metaphor, Translation, and the Construction of Kingship in the Scripture for Humane Kings and the Mahāmāyūrī Vidyārājñī Sūtra." *Cahiers d'Extrême Asie* 13: 55–83.

———. 2006. "Looking for Bhairava: Exploring the Circulation of Esoteric Texts Produced by the Song Institute for Canonical Translation." *Pacific World* 8: 139–66.

———. 2011. "On the Subject of Abhiṣeka." *Pacific World* 13: 113–28.

———. 2012. "The Trouble with Tantra in China: Reflections on Method and History." In István Keul (ed.), *Transformations and Transfer of Tantra in Asia and Beyond.* Berlin: De Gruyter.

Overbey, Ryan Richard. 2008. "'Why Don't We Translate Spells in Our Scriptures?' Chinese Exegesis on the Untranslatable Dhāraṇī of the Lotus Sūtra." Paper presented at the Fifteenth Congress of the International Association of Buddhist Studies, Emory University, Atlanta, 28 June.

Ownby, David. 1999. "Chinese Millenarian Traditions: The Formative Years." *American Historical Review* 104 (5): 1513–30.

Park, Jungnok. 2012. *How Buddhism Acquired a Soul on the Way to China.* Sheffield: Equinox.

Paul, Diana Y. 1984. *Philosophy of Mind in Sixth-Century China: Paramārtha's "Evolution of Consciousness."* Stanford, Calif.: Stanford University Press.

Payne, Richard Karl. 2006. *Tantric Buddhism in East Asia.* Boston: Wisdom Publications.

Pearce, Scott, Audrey G. Spiro, and Patricia Buckley Ebrey. 2001. *Culture and Power in the Reconstitution of the Chinese Realm, 200–600.* Cambridge, Mass.: Harvard University Press.

Pelling, Margaret. 1987. "Medical Practice in Early Modern England: Trade or Profession?" In Wilfrid Prest (ed.), *The Professions in Early Modern England.* London: Croom Helm.

Pelliot, Paul. 1912. "Autour d'une traduction sanscrite du Tao tö king." *T'oung Pao* 13: 351–430.

Penny, Benjamin (ed.) 2006. *Daoism in History: Essays in Honour of Liu Ts'un-yan.* London: Routledge.

Pollock, Sheldon. 2006. *The Language of the Gods in the World of Men: Sanskrit, Culture, and Power in Premodern India.* Berkeley: University of California Press.

Poo, Mu-chou. 1995. "The Images of Immortals and Eminent Monks: Religious Mentality in Early Medieval China (4–6 c. A.D.)." *Numen* 42 (2): 172–96.

———. 2000. "Ghost Literature: Exorcistic Ritual Texts or Daily Entertainment?" *Asia Major* 13 (1): 43–64.

———. 2004. "The Concept of Ghost in Ancient China." In Lagerwey 2004.

———. 2010. "Images and Ritual Treatment of Dangerous Spirits." In Lagerwey and Lü 2010.

Porter, Roy. 1989. *Health for Sale: Quackery in England, 1660–1850.* Manchester: Manchester University Press.

Powers, John. 2009. *A Bull of a Man: Images of Masculinity, Sex, and the Body in Indian Buddhism.* Cambridge, Mass.: Harvard University Press.

Pregadio, Fabrizio. 2000. "Elixirs and Alchemy." In Kohn 2000.

———. 2006a. "Early Daoist Meditation and the Origins of Inner Alchemy." In Penny 2006.

———. 2006b. *Great Clarity: Daoism and Alchemy in Early Medieval China.* Stanford, Calif.: Stanford University Press.

Pritzker, Sonya. Forthcoming. *Living Translation: Language and the Search for Resonance in Chinese Medicine.* Oxford: Berghahn Books.

Puente-Ballesteros, Beatriz. 2011. "Jesuit Medicine in the Kangxi Court (1662–1722): Imperial Networks and Patronage." *EASTM* 34: 86–162.

Puett, Michael J. 2002. *To Become a God: Cosmology, Sacrifice, and Self-Divinization in Early China.* Cambridge, Mass.: Harvard University Press.

Pulleyblank, Edwin G. 1983. "Stages in the Transcription of Indian Words in Chinese from Han to Tang." In K. Röhrborn and W. Veenker (eds.), *Sprachen des Buddhismus in Zentralasien: Vorträge des Hamburger Symposions vom 2.* Wiesbaden: Harrassowitz.

Punjani, B. L. 1998. "Plants Used as Tooth Brush by Tribes of District Sabarkantha (North Gujarat)." *Ethnobotany* 10 (1–2): 133–35.

Pym, Anthony, Miriam Shlesinger, and Zuzana Jettmarová (eds.). 2006. *Sociocultural Aspects of Translating and Interpreting.* Amsterdam: Benjamins.

Quine, Willard Van Orman. 1960. *Word and Object.* Cambridge, Mass.: MIT Press.

Radich, Michael. 2007. "The Somatics of Liberation: Ideas About Embodiment in Buddhism from Its Origins to the Fifth Century C.E." Ph.D. diss., Harvard University.

Rahman, A. (ed.). 2002. *History of Science, Philosophy and Culture in Indian Civilization.* Vol. 3, part 2, *India's Interaction with China, Central, and West Asia.* Oxford: Oxford University Press.

Rao, B. Rama. 1982. "Bath in Ayurveda, Yoga, and Dharmasastra." *Bulletin of the Indian Institute of History of Medicine* 12: 13–21.

Rawlinson, Andrew. 1986. "Nāgas and the Magical Cosmology of Buddhism." *Religion* 16: 135–53.

Reddy, Subba. 1938. "Glimpses into the Practice and Principles of Medicine in Buddhistic India in the 7th Century A.D. Gleaned from 'The Records of Buddhist Religion' by the Chinese Monk I-tsing.'" *Bulletin of the Indian Institute of History of Medicine* 17: 155–67.

Reddy, Sujata. 2002. "India-China Cultural Synthesis—Contributions to Medicine." In Rahman 2002.

Redfield, Robert. 1956. *Peasant Society and Culture: An Anthropological Approach to Civilization.* Chicago: University of Chicago Press.

Rhie, Marylin Martin. 1999. *Early Buddhist Art of China and Central Asia.* Vol. 1, *Later Han, Three Kingdoms and Western Chin in China and Bactria to Shan-shan in Central Asia.* Leiden: Brill.

Richards, I. A. 1953. "Toward a Theory of Translating." In Wright 1953b.

Robinet, Isabelle. 1993. *Taoist Meditation: The Mao-shan Tradition of Great Purity*. Albany: State University of New York Press.

Robinson, Richard H. 1976. *Early Mādhyamika in India and China*. Delhi: Motilal Banarsidass.

Robson, James. 2008. "Signs of Power: Talismanic Writing in Chinese Buddhism." *History of Religions* 48 (2): 130–69.

———. 2009. *Power of Place: The Religious Landscape of the Southern Sacred Peak (Nanyue) in Medieval China*. Cambridge, Mass.: Harvard University Asia Center.

Rong Xinjiang. 2004. "Land Road or Sea Route? Commentary on the Studies of the Path of Transmission and Areas in Which Buddhism Was Disseminated During the Han Period." *Sino-Platonic Papers* 144: 320–42.

Rotman, Andy. 2008. *Divine Stories: Divyāvadāna (Part 1)*. Boston: Wisdom.

Sakade Yoshinobu. 1998. "Sun Simiao et le Bouddhisme." *Kansai daigaku bunka ronshū* 42 (1): 81–98.

———. 2005. "Daoism and the Dunhuang Regimen Texts." In Lo and Cullen 2005.

———. 2007. *Taoism, Medicine and Qi in China and Japan*. Osaka: Kansai University Press.

Samuel, Geoffrey. 2008. *The Origins of Yoga and Tantra: Indic Religions to the Thirteenth Century*. Cambridge: Cambridge University Press.

Salguero, C. Pierce. 2009. "The Buddhist Medicine King in Literary Context: Reconsidering an Early Example of Indian Influence on Chinese Medicine and Surgery." *History of Religions* 48 (3): 183–210.

———. 2010. "'A Flock of Ghosts Bursting Forth and Scattering': Healing Narratives in a Sixth-Century Chinese Buddhist Hagiography." *EASTM* 32: 89–120.

———. 2010–11. "Mixing Metaphors: Translating the Indian Medical Doctrine Tridoṣa in Chinese Buddhist Sources." *Asian Medicine* 6 (1): 55–74.

———. 2012. "'Treating Illness': Translation of a Chapter from a Medieval Chinese Buddhist Meditation Manual by Zhiyi (538–597)." *Asian Medicine* 7 (2): 461–73.

———. 2013. "'On Eliminating Disease': Translations of the Medical Chapter from the Chinese Versions of the Sutra of Golden Light." *eJournal of Indian Medicine* 6 (1): 21–43.

Sasson, Vanessa R. 2009. "A Womb with a View: The Buddha's Final Fetal Experience." In Sasson and Law 2009.

Sasson, Vanessa R., and Jane Marie Law (eds.). 2009. *Imagining the Fetus: The Unborn in Myth, Religion, and Culture*. Oxford: Oxford University Press.

Satō Tatsugen. 1986. *Chūgoku bukkyō ni okeru kairitsu no kenkyū*. Tokyo: Mokujisha.

Schafer, Edward H. 1956. "The Development of Bathing Customs in Ancient and Medieval China and the History of the Floriate Clear Palace." *JAOS* 76 (2): 57–82.

———. 1963. *The Golden Peaches of Samarkand: A Study of T'ang Exotics*. Berkeley: University of California Press.

———. 1967. *The Vermilion Bird: T'ang Images of the South*. Berkeley: University of California Press.

Scharfe, Hartmut. 1999. "The Doctrine of the Three Humors in Traditional Indian Medicine and the Alleged Antiquity of Tamil Siddha Medicine." *JAOS* 119 (4): 609–29.

Scheid, Volker. 2006. "Chinese Medicine and the Problem of Tradition." *Asian Medicine* 2 (1): 59–71.

———. 2007. *Currents of Tradition in Chinese Medicine, 1626–2006.* Seattle: Eastland Press.

Schmidt, F. R. A. 2006. "The Textual History of the Materia Medica in the Han Period: A System-Theoretical Reconsideration." *T'oung Pao* 92: 293–324.

Schober, Juliane (ed.). 1997. *Sacred Biography in the Buddhist Traditions of South and Southeast Asia.* Honolulu: University of Hawai'i Press.

Schopen, Gregory. 2004. *Buddhist Monks and Business Matters: Still More Papers on Monastic Buddhism in India.* Honolulu: University of Hawai'i Press.

Scogin, Hugh. 1978. "Poor Relief in Northern Sung China." *Oriens Extremus* 25 (1): 30–46.

Scott, David. 1985. "Ashokan Missionary Expansion of Buddhism Among the Greeks (in N.W. India, Bactria and the Levant)." *Religion* 15: 131–41.

Seidel, Anna. 1984. "Taoist Messianism." *Numen* 31 (2): 161–74.

———. 1987. "Traces of Han Religion in Funeral Texts Found in Tombs." In Akizuki Kan'ei (ed.), *Dōkuō to shūkyō bunka.* Tokyo: Hirakawa shuppansha.

Sekiguchi Shindai. 1954. *Tendai shōshikan no kenkyō.* Tokyo: Sankibō busshorin.

Selby, Martha Ann. 2005. "Narratives of Conception, Gestation, and Labour in Sanskrit Āyurveda." *Asian Medicine* 1 (2): 254–75.

Sen, Satiranjan. 1945. "Two Medical Texts in Chinese Translation." *Visva-Bharati Annals* 1: 70–95.

Sen, Tansen. 1995. "Gautama Zhuan: An Indian Astronomer at the Tang Court." *China Report* 31 (2): 197–208.

———. 2001. "In Search of Longevity and Good Karma: Chinese Diplomatic Missions to Middle India in the Seventh Century." *Journal of World History* 12 (1): 1–28.

———. 2002. "The Revival and Failure of Buddhist Translations During the Song Dynasty." *T'oung Pao* 88: 27–80.

———. 2003. *Buddhism, Diplomacy, and Trade: The Realignment of Sino-Indian Relations, 600–1400.* Honolulu: Association for Asian Studies and University of Hawai'i Press.

Sered, Susan. 2007–8. "Taxonomies of Ritual Mixing: Ritual Healing in the Contemporary United States." *History of Religions* 47 (2–3): 221–38.

Sewell, William H., Jr. 1999. "Concept(s) of Culture." In Victoria E. Bonnell and Lynn Hunt (eds.), *Beyond the Cultural Turn: New Directions in the Study of Society and Culture.* Berkeley: University of California Press.

Sharf, Robert H. 2002. *Coming to Terms with Chinese Buddhism: A Reading of the Treasure Store Treatise.* Honolulu: University of Hawai'i Press.

Sharma, Priya Vrat (trans.). 2004–5. *Suśruta-saṃhitā*. Varanasi: Chaukhambha Visvabharati.

———— (trans.). 2007–8. *Caraka-saṃhitā*. Varanasi: Chaukhambha Orientalia.

Shen Julong. 2001. "Fojiao sida shuo dui chuantong yixue de yingxiang." *Nanjing daxue xuebao (Zhexue renwen kexue shehui kexue)* 38 (141): 73–78.

Shi Wangcheng. 1992. "Lüelun fojiao yixue dui zhong yiyaoxue de yingxiang." *Wutaishan yanjiu* 3.

Shi Yongxin and Li Liangsong (eds.). 2011. *Zhongguo fojiao yiyao quanshu*. Beijing: Zhongguo shudian.

Shi Zhiru. 2013. "Lighting Lamps to Prolong Life: Venerating Bhaiṣajyaguru and Popular Ritual Conceptions of Healing and Longevity in Fifth- and Sixth-Century China." In *The Cult of the Healing Buddha in East Asia: Donghwasa Temple & Columbia Center for Buddhism, East Asian Religions (C-BEAR) International Conference (May 29–30, 2013)*. Daegu: Donghwasa Temple.

Shih, Robert. 1968. *Biographies des moines éminents (Kao seng tchouan) de Houei-Kiao*. Louvain: Institut Orientaliste.

Shinohara, Koichi. 1990. "Daoxuan's Collection of Miracle Stories About 'Supernatural Monks' (Shenseng gantong lu): An Analysis of Its Sources." *Chung-hwa Buddhist Journal* 3: 319–79.

————. 1991. "The Ji shenzhou sanbao gantong lu: Exploratory Notes." In V. N. Jha (ed.), *Kalyāṇa-Mitta: Professor Hajime Nakamura Felicitation Volume*. Delhi: Sri Satguru.

————. 1994. "Biographies of Eminent Monks in a Comparative Perspective: The Function of the Holy in Medieval Chinese Buddhism." *Chung-hwa Buddhist Journal* 7: 477–500.

————. 1998. "Changing Roles for Miraculous Images in Medieval Chinese Buddhism: A Study of the Miracle Image Section in Daoxuan's 'Collected Records.'" In Richard H. Davis 1998.

————. 2007. "The Moment of Death in Daoxuan's Vinaya Commentary." In Cuevas and Stone 2007.

Shinohara, Koichi, and Gregory Schopen (eds.). 1991. *From Benares to Beijing: Essays on Buddhism and Chinese Religion*. New York: Mosaic.

Silk, Jonathan A. 1989. "A Note on the Opening Formula of Buddhist Sūtras." *JIABS* 12 (1): 158–63.

Sinor, Denis. 1995. "Languages and Cultural Interchange Along the Silk Road." *Diogenes* 43 (171): 1–13.

Sivin, Nathan. 1967. "A Seventh-Century Chinese Medical Case History." *Bulletin of the History of Medicine* 41 (3): 267–73.

————. 1968. *Chinese Alchemy: Preliminary Studies*. Cambridge, Mass.: Harvard University Press.

————. 1978. "On the Word 'Taoist' as a Source of Perplexity: With Special Reference to the Relations of Science and Religion in Traditional China." *History of Religions* 17 (3–4): 303–30.

————. 1987. *Traditional Medicine in Contemporary China*. Ann Arbor: Center for Chinese Studies, University of Michigan.

————. 1993. "Huang Ti Nei Ching." In Michael Loewe (ed.), *Early Chinese Texts: A Bibliographical Guide*. Berkeley: University of California.

————. 1995a. "State, Cosmos and Body in the Last Three Centuries B.C." *HJAS* 55 (1): 5–37.

————. 1995b. "Taoism and Science." In Nathan Sivin, *Medicine, Philosophy and Religion in Ancient China: Researches and Reflections*. Aldershot: Variorum.

————. 1995c. "Text and Experience in Classical Chinese Medicine." In Donald Bates (ed.), *Knowledge and the Scholarly Medical Traditions*. Cambridge: Cambridge University Press.

————. 2011. "Health Care and Daoism." *Daoism: Religion, History and Society* 3: 1–16.

Skonicki, Douglas. 2011. "A Buddhist Response to Ancient-Style Learning: Qisong's Conception of Political Order." *T'oung Pao* 97 (1–3): 1–36.

Slouber, Michael James. "Gāruḍa Medicine: A History of Snakebite and Religious Healing in South Asia." Ph.D. diss., University of California, Berkeley.

Smith, Frederick M. 2006. *The Self Possessed: Deity and Spirit Possession in Classical Indian Literature and Civilization*. New York: Columbia University Press.

Snell-Hornby, Mary. 1995. *Translation Studies: An Integrated Approach*. Amsterdam: Benjamins.

Song Xian. 2001. *Gudai bosi yixue yu Zhongguo*. Beijing: Jingji ribao chubanshe.

Stanley-Baker, Michael. 2013. "Daoists and Doctors: The Role of Medicine in Six Dynasties Shangqing Daoism." Ph.D. diss., University College London.

Stein, Rolf A. 1979. "Religious Taoism and Popular Religion from the Second to Seventh Centuries." In Welch and Seidel 1979.

Sterckx, Roel. 2002. *The Animal and the Daemon in Early China*. Albany: State University of New York Press.

Stewart, Tony K. 2001. "In Search of Equivalence: Conceiving Muslim-Hindu Encounter Through Translation Theory." *History of Religions* 40 (3): 260–87.

Storch, Tanya. 1993. "Chinese Buddhist Historiography and Orality." *Sino-Platonic Papers* 37: 1–16.

Strange, Mark. 2011. "Representations of Liang Emperor Wu as a Buddhist Ruler in Sixth- and Seventh-Century Texts." *Asia Major* 24 (2): 53–112.

Strickmann, Michel. 1978. "The Longest Taoist Scripture." *History of Religions* 17 (3–4): 331–54.

————. 1979. "On the Alchemy of T'ao Hung-ching." In Welch and Seidel 1979.

————. 1988. "Dreamwork of Psycho-Sinologists: Doctors, Taoists, Monks." In Carolyn T. Brown 1988.

————. 1990. "The Consecration Sutra: A Buddhist Book of Spells." In Buswell 1990.

————. 1990–91. "Buddhas in and out of Bodies." *Discours social / Social Discourse* 3: 107–20.

————. 1991. "Histoire des syncrétismes religieux taoîstes et bouddhistes en Chine et au Japon." Vol. 3, "Chinese Magical Medicine: Therapeutic Rituals." Ph.D. diss., Université Paris.

————. 1993. "The Seal of the Law: A Ritual Implement and the Origins of Printing." *Asia Major* 6 (2): 1–83.

————. 1995. "The Seal of the Jungle Woman." *Asia Major* 8 (2): 147–53.

————. 1996. *Mantras et mandarins: Le bouddhisme tantrique en Chine*. Paris: Gallimard.

————. 2002. *Chinese Magical Medicine*. Stanford, Calif.: Stanford University Press.

Strong, John S. 1983. *The Legend of King Aśoka: A Study and Translation of the Aśokāvadāna*. Princeton, N.J.: Princeton University Press.

Swanson, Paul L. 1997. "What's Going on Here? Chih-i's Use (and Abuse) of Scripture." *JIABS* 20 (1): 1–30.

————. 2007. "Ch'an and Chih-kuan: T'ien-t'ai Chih-i's View of 'Zen' and the Practice of the Lotus Sutra." *Tiantai xuebao*, special issue, 143–64.

Takakusu Junjirō. 1966 [1896]. *A Record of the Buddhist Religion as Practiced in India and the Malay Archipelago (AD 671–695) by I-tsing*. Delhi: Munshiram Manoharlal.

Tambiah, Stanley Jeyaraja. 1990. *Magic, Science and Religion and the Scope of Rationality*. Cambridge: Cambridge University Press.

Tan Zhihui. 2002. "Daoxuan's Vision of Jetavana: Imagining a Utopian Monastery in Early Tang." Ph.D. diss., University of Arizona.

Tang Jian. 1992. "Medieval Chinese and Sanskrit: Historical Linguistic Contacts Through Translation of Mahayana Buddhist Scriptures." In Bernard Hung-Kay Luk and Barry D. Steben (eds.), *Contact Between Cultures, Eastern Asia: Literature and Humanities*. Lewiston, N.Y.: Edwin Mellen.

Tang Yijie. 1991. "The Development of Chinese Culture: Some Comments in Light of the Study of the Introduction of Indian Buddhism into China." In Shinohara and Schopen 1991

T'ang Yung-t'ung. 1962. *Han Wei Liang Jin Nanbeichao fojiao shi*. Taipei: Dingwen shuju.

————. 1968. "On 'Ko-yi,' the Earliest Method by Which Indian Buddhism and Chinese Thought Were Synthesized." In W. R. Inge et al. (eds.), *Radhakrishnan: Comparative Studies in Philosophy Presented in Honour of His Sixtieth Birthday*. London: Allen & Unwin; and New York: Humanities Press.

Taylor, Kim. 2005. *Chinese Medicine in Early Communist China, 1945–63: A Medicine of Revolution*. London: RoutledgeCurzon.

Teiser, Stephen F. 1985. "T'ang Buddhist Encyclopedias: An Introduction to *Fa-yüan chu-lin* and *Chu-ching yao-chi*." *T'ang Studies* 3: 109–28.

————. 1988. *The Ghost Festival in Medieval China*. Princeton, N.J.: Princeton University Press.

————. 1994. *The Scripture on the Ten Kings and the Making of Purgatory in Medieval Chinese Buddhism*. Honolulu: University of Hawai'i Press.

———. 2006. *Reinventing the Wheel: Paintings of Rebirth in Medieval Buddhist Temples.* Seattle: University of Washington Press.

———. 2009. "Healing Rituals in Northwest China, 9th–10th Centuries." Paper presented at "Monk and Medicine: A Monk's Roles and Image as a Physician," People's University, Tangshan, 11 December.

Ṭhānissaro Bhikkhu. 2007. *The Buddhist Monastic Code II: The Khandaka Training Rules Translated and Explained.* 2nd ed., rev. Valley Center, Calif.: Metta Forest Monastery.

Thapar, Romila. 1975. "Aśokan India and the Gupta Age." In A. L. Basham (ed.), *A Cultural History of India.* Oxford: Oxford University Press.

———. 2004. *Early India: From the Origins to AD 1300.* Berkeley: University of California Press.

Thompson, Laurence G. 1990. "Medicine and Religion in Late Ming China." *Journal of Chinese Religions* 18: 45–59.

Ting, Joseph S. P. (ed.). 1996. *The Maritime Silk Route: 2000 Years of Trade on the South China Sea.* Hong Kong: Urban Council.

Tokuno, Kyoko. 1994. "Byways in Chinese Buddhism: The 'Book of Trapusa' and Indigenous Scriptures." Ph.D. diss., University of California, Berkeley.

Toury, Gideon. 1995. *Descriptive Translation Studies and Beyond.* Amsterdam: Benjamins.

———. 2004 [1978]. "The Nature and Role of Norms in Literary Translation." In Venuti 2004.

Trivedi, Harish. 2007. "Translating Culture vs. Cultural Translation." In Paul St-Pierre and Prafulla C. Kar (eds.), *In Translation: Reflections, Refractions, Transformations.* Amsterdam: John Benjamins.

Tryjarski, Edward. 1995. "The Geographic and Linguistic Status of the Silk Roads." *Diogenes* 43 (171): 15–24.

Tsai, Kathryn Ann. 1994. *Lives of the Nuns: Biographies of Chinese Buddhist Nuns from the Fourth to Sixth Centuries; A Translation of the Pi-ch'iu-ni chuan; Compiled by Shih Pao-ch'ang.* Honolulu: University of Hawai'i Press.

Tsiang, Katherine R. 1996. "Monumentalization of Buddhist Texts in the Northern Qi Dynasty: The Engraving of Sutras at the Xiangtangshan Caves and Other Sites in the Sixth Century." *Artibus Asiae* 56 (3–4): 233–61.

———. 2002. "Changing Patterns of Divinity and Reform in the Late Northern Wei." *Art Bulletin* 84 (2): 222–45.

Tso Sze-bong. 1980. "Sifen lü zhong youguan yiliao de ziliao." *Nanyang fojiao* 139: 11–14

———. 1982. "The Transformation of Buddhist Vinaya in China." Ph.D. diss., Australian National University.

———. 1994. "Zhongguo shamen de yiyao zhishi jiqi chengjiu." In Tso Sze-bong (ed.), *Zhongguo shamen waixue de yanjiu: Hanmo zhi wudai.* Taipei: Dongchu.

Tsukamoto, Zenryu. 1985 [1942]. *A History of Early Chinese Buddhism: From Its Introduction to the Death of Hui-yüan*. Tokyo: Kodansha.

Tu Zhimao. 2001. "Fojiao yifangming de yinshi yaowu liaofa." Ph.D. diss., Faguang fojiao wenhua yanjiusuo.

Twitchett, Denis C. 1979a. *The Cambridge History of China*. Vol. 3, *Sui and Tang China, 589–906*. Cambridge: Cambridge University Press.

————. 1979b. "Population and Pestilence in T'ang China." In Wolfgang Bauer (ed.), *Studia Sino-Mongolica: Festschrift fur Herbert Frank*. Wiesbaden: Franz Steiner Verlag.

Tymoczko, Maria. 2012. "The Neuroscience of Translation." *Target* 42 (1): 83–102.

Ui Hakuju. 1956. *Shaku Dōan kenyū*. Tokyo: Iwanami shoten.

Unschuld, Paul U. 1979a. "The Chinese Reception of Indian Medicine in the First Millennium A.D." *Bulletin of the History of Medicine* 53 (3): 329–45.

————. 1979b. *Medical Ethics in Imperial China: A Study in Historical Anthropology*. Berkeley: University of California Press.

————. 1986. *Medicine in China: A History of Pharmaceutics*. Berkeley: University of California Press.

————. 1994. "Der chinesische 'Arzneikönig' Sun Simiao: Geschichte—Legende—Ikonographie; Zur Plausibilität naturkundlicher and übernatürlicher Erklärungsmodelle." *Monumenta Serica* 42: 217–57.

————. 2003. *Huang Di Nei Jing Su Wen: Nature, Knowledge, Imagery in an Ancient Chinese Medical Text*. Berkeley: University of California Press.

————. 2006. "The Limits of Individualism and the Advantages of Modular Therapy: Concepts of Illness in Chinese Medicine." *Asian Medicine* 2 (1): 14–37.

————. 2010 [1985]. *Medicine in China: A History of Ideas*. Berkeley: University of California Press.

Unschuld, Paul U., and Hermann Tessenow. 2011. *Huang Di Nei Jing Su Wen: An Annotated Translation of Huang Di's Inner Classic—Basic Questions*. Berkeley: University of California Press.

van Gulik, Robert H. 1980 [1956]. *Siddham: An Essay on the History of Sanskrit Studies in China and Japan*. New Delhi: International Academy of Indian Culture.

Veith, Ilza, and Atsumi Minami. 1966. "A Buddhist Prayer Against Sickness." *History of Religions* 5 (2): 239–49.

Venuti, Lawrence (ed.). 1992. *Rethinking Translation: Discourse, Subjectivity, Ideology*. London: Routledge.

———— (ed.). 2004. *The Translation Studies Reader*. London: Routledge.

————. 2008. *The Translator's Invisibility: A History of Translation*. 2nd ed. New York: Routledge.

Verellen, Franciscus. 1992. " 'Evidential Miracles in Support of Taoism': The Inversion of a Buddhist Apologetic Tradition in Late Tang China." *T'oung Pao* 78: 217–63.

von Falkenhausen, Lothar. 1995. "Reflections on the Political Role of Spirit Mediums in Early China: The Wu Officials in the Zhou Li." *Early China* 20: 279–300.

von Glahn, Richard. 2004. *The Sinister Way: The Divine and the Demonic in Chinese Religious Culture*. Berkeley: University of California Press.

Wagner, Robin Beth. 1995. "Buddhism, Biography and Power: A Study of Daoxuan's *Continued Lives of Eminent Monks*." Ph.D. diss., Harvard University.

Wagner, Rudolf G. 2003. *Language, Ontology, and Political Philosophy in China: Wang Bi's Scholarly Exploration of the Dark (Xuanxue)*. Albany: State University of New York Press.

Wales, H. G. Quaritch. 1967. *The Indianization of China and of South-East Asia*. London: Quaritch.

Waley, Arthur. 1952. *The Real Tripitaka and Other Pieces*. New York: Macmillian.

Wang Gungwu. 1998 [1958]. *The Nanhai Trade: The Early History of Chinese Trade in the South China Sea*. Singapore: Times Academic Press.

Wang Shumin. 2005a. "Abstracts of the Medical Manuscripts from Dunhuang." In Lo and Cullen 2005.

———. 2005b. "A General Survey of Medical Works Contained in the Dunhuang Medical Manuscripts." In Lo and Cullen 2005.

Wang Xiaoxian. 1994. *Sichouzilu yiyaoxue jiaoliu yanjiu*. Urumqi: Xinjiang renmin chubanshe.

Watson, Burton (trans.). 1993a. *The Lotus Sutra*. New York: Columbia University Press.

——— (trans.). 1993b. *Records of the Grand Historian: Han Dynasty*. Rev. ed., 2 vols. Hong Kong: Columbia University Press.

——— (trans.). 1997. *The Vimalakirti Sutra*. New York: Columbia University Press.

Wei Zheng. 1973. *Suishu*. Beijing: Zhonghua shuju.

Weinstein, Stanley. 1973. "Imperial Patronage in the Formation of T'ang Buddhism." In Arthur F. Wright and Denis Twitchett (eds.), *Perspectives on the T'ang*. New Haven, Conn.: Yale University Press.

———. 1987. *Buddhism Under the T'ang*. Cambridge: Cambridge University Press.

Weinstein, Stanley, and William M. Bodiford (eds.). 2005. *Going Forth: Visions of Buddhist Vinaya: Essays Presented in Honor of Professor Stanley Weinstein*. Honolulu: University of Hawai'i Press.

Welch, Holmes, and Anna Seidel (eds.). 1979. *Facets of Taoism: Essays in Chinese Religion*. New Haven, Conn.: Yale University Press.

White, David Gordon. 1996. *The Alchemical Body: Siddha Traditions in Medieval India*. Chicago: University of Chicago Press.

——— (ed.). 2000. *Tantra in Practice*. Princeton, N.J.: Princeton University Press.

Whitfield, Susan. 2005. "The Dunhuang Collections and International Collaboration." In Lo and Cullen 2005.

———. 2007. "Was There a Silk Road?" *Asian Medicine* 3 (2): 201–13.

Wile, Douglas. 1992. *Art of the Bedchamber: The Chinese Sexual Yoga Classics Including Women's Solo Meditation Texts*. Albany: State University of New York Press.

Wilkinson, Endymion. 2012. *Chinese History: A New Manual.* Cambridge, Mass.: Harvard University Asia Center.

Wilms, Sabine. 2005. "The Transmission of Medical Knowledge on 'Nurturing the Fetus' in Early China." *Asian Medicine* 1 (2): 276–314.

———. 2008. *Bei Ji Qian Jin Yao Fang: Essential Prescriptions Worth a Thousand in Gold for Every Emergency, Volumes 2–4 on Gynecology.* Portland, Ore.: Chinese Medicine Database.

Wong, Dorothy C. 2004. *Chinese Steles: Pre-Buddhist and Buddhist Use of a Symbolic Form.* Honolulu: University of Hawai'i Press.

Wriggins, Sally Hovey. 1996. *Xuanzang: A Buddhist Pilgrim on the Silk Road.* Oxford: Westview Press.

Wright, Arthur F. 1948. "Fo-tu-têng: A Biography." *HJAS* 11 (3–4): 312–71.

———. 1953a. "The Chinese Language and Foreign Ideas." In Wright 1953b.

——— (ed.). 1953b. *Studies in Chinese Thought.* Chicago: University of Chicago Press.

———. 1954. "Biography and Hagiography: Hui-chiao's Lives of Eminent Monks." In *Silver Jubilee Volume of the Zinbun-kagaku-kenkyusyo.* Kyoto: Kyoto University.

———. 1957. "The Formation of Sui Ideology, 581–604." In Fairbank 1957.

———. 1959. *Buddhism in Chinese History.* Stanford, Calif.: Stanford University Press; and London: Oxford University Press.

Wu Hung. 1986. "Buddhist Elements in Early Chinese Art (2nd and 3rd Centuries A.D.)." *Artibus Asiae* 47 (3–4): 263–352.

Wu, Pei-yi. 1979. "Self-Examination and Confession of Sins in Traditional China." *HJAS* 39 (1): 5–38.

Wu, Yi-Li. 2000. "The Bamboo Grove Monastery and Popular Gynecology in Qing China." *Late Imperial China* 21 (1): 41–76.

———. 2010. *Reproducing Women: Medicine, Metaphor, and Childbirth in Late Imperial China.* Berkeley: University of California Press.

Wujastyk, Dominik. 2003 [1998]. *The Roots of Ayurveda.* London: Penguin Books.

———. 2009. "Interpreting the Image of the Human Body in Premodern India." *International Journal of Hindu Studies* 13 (2): 189–228.

Xiao Fan. 1993. "Han-Song jian wenxian suojian gudai Zhongguo nanfang de dili huanjing yu difangbing ji qi yingxiang." *Bulletin of the Institute for History and Philology, Academia Sinica* 63 (1): 67–171.

Xiong, Victor Cunrui. 2005. "Han Yu, 'A Memorial on the Relic of the Buddha.'" In Mair, Steinhardt, and Goldin 2005.

———. 2006. *Emperor Yang of the Sui Dynasty: His Life, Times, and Legacy.* Albany: State University of New York Press.

Xue Gongchen. 2002. *Ru dao fo yu zhongyiyao xue.* Beijing: Zhongguo shudian.

Yamabe Nobuyoshi. 1999. "The Sūtra on the Ocean-Like Samādhi of the Visualization of the Buddha: The Interfusion of the Chinese and Indian Cultures in Central Asia as Reflected Upon a Fifth Century Apocryphal Sūtra." Ph.D. diss., Yale University.

———. 2005. "Visionary Repentance and Visionary Ordination in the Brahmā Net Sūtra." In Weinstein and Bodiford 2005.

Yamada, Keiji. 1979. "The Formation of the Huang-ti Nei-ching." *Acta Asiatica* 36: 67–89.

———. 1991. "Anatometrics in Ancient China." *Chinese Science* 10: 39–52.

———. 1998. *The Origins of Acupuncture, Moxibustion, and Decoction.* Kyoto: Nichibunken.

Yamano Toshirou. 1985. "Tendai Chigi no igaku shisō josetsu." *Shinshū sōgō kenkyūjo kenkyū kiyō* 3: 115–42.

Yang, Lien-sheng. 1957. "The Concept of Pao as a Basis for Social Relations in China." In Fairbank 1957.

Yao Chongxin. 2013. "Yearning for the Pure Land or Cherishing This Life: The Connotations of the Healing Buddha Cult in Medieval China." In *The Cult of the Healing Buddha in East Asia: Donghwasa Temple & Columbia Center for Buddhism, East Asian Religions (C-BEAR) International Conference (May 29–30, 2013).* Daegu: Donghwasa Temple.

Yifa. 2002. *The Origins of Buddhist Monastic Codes in China: An Annotated Translation and Study of the Chanyuan Qinggui.* Honolulu: University of Hawai'i Press. .

Yoshikawa Tadao and Funayama Tōru. 2009–10. *Kōsō-den.* Tokyo: Iwanami Shoten.

Young, Stuart H. Forthcoming. *Conceiving the Indian Buddhist Patriarchs in China.* Honolulu: University of Hawai'i Press.

Yü, Chün-fang. 2001. *Kuan-yin: The Chinese Transformation of Avalokiteśvara.* New York: Columbia University Press.

Zhan, Mei. 2009. *Other-Wordly: Making Chinese Medicine Through Transnational Frames.* Durham, N.C.: Duke University Press.

Zhang Ruixian. 1999. *Longmen yaofang shiyi.* Zhengzhou: Henan yike daxue chubanshe.

Zhang Xueming and Liang Yuansheng (eds.). 2005. *Lishishang de cishan huodong yu shehui dongli.* Hong Kong: Xianggang jiaoyu tushu gongsi.

Zhou Minhui. 2003. "'Jin guangmin jing' wenxue tezhi zhi yanjiu." Ph.D. diss., Guoli zhengzhi daxue.

Zhu Jianping. 1999. "Sun Simiao 'Qianjin fang' zhong de fojiao yingxiang (English Title: Buddhist Influences on Sun Simiao's Precious Prescriptions for Emergency [Qian jin fang])." *Zhonghua yishi zazhi* 4: 220–22.

Zhu Qingzhi. 1992. *Fodian yu zhonggu hanyu cihui yanjiu.* Taipei: Wenjin chubanshe.

———. 1995. "Some Linguistic Evidence for Early Cultural Exchange Between China and India." *Sino-Platonic Papers* 66: 1–7.

Zieme, Peter, and Kōgi Kudara. 2008. *Aspects of Research into Central Asian Buddhism: In Memoriam Kōgi Kudara.* Turnhout: Brepols.

Zürcher, Erik. 1977. "Late Han Vernacular Elements in the Earliest Buddhist Translations." *Journal of the Chinese Language Teachers Association* 13 (3): 177–203.

———. 1980. "Buddhist Influence on Early Taoism: A Survey of Scriptural Evidence." *T'oung Pao* 66: 84–147.

———. 1981. "Eschatology and Messianism in Early Chinese Buddhism." In W. L. Idema (ed.), *Leyden Studies in Sinology.* Leiden: Brill.

———. 1982a. "Perspectives in the Study of Chinese Buddhism." *Journal of the Royal Asiatic Society* 2: 161–76.

———. 1982b. "'Prince Moonlight': Messianism and Eschatology in Early Medieval Chinese Buddhism." *T'oung Pao* 68 (1–3): 1–75.

———. 1989. "Buddhism and Education in T'ang Times." In William Theodore de Bary and John W. Chaffee (eds.), *Neo-Confucian Education: The Formative Stage*. Berkeley: University of California Press.

———. 1990. "Han Buddhism and the Western Regions." In Idema and Zürcher 1990.

———. 1991. "A New Look at the Earliest Chinese Buddhist Texts." In Shinohara and Schopen 1991.

———. 1996. "Vernacular Elements in Early Buddhist Texts: An Attempt to Define the Optimal Source Materials." *Sino-Platonic Papers* 71: 1–31.

———. 2007. *The Buddhist Conquest of China: The Spread and Adaptation of Buddhism in Early Medieval China*. 3rd ed. Leiden: Brill.

———. 2012 [1999]. "Buddhism Across Boundaries: The Foreign Input." *Sino-Platonic Papers* 222: 1–25.

Zysk, Kenneth G. 1986. "The Evolution of Anatomical Knowledge in Ancient India, with Special Reference to Cross-Cultural Influences." *JAOS* 106 (4): 687–705.

———. 1993 [1985]. *Religious Medicine: The History and Evolution of Indian Medicine*. New Brunswick, N.J.: Transaction.

———. 1998 [1991]. *Asceticism and Healing in Ancient India: Medicine in the Buddhist Monastery*. Delhi: Motilal Banarsidass.

———. 2007. "The Bodily Winds in Ancient India Revisited." *Journal of the Royal Anthropological Institute* 13, Supp. 1: 105–15.

ACKNOWLEDGMENTS

Alexander Hsu   Amy Langenberg   **Bill Rowe**   Catherine Despeux

Chen Ming   Colavita Publishing Support Fund at Penn State Abington

Dan Lusthaus   **Daniel Todes**   Dmytro Byelmac   Eric Greene

Erica Ginsburg   Geoffrey Goble   James Benn   James Robson

Janet Gyatso   **Jonathan Pettit**   **Marcie Salguero**   Marcus Bingenheimer

Marta Hanson   **Mary Fissell**   **Michael Stanley-Baker**   Natalie Köhle

Nathan Sivin   Paul Swanson   Penn Humanities Forum

Philadelphia Area Buddhist Studies Work Group   **Richard Jaffe**

Rob Campany   Shayne Clarke   Sonya Pritzker   **Stephen Teiser**

Stuart Young   TJ Hinrichs   **Tobie Meyer-Fong**

Ven. Jianrong   Ven. Yifa   **Victor Mair**